Edition 11

Medical Dosage Calculations

A Dimensional Analysis Approach

June L. Olsen, MS, RN
Professor of Nursing (Emerita)
College of Staten Island
Staten Island, NY

Anthony Patrick Giangrasso, PhD
Professor of Mathematics
LaGuardia Community College
Long Island City, NY

Dolores M. Shrimpton, MA, RN
Professor of Nursing (Emerita)
Kingsborough Community College
Brooklyn, NY

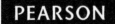

Boston   Columbus   Indianapolis   New York   San Francisco   Hoboken
Amsterdam   Cape Town   Dubai   London   Madrid   Milan   Munich   Paris   Montréal   Toronto
Delhi   Mexico City   São Paulo   Sydney   Hong Kong   Seoul   Singapore   Taipei   Tokyo

Publisher: Julie Levin Alexander
Executive Editor: Kelly Trakalo
Program Manger: Melissa Bashe
Editorial Assistant: Kevin Wilson
Director of Marketing: David Gesell
Senior Product Marketing Manager: Phoenix Harvey
Field Marketing Manager: Debi Doyle
Director, Product Management Services: Etain O'Dea

Project Management Team Lead: Cynthia Zonneveld
Project Manager: Michael Giacobbe
Manufacturing Manager: Maura Zaldivar-Garcia
Senior Interior and Cover Design: Maria Guglielmo
Full-Service Project Management and Composition: Integra Software Services Pvt Ltd.
Printer/Binder: LSC Communications
Cover Printer: LSC Communications

Notice: Care has been taken to confirm the accuracy of information presented in this book. The authors, editors, and the publisher, however, cannot accept any responsibility for errors or omissions or for consequences from application of the information in this book and make no warranty, express or implied, with respect to its contents. The authors and publisher have exerted every effort to ensure that drug selections and dosages set forth in this text are in accord with current recommendations and practice at time of publication. However, in view of ongoing research, changes in government regulations, and the constant flow of information relating to drug therapy and drug reactions, the reader is urged to check the package inserts of all drugs for any change in indications of dosage and for added warnings and precautions. This is particularly important when the recommended agent is a new and/or infrequently employed drug.

Library of Congress Cataloging-in-Publication Data

Olsen, June Looby, author.
    Medical dosage calculations: a dimensional analysis approach / June L. Olsen, Anthony Patrick Giangrasso, Dolores M. Shrimpton. — 11th edition.
        p. ; cm.
    Includes index.
    ISBN 978-0-13-394071-8 — ISBN 0-13-394071-3
    I. Giangrasso, Anthony Patrick, author. II. Shrimpton, Dolores M., author. III. Title.
    [DNLM: 1. Drug Dosage Calculations—Nurses' Instruction. 2. Pharmaceutical
Preparations—administration & dosage—Nurses' Instruction.   QV 748]
    RS57
    615'.1401513—dc23
                                                            2014034132

17 2021

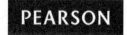
www.pearsonhighered.com

ISBN 10:   0-13-394071-3
ISBN 13: 978-0-13-394071-8

About the Authors

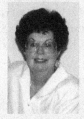

JUNE LOOBY OLSEN began her nursing career in Burlington, Vermont, at Bishop De Goesbriand Memorial Hospital, where she graduated from its nursing program. She obtained her BS and MS degrees in nursing from St. John's University, New York. She was a staff nurse, as well as a nurse supervisor, and became head nurse at the Veterans Administration Hospital in Brooklyn, New York.

Her teaching career began at Staten Island Community College, and she retired as full professor emeritus from the College of Staten Island of the City University of New York. In addition to this textbook, Professor Olsen has written *Fundamentals of Nursing Review* and *Dosage Calculation*, both published by Springhouse. She was a recipient of the Mu Epsilon Leadership in Nursing award.

Dedication
For my grandson Daniel James Olsen, who has added much happiness to our lives.

—June Looby Olsen

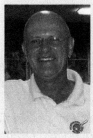

ANTHONY GIANGRASSO was born and raised in Maspeth, New York. He attended Rice High School on a scholarship and in his senior year was named in an annual citywide contest by the *New York Journal-American* newspaper as New York City's most outstanding high school scholar-athlete. He was also awarded a full-tuition scholarship to Iona College, from which he obtained a BA in mathematics, magna cum laude, with a ranking of sixth in his graduating class.

Anthony began his teaching career as a fifth-grade teacher in Manhattan, as a member of the Christian Brothers of Ireland, and taught high school mathematics and physics in Harlem and Newark, New Jersey. He holds an MS and PhD from New York University and has taught at all levels from elementary school through graduate school. He is currently teaching at Adelphi University and LaGuardia Community College, where he was chairman of the mathematics department. He has authored nine college textbooks through twenty-five editions.

Anthony's community service has included membership on the boards of directors of the Polish-American Museum Foundation, Catholic Adoptive Parents Association, and Family Focus Adoptive Services. He was the president of the Italian-American Faculty Association of the City University of New York and the founding chairman of the board of the Italian-American Legal Defense and Higher Education Fund, Inc. He and his wife, Susan, are proud parents of three children—Anthony, Michael, and Jennifer—and grandparents of Calvin and Jackson. He enjoys tennis and twice has been ranked #1 for his age group in the Eastern Section by the United States Tennis Association.

Dedication
For my lovely wife, Susan. Thanks for your love and support for over four decades.

—Anthony Giangrasso

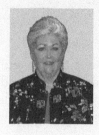

DOLORES M. SHRIMPTON is Professor emerita of Nursing at Kingsborough Community College (CUNY), where she was Chairperson of the department for thirteen years. She received a diploma in nursing from Kings Country Hospital Center School of Nursing, a BS from C.W. Post College, an MA in nursing administration from New York University, and a post-Master's certificate in nursing education from Adelphi University. She is a member of the Upsilon and Mu Upilson Chapters of Sigma Theta Tau. She has taught a wide variety of courses in practical nursing, diploma, and associate degree nursing programs. She has authored three college nursing books through seven editions.

Dolores has held many leadership positions in nursing, including Board Member, Vice-President, and President of the NYS Associate Degree Nursing Council. She was the Co-Chair of the CUNY Nursing Discipline Council, and Member of the Board of Directors and Co-President of the Brooklyn Nursing Partnership. She has served on a number of Advisory Boards of LPN, associate degree, and baccalaureate degree nursing programs. She is a recipient of the Presidential Award in Nursing Leadership from the Nurses Association of Long Island (NACLI) as well as of the Mu Upsilon award for Excellence in Nursing Education and Excellence in Nursing Leadership. She has also been recognized for her commitment to nursing by the Brooklyn Nursing Partnership.

Dolores lives in Brooklyn, New York, and enjoys cooking and spending time with her grandchildren, Brooke Elizabeth, Paige Dolores, Jack Paul, and their parents, Kim and Shawn. She also enjoys traveling and spending time with friends and family in Harwich Port, Cape Cod, Massachusetts.

Dedication

In loving memory of Dr. Margaret (Peggy) Doell Budnik, RN.

The true meaning of success lies not so much in what you have achieved, but in whether you have made a difference. It's knowing you have touched the lives of others and have in some way made the world a little bit brighter and better.

Loved and missed dearly by numerous colleagues, friends, and family—most especially her children, Michael and Jimmy Budnik and Kerri Budnik Kochevar, as well as "Nana's eight," Nicholas, Drew, Michael, and Jack Welch; Bianca, Brea, and Michael Jr. Budnik; and Zoe Budnik.

—Dolores M. Shrimpton

Preface

In 1995, the Institute of Medicine issued its landmark report, "To Err Is Human: Building a Safer Health System," which claimed that nearly 100,000 people died annually due to medical errors. Since that report, greater emphasis has been placed on improving safety in medication administration. One aspect of that safety is accuracy in drug calculations. *Medical Dosage Calculations* is not merely a textbook about math skills; it is also an introduction to the professional context of safe drug administration. Calculation skills and the rationales behind them are emphasized throughout.

This book uses the dimensional analysis method for dosage calculations, a time-tested approach based on simple mathematical concepts. It helps the student develop a number sense, and largely frees the student from the need to memorize formulas. Once the technique is mastered, students will be able to calculate drug dosages quickly and safely.

Medical Dosage Calculations is a combined text- and workbook. Its consistent focus on safety, accuracy, and professionalism make it a valuable part of a course for nursing or allied health programs. It is also highly effective for independent study and may be used as a refresher for dosage calculation skills and as a professional reference.

Medical Dosage Calculations is arranged into four basic learning units:

Unit 1: Basic Calculation Skills and Introduction to Medication Administration
Chapter 1 includes a diagnostic test of arithmetic and reviews the necessary basic mathematics skills. Chapter 2 introduces the student to the essentials of the medication administration process. Chapter 3 introduces the dimensional analysis method in small increments using a simple, step-by-step, common-sense approach.

Unit 2: Systems of Measurement
Chapters 4 and 5 present the metric and household systems of measurement that nurses and other allied health professionals must understand in order to interpret medication orders and calculate dosages. Students learn to convert measurements between and within measurement systems.

Unit 3: Oral and Parenteral Medications
This unit prepares students to calculate oral and parenteral dosages and introduces them to the essential equipment needed for administration and preparation of solutions. Chapter 6 introduces oral drug dosage calculations. It also includes dosages based on patient size. Chapter 7 discusses syringes and insulin. Chapter 8 deals with solutions, and Chapter 9 introduces parenteral medications and heparin.

Unit 4: Infusions and Pediatric Dosages
Chapters 10 and 11 provide a solid foundation for calculating intravenous and enteral dosage rates and flow rates and include titrating IV medications. Pediatric dosages and daily fluid maintenance needs are also discussed in Chapter 12.

What's New in the 11th Edition

- Keystroke Sequences in Chapter 1. This enables students to check their calculations and ensure safety.
- Updated and revised drug labels and drug examples throughout the text that contain both trade and generic drug names.
- Increased emphasis on the safety in medication administration following the Joint Commission National Patient Safety Goals, the Institute for Safe Medical Practice, and the CDC One and Only Campaign.
- Dosage Calculation Online Application provides diagnostic testing and student remediation with hundreds of additional practice questions.
- Updated information on insulin administration and calculations.
- Enhanced information on heparin administration and calculations.
- Expanded content on both titration tables and IV push.
- A more visual approach is employed for computations concerning solutions and IV calculations.
- All new questions in the Exercises.
- Many new illustrative examples are included throughout all the chapters.
- Chapter 12, Pediatric Dosages, includes an expanded discussion of the volume-control chamber.

Features and Benefits of *Medical Dosage Calculations*

- Throughout the textbook there are worked-out solutions to all illustrated examples. Care is taken to show each step in the process.
- Constant skill reinforcement through frequent practice opportunities.
- More than 1,000 problems for students to solve.
- Actual drug labels, syringes, drug package inserts, prescriptions, and medication administration records (MARs) are illustrated throughout the text.
- Ample work space on every page for note taking and problem solving.
- All medication orders in this book contain actual safe recommended doses.
- The Illustrative Examples and Practice Sets provide ample opportunity for student development of critical decision making/critical thinking when calculating dosages.
- Answers to Try These for Practice, Exercises, and Cumulative Review questions are found in Appendix A.
- Answers to the Additional Exercises are found in the Instructor's Resource Manual.

Acknowledgments

Our special thanks to the nursing and mathematics faculty and the students at LaGuardia Community College and Kingsborough Community College. Also, a special thank you to our editor, Kelly Trakalo, and development editor, Michael Giacobbe, and to the production and marketing teams at Pearson.

Thank you also to the following manufacturers for supplying labels and art for this textbook:

Courtesy of Abbott Laboratories

Courtesy of AbbVie

ADD-Vantage®/Courtesy of Hospira, Inc
© Copyright El Lily & Company. All rights reserved. Used with permission
Forest Pharmaceuticals
Courtesy of JHP Pharmaceuticals and Par Pharmaceutical, Inc.

Reproduced with permission of Merck Sharp & Dohme Corp., a subsidiary of Merck & Co, Inc., Whitehouse Station, New Jersey, USA. All Rights Reserved.

Courtesy of Norvartis AG

Novo Nordisk

Courtesy of Pfizer, Inc.

© Purdue, used with permission

Teva North America

Valeant Pharmaceuticals International, Inc.

Reviewers for *Medical Dosage Calculations*

Michele Bach
Kansas City Kansas Community College

Karen S. Bloomfield, RN, MSN, PMHCBS-BC
Piedmont Virginia Community College

Eileen O. Costello, RN, MSN
Mount Wachusett Community College

Dr. Jennifer L. Ellis DNP, RN
University of Cincinnati

Dr. Jim Hodge Ed.D.
University of Charleston

Jennifer Hoxsey MSN
Southern Illinois University Edwardsville

Carol A. Penrosa RN, MSN
Southeast Community College

Sonia Rudolph, RN, MSN, APRN, FNP-BC
Jefferson Community & Technical College

Mary G. Tan PhD MSN RN
South University

Debra D Terry, RN MSN
Jefferson Community & Technical College

Learn to Calculate Dosages Safely and Accurately!

The Ease of Learning with Dimensional Analysis

Medical Dosage Calculations provides the ease of learning the dimensional analysis method of calculation with a building block approach of the basics.

Name: _____   Date: _____

Diagnostic Test of Arithmetic

The following Diagnostic Test illustrates *all* the arithmetic skills needed to do the computations in this textbook. Take the test and compare your answers with the answers found in Appendix A. If you discover areas of weakness, carefully review the relevant review materials in this chapter so that you will be mathematically prepared for the rest of the textbook.

1. Write 0.375 as a fraction in lowest terms. _____

2. Write $\frac{28,500}{100,000}$ as a decimal number. _____

3. Round off 6.492 to the nearest tenth. _____

4. Write $\frac{5}{6}$ as a decimal number rounded off to the nearest hundredth. _____

5. Simplify $\frac{0.63}{0.2}$ to a decimal number rounded off to the nearest tenth. _____

6. $0.038 \times 100 =$ _____

7. $4.26 \times 0.015 =$ _____

8. $55 \div 0.11 =$ _____

9. $90 \times \frac{1}{300} \times \frac{20}{3} =$ _____

10. Write $5\frac{3}{4} \div 23$ as a fraction and as a decimal number. _____

11. Write $\frac{7}{100} \div \frac{3}{100}$ as a mixed number. _____

12. Write $\frac{\frac{4}{5}}{20}$ as a simple fraction in lowest terms. _____

The Diagnostic Test of Arithmetic helps students rediscover their understanding of basic math concepts and guides them in identifying areas for review.

EXAMPLE 5.5

A patient weighs 150 *pounds*. What is the patient's weight measured in kilograms?

$$150 \ pounds = ? \ kilograms$$

You want to cancel the *pounds* and get the answer in *kilograms*, so choose a fraction with *pounds* on the bottom and *kilograms* on top.

You need a fraction in the form of $\frac{? \ kg}{? \ lb}$

Because 2.2 *pounds* = 1 *kilogram*, the fraction you need is $\frac{1 \ kg}{2.2 \ lb}$

$$\frac{150 \ lb}{1} \times \frac{1 \ kg}{2.2 \ lb} \approx 68.1818 \ kg$$

So, the patient weighs about 68 *kilograms*.

Learn by Example. Each chapter unfolds basic concepts and skills through completely worked-out questions with solutions.

EXAMPLE 6.2

The prescriber orders *Zoloft (sertraline HCl) 50 mg PO B.I.D.* Read the drug label in • Figure 6.2 and determine how many tablets of this antipsychotic drug you would give to the patient.

You must convert the order of 50 *milligrams* to tablets.

$$50 \ mg = ? \ tab$$

Cancel the milligrams and obtain the equivalent amount in tablets.

$$\frac{50 \ mg}{1} \times \frac{? \ tab}{? \ mg} = ? \ tab$$

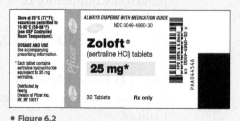

• Figure 6.2
Drug label for Zoloft.

Safe and Accurate Dosage Calculation

Safe and accurate dosage calculation comes from practice and critical thinking.

Try These for Practice, Exercises, and **Additional Exercises.** found in every chapter, tests your comprehension of material.

Workspace

Practice Sets

The answers to *Try These for Practice* and *Exercises* are found in Appendix A. Ask your instructor for the answers to the *Additional Exercises*.

Try These for Practice

Test your comprehension after reading the chapter.

1. Write $\frac{7}{16}$ as a decimal number rounded off to the hundredths place.

2. Find 23% of 59 and round down the answer to the tenths place.

3. Fill in the missing numbers in this chart.

Fraction	Decimal	Percent
$\frac{1}{2}$	0.5	50%
$\frac{3}{4}$		
	0.45	
		3%

4. Perform the multiplication: $\frac{6}{33} \times \frac{55}{6} \times 14$

5. Write the value of this expression as an ordinary fraction: $\frac{\frac{21}{80}}{\frac{7}{8}}$

Exercises

Reinforce your understanding in class or at home.

Convert to whole numbers, proper fractions, or mixed numbers (Questions 1–7).

Workspace

1. $0.55 =$ _____
2. $4\frac{1}{4} + 3\frac{3}{4} =$ _____
3. $15 \times \frac{3}{5} \times \frac{4}{27} =$ _____
4. $2\frac{3}{4} \div 7 =$ _____
5. $36 \div \frac{9}{10} =$ _____
6. $0.72 + \frac{9}{20} =$ _____
7. $20,000 \times \frac{7}{15,000} \times \frac{1}{56} =$ _____

Additional Exercises

Now, test yourself!

Convert to proper fractions or mixed numbers (Questions 1–7).

1. $0.65 =$ _____
2. $3\frac{1}{4} + 4\frac{1}{4} =$ _____
3. $50 \times \frac{3}{5} \times \frac{1}{30} =$ _____
4. $6\frac{3}{5} \div 11 =$ _____
5. $60 + \frac{13}{5} =$ _____
6. $6.3 + \frac{3}{4} =$ _____
7. $52 \times \frac{5}{8,400} \times \frac{21}{0.13} =$ _____

Cumulative Review Exercises begin in Chapter 4 and review mastery of earlier chapters.

Workspace

Cumulative Review Exercises

Reinforce your mastery of previous chapters.

1. $88 \; mm =$ _____ cm
2. $40 \; oz =$ _____ lb
3. $3.7 \; L =$ _____ mL
4. $5 \; T =$ _____ t
5. $5 \; ft =$ _____ in
6. $2\frac{1}{2}$ *cups per day* = ? *ounces per week*
7. Order: *Dilantin (phenytoin) 300 mg po t.i.d.* How many *grams* are to be administered to the patient in the course of one day?
8. A patient must drink 16 *ounces* of the laxative GoLYTELY. How many *cups* must the patient drink?
9. Order: *Ritalin (methylphenidate hydrochloride) 20 mg po daily in 2 divided doses.* How many *mg* of this psychostimulant drug will you administer to the patient with attention-deficit hyperactivity disorder (ADHD)?
10. What is missing from this order? *Sitavig (acyclovir) 50 mg apply within one hour after the onset of symptoms and before the appearance of any signs of herpes labialis lesions.*
11. If a patient receives a drug *40 mg po b.i.d.*, how many *mg* would be administered in a 24-hour period?
12. If a patient receives a drug *40 mg po q12h*, how many *mg* would be administered in a 24-hour period?
13. If a patient receives a drug *40 mg po daily in two divided doses*, how many *mg* would be administered in a 24-hour period?

Case Studies. Clinical case scenarios provide opportunities for critical thinking as you apply concepts and techniques presented in the text.

Case Study 8.1

Read the Case Study and answer the questions. Answers can be found in Appendix A.

A 65-year-old male is admitted to a rehab facility, status post right-sided cerebral vascular accident (CVA). He has a past medical history of hypertension, hyperlipidemia, atrial fibrillation, osteoarthritis, and insulin-dependent diabetes mellitus. He is alert and oriented to person, place, time, and recent memory. He has left-sided weakness, needs assistance with activities of daily living (ADL), and has a 3 cm wound on his left heel. He rates his pain level as 8 on a scale of 0–10. Vital signs are: T 98.7° F; P 88; R 24; B/P 134/82. His orders are as follows:

- diltiazem LA 120 *mg* po daily
- nabumetone 1,000 *mg* po at bedtime

- warfarin 2.5 *mg* po daily
- Lipitor 40 *mg* po at bedtime
- Sustacal 2 *oz* po with each oral medication administration
- Humulin R insulin 10 *units* and Humulin N insulin 34 *units* subcut 30 *minutes* ac breakfast
- Humulin R insulin 10 *units* and Humulin N insulin 28 *units* subcut 30 *minutes* ac dinner
- Pneumovax 0.5 *mL* IM stat for 1 dose
- Cleanse left heel with NS solution (0.9% Na Cl) and apply DSD daily

Refer to the labels below when necessary to answer the following questions.

1. Select the correct label for the diltiazem dose. How many tablets will you administer?
2. Select the correct label for the warfarin dose. How many tablets will you administer?
3. How many tablets of atorvastatin will you administer?
4. How many tablets of nabumetone will you administer?
5. How many *mL* of Sustacal will the patient receive daily?

ALERT

The same insulin pen should not be used for multiple patients.

Notes and **Alerts** highlight concepts and principles for safe medication calculation and administration.

NOTE

When you are mixing two types of insulin, think: "Clear, then Cloudy."

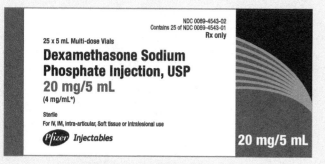

NDC 0069-4543-02
Contains 25 of NDC 0069-4543-01
Rx only

25 x 5 mL Multi-dose Vials

Dexamethasone Sodium Phosphate Injection, USP
20 mg/5 mL
(4 mg/mL*)

Sterile
For IV, IM, intra-articular, Soft tissue or intralesional use

Pfizer Injectables

20 mg/5 mL

Realistic Illustrations. Real drug labels and realistic syringes aid in identifying and practicing with what you will encounter in actual clinical settings.

Additional Student Resources!
Go to nursing.pearsonhighered.com for additional practice questions.

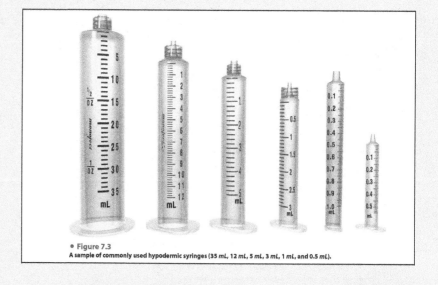

• Figure 7.3
A sample of commonly used hypodermic syringes (35 mL, 12 mL, 5 mL, 3 mL, 1 mL, and 0.5 mL).

Contents

CHAPTER 3   Dimensional Analysis   77

Unit 2   Systems of Measurement   97

CHAPTER 4   The Household and Metric Systems   98

Unit

1

Basic Calculation Skills and Introduction to Medication Administration

Chapter

1

Review of Arithmetic for Dosage Calculations

Learning Outcomes

$$5\tfrac{3}{4} \div 23$$

After completing this chapter, you will be able to

1. Reduce and build fractions into equivalent forms.
2. Add, subtract, multiply, and divide fractions.
3. Simplify complex fractions.
4. Convert between decimal numbers and fractions.
5. Add, subtract, multiply, and divide decimal numbers.
6. Round decimal numbers to a desired number of decimal places.
7. Write percentages as decimal numbers and fractions.
8. Find the percent of a number and the percent of change.
9. Estimate answers.
10. Use a calculator to verify answers.

Medical dosage calculations can involve whole numbers, fractions, decimal numbers, and percentages. Your results on the *Diagnostic Test of Arithmetic*, found on the next page, will identify your areas of strength and weakness. You can use this chapter to improve your math skills or simply to review the kinds of calculations you will encounter in this text.

Name: _____   Date: _____

Diagnostic Test of Arithmetic

The following Diagnostic Test illustrates *all* the arithmetic skills needed to do the computations in this textbook. Take the test and compare your answers with the answers found in Appendix A. If you discover areas of weakness, carefully review the relevant review materials in this chapter so that you will be mathematically prepared for the rest of the textbook.

1. Write 0.375 as a fraction in lowest terms. _____

2. Write $\frac{28,500}{100,000}$ as a decimal number. _____

3. Round off 6.492 to the nearest tenth. _____

4. Write $\frac{5}{6}$ as a decimal number rounded off to the nearest hundredth.

   _____

5. Simplify $\frac{0.63}{0.2}$ to a decimal number rounded off to the nearest tenth.

   _____

6. $0.038 \times 100 =$ _____

7. $4.26 \times 0.015 =$ _____

8. $55 \div 0.11 =$ _____

9. $90 \times \frac{1}{300} \times \frac{20}{3} =$ _____

10. Write $5\frac{3}{4} \div 23$ as a fraction and as a decimal number. _____

11. Write $\frac{7}{100} \div \frac{3}{100}$ as a mixed number. _____

12. Write $\frac{\frac{4}{5}}{20}$ as a simple fraction in lowest terms. _____

13. Write 45% as a fraction in lowest terms. _____

14. Write $2\frac{1}{2}\%$ as a decimal number. _____

15. Write $2\frac{4}{7}$ as an improper fraction. _____

16. 30% of 40 = _____

17. $4.1 + 0.5 + 3 =$ _____

18. $\frac{3}{4} = \frac{?}{8}$ _____

19. Which is larger, 0.4 or 0.21? _____

20. Express the ratio *15 to 20* as a fraction in lowest terms. _____

Workspace

Changing Decimal Numbers and Whole Numbers to Fractions

A decimal number represents a fraction with a denominator of 10; 100; 1,000; and so on. Each decimal number has three parts: the whole-number part, the decimal point, and the fraction part. Table 1.1 shows the names of the decimal positions (places values).

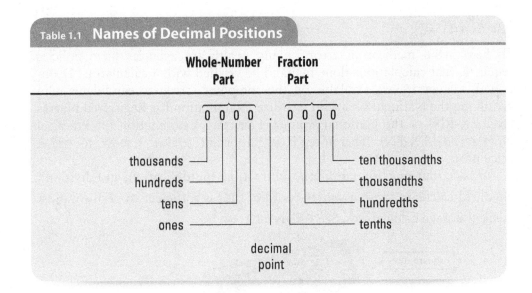

Table 1.1 Names of Decimal Positions

Reading a decimal number will help you write it as a fraction.

Decimal Number	$\longrightarrow$	Read	$\longrightarrow$	Fraction
4.1	$\longrightarrow$	four and one tenth	$\longrightarrow$	$4\frac{1}{10}$
0.3	$\longrightarrow$	three tenths	$\longrightarrow$	$\frac{3}{10}$
6.07	$\longrightarrow$	six and seven hundredths	$\longrightarrow$	$6\frac{7}{100}$
0.231	$\longrightarrow$	two hundred thirty-one thousandths	$\longrightarrow$	$\frac{231}{1,000}$
0.0025	$\longrightarrow$	twenty-five ten thousandths	$\longrightarrow$	$\frac{25}{10,000}$

NOTE

A decimal number that is less than 1 is written with a leading zero—for example, 0.3 and 0.0025.

A number can be written in different forms. A decimal number *less than 1,* such as 0.9, is read as *nine tenths* and also can be written as the *proper fraction* $\frac{9}{10}$. In a **proper fraction,** the **numerator** (the number on the top) of the fraction is smaller than its **denominator** (the number on the bottom).

A decimal number *greater than 1,* such as 3.5, is read as *three and five tenths* and can also be written as the *mixed number* $3\frac{5}{10}$ or reduced to lowest terms as $3\frac{1}{2}$. A **mixed number** combines a whole number and a proper fraction. The *mixed number* $3\frac{1}{2}$ can be changed to an *improper fraction* as follows:

$$3\frac{1}{2} = \frac{3 \times 2 + 1}{2} = \frac{7}{2}$$

The numerator of an **improper fraction** is larger than or equal to its denominator.

Any number can be written as a fraction by writing it over 1. For example, 9 can be written as the improper fraction $\frac{9}{1}$.

Calculator

To help avoid medication errors, many healthcare agencies have policies requiring that calculations done by hand be verified with a calculator. "Drop-down" calculators are available on the computer screen to candidates who are taking the National Council Licensure Examination for Registered Nurses (NCLEX-RN) or the National Council Licensure Examination for Practical Nurses (NCLEX-PN). Therefore, it is important to know how to use a calculator.

A basic four-function (addition, subtraction, multiplication, and division), handheld calculator with a square-root key $\sqrt{}$ is sufficient to perform most medical dosage calculations. See • **Figure 1.1**.

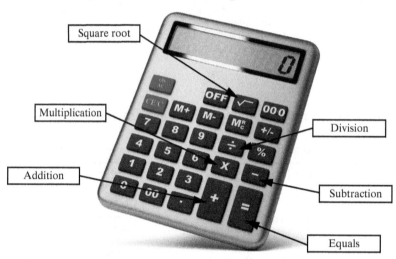

• **Figure 1.1**
Basic handheld calculator.

Some students might prefer a calculator that also has a percent key %, a fraction key a^b/c, and parentheses keys (and).

To change the improper fraction $\frac{7}{2}$ to a decimal number with a calculator:

First press 7
Then press ÷
Then press 2
Then press =
The display shows 3.5

This keystroke sequence will be abbreviated as 7 ÷ 2 = 3.5

If the calculator has a fraction key, the mixed-number form of $\frac{7}{2}$ will be obtained by the following keystroke sequence:

$$7 \boxed{a^{b}/_{c}} \ 2 \ \boxed{=} \quad \boxed{3\frac{1}{2}}$$

Throughout this chapter, keystroke sequences will be shown for selected examples. The calculator icon, , will indicate where this occurs.

EXAMPLE 1.1

Write 2.25 as a mixed number and as an improper fraction.

The number 2.25 is read *two and twenty-five hundredths* and is written $2\frac{25}{100}$. You can simplify:

$$2\frac{25}{100} = 2\frac{\overset{1}{\cancel{25}}}{\underset{4}{\cancel{100}}} = 2\frac{1}{4} = \frac{2 \times 4 + 1}{4} = \frac{9}{4}$$

So, 2.25 can be written as the mixed number $2\frac{1}{4}$ or as the improper fraction $\frac{9}{4}$.

Keystroke Sequence for Example 1.1:

To obtain the simplified mixed number, enter the following keystroke sequence.

$$2 \boxed{a^{b}/_{c}} \ 25 \boxed{a^{b}/_{c}} \ 100 \ \boxed{=}$$
$$\boxed{2\frac{1}{4}}$$

Ratios

A **ratio** is a comparison of two numbers.

The ratio of *5 to 10* can also be written as *5:10* or in fractional form as $\frac{5}{10}$. This fraction may be *reduced by cancelling* by a number that evenly divides both the numerator and the denominator. Because *5* evenly divides both *5* and 10, divide as follows:

$$\frac{5}{10} = \frac{5 \div 5}{10 \div 5} = \frac{1}{2}$$

The fraction $\frac{5}{10}$ is *reduced to lowest terms* as $\frac{1}{2}$.

So, the ratio of *5 to 10* can also be written as the ratio of *1 to 2* or *1:2*.

EXAMPLE 1.2

Express 6:18 as an equivalent fraction and ratio in lowest terms.

The ratio *6:18*, also written as *6 to 18*, can be written in fractional form as $\frac{6}{18}$. This fraction may be *reduced by cancelling* by a number that evenly divides both the numerator and the denominator. Because 6 divides both 6 and 18, divide as follows:

$$\frac{6}{18} = \frac{6 \div 6}{18 \div 6} = \frac{1}{3}$$

So, the ratio 6 to 18 equals the fraction $\frac{1}{3}$ and the ratio 1:3.

Keystroke Sequence for Example 1.2:

$$6 \boxed{a^{b}/_{c}} \ 18 \ \boxed{=} \ \boxed{\frac{1}{3}}$$

Keystroke Sequence for Example 1.3:

To check the answer use

 12 $a^{b}/_{c}$ 120 = $\frac{1}{10}$

NOTE

When *reducing* a fraction, you *divide* both numerator and denominator by the same number. This process is called *cancelling*.

When *building* a fraction, you *multiply* both numerator and denominator by the same number.

EXAMPLE 1.3

Write the ratio 1:10 as an equivalent fraction with 120 in the denominator.

Because 1:10 as a fraction is $\frac{1}{10}$, you need to write this fraction with the larger denominator of 120. Such processes are called **building fractions.**

$$\frac{1}{10} = \frac{?}{120}$$

$\frac{1}{10}$ may be built up by *multiplying numerator and denominator of the fraction by the same number* (12 in this case) as follows:

$$\frac{1}{10} = \frac{1 \times 12}{10 \times 12} = \frac{12}{120}$$

So, 1:10 is equivalent to $\frac{12}{120}$.

Changing Fractions to Decimal Numbers

To change a fraction to a decimal number, think of the fraction as a division problem. For example:

$$\frac{2}{5} \quad \text{means} \quad 2 \div 5 \quad \text{or} \quad 5\overline{)2}$$

Here are the steps for this division.

Step 1   Replace 2 with 2.0, and then place a decimal point directly above the decimal point in 2.0.

$$5\overline{)\overset{.}{2.0}}$$

Step 2   Perform the division *twenty divided by five = four.*

$$\begin{array}{r} 0.4 \\ 5\overline{)2.0} \\ \underline{2\ 0} \\ 0 \end{array}$$

Keystroke sequence:

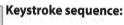 2 ÷ 5 = 0.4   So, $\frac{2}{5} = 0.4$

EXAMPLE 1.4

Write $\frac{5}{2}$ as a decimal number.

$$\frac{5}{2} \quad \text{means} \quad 5 \div 2 \quad \text{or} \quad 2\overline{)5}$$

Step 1 $2\overline{)5.0}$

Step 2 $\begin{array}{r} 2.5 \\ 2\overline{)5.0} \\ \underline{4} \\ 1\ 0 \\ \underline{1\ 0} \end{array}$

So, $\dfrac{5}{2} = 2.5$.

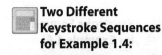

Two Different Keystroke Sequences for Example 1.4:

● 5 ÷ 2 = 2.5

If your calculator has a fraction key, you can also use the keystroke sequence:

● 5 $a^{b}\!/_{c}$ 2 = $2\frac{1}{2}$

EXAMPLE 1.5

Write $\dfrac{193}{10}$ as a decimal number.

$$\dfrac{193}{10} \quad \text{means} \quad 193 \div 10 \quad \text{or} \quad 10\overline{)193}$$

Step 1 $10\overline{)193.0}$

Step 2 $\begin{array}{r} 19.3 \\ 10\overline{)193.0} \\ \underline{10} \\ 93 \\ \underline{90} \\ 30 \\ \underline{30} \\ 0 \end{array}$

So, $\dfrac{193}{10} = 19.3$.

Two Different Keystroke Sequences for Example 1.5:

● 193 ÷ 10 = 19.3

If your calculator has a fraction key, you can also use:

● 193 $a^{b}\!/_{c}$ 10 = $19\frac{3}{10}$

There is a quicker way to do Example 1.5. To divide a *decimal number by 10*, *move* the decimal point in the number *one place to the left*. Notice that there is one zero in 10.

$$\dfrac{193}{10} = \dfrac{193.}{10} = 19\overset{\curvearrowleft}{3.} = 19.3$$

To *divide a number by 100*, *move* the decimal point in the number *two places to the left* because there are two zeros in 100. So, the quick way to divide by 10; 100; 1,000; and so on is to count the zeros and then move the decimal point to the left the same number of places; the answer should always be a *smaller* number than the original number. Check your answer to be sure.

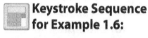

Keystroke Sequence for Example 1.6:

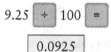

9.25 ÷ 100 =

0.0925

EXAMPLE 1.6

Write $\frac{9.25}{100}$ as a decimal number.

This fraction means $9.25 \div 100$. There are two zeros in 100, so move the decimal point in 9.25 two places to the left, and fill the empty position with a zero.

$$\frac{9.25}{100} = \underset{\smile\smile}{}9.25 = 0.0925$$

Rounding Decimal Numbers

Sometimes it is convenient to round an answer—that is, to use an approximate answer rather than an exact one.

Rounding Off

To round off 1.267 to the *nearest tenth*—that is, to round off the number to one decimal place—do the following:

Look at the digit after the tenths-place (the hundredths-place digit). Because this digit (6) is 5 or more, round off 1.267 by adding 1 to the tenths-place digit. Finally, drop all the digits after the tenths-place.

So, 1.267 is approximated by 1.3 when rounded off to the nearest tenth.

To round off 0.8345 to the *nearest hundredth*—that is, to round off the number to two decimal places—do the following:

Look at the digit after the hundredths-place (the thousandths-place digit). Because this digit (4) is less than 5, round off 0.8345 by leaving the hundredths digit alone. Finally, drop all the digits after the hundredths-place.

So, 0.8345 is approximated by 0.83 when rounded off to the nearest hundredth.

EXAMPLE 1.7

Round off 4.8075 to the nearest hundredth, tenth, and whole number.

4.8075 rounded off to the nearest: hundredth → 4.81

tenth → 4.8

whole number → 5

Rounding Down and Rounding Up

NOTE

Rounding down is also referred to as *truncating,* which means "cutting off" digits.

In the *rounding off* process, either 0 or 1 is added to the appropriate digit of a given number; therefore, the rounded result can be either smaller or larger than the given number. In healthcare, two other types of rounding are also used. **Rounding down** and **rounding up** are similar to rounding off. The only difference is that in *rounding down, 0 is always added* to the appropriate digit, whereas in *rounding up, 1 is always added* to the appropriate digit.

When rounding down both 2.34 and 2.36 to the tenths place, *add 0* to the tenths-place digit and delete the remaining digits. Thus, both 2.34 and 2.36 round down to 2.3.

When rounding up 2.34 and 2.36 to the tenths place, *add 1* to the tenths-place digit and delete the remaining digits. Thus, both 2.34 and 2.36 round up to 2.4.

Generally speaking, rounding down results in a smaller quantity, whereas rounding up results in a larger quantity. So, *rounding down* a dosage helps to avoid an overdose, and *rounding up* a dosage helps to avoid an underdose. When rounding a dosage calculation, most of the time rounding off is used. However, sometimes rounding down is used, whereas rounding up is very rarely used.

EXAMPLE 1.8

Fill in the table with the indicated rounded numbers.

Number	Round to	Rounded Off	Rounded Down	Rounded Up
0.123	hundredths			
0.129	hundredths			
3.87	tenths			
3.84	tenths			

You should have gotten the following answers:

Number	Round to	Rounded Off	Rounded Down	Rounded Up
0.123	hundredths	0.12	0.12	0.13
0.129	hundredths	0.13	0.12	0.13
3.87	tenths	3.9	3.8	3.9
3.84	tenths	3.8	3.8	3.9

Adding Decimal Numbers

When adding decimal numbers, write the numbers in a column with the *decimal points lined up under each other*.

EXAMPLE 1.9

$$3.4 + 0.07 + 6 = ?$$

Write the numbers in a column with the decimal points lined up. *Trailing zeros* may be included to give each number the same amount of decimal places. Therefore, write 6 as 6.00 [Think: $6 is equivalent to $6.00].

$$
\begin{array}{r}
3.40 \\
0.07 \\
+ \ 6.00 \\
\hline
9.47
\end{array}
$$

So, the sum of 3.4, 0.07, and 6 is 9.47.

Keystroke Sequence for Example 1.9:

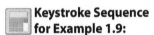

3.4 [+] .07 [+] 6 [=]

9.47

Subtracting Decimal Numbers

When adding or subtracting decimal numbers, write the numbers in a column with the *decimal points lined up under each other*.

Keystroke Sequence for Example 1.10:

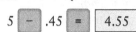

5 [−] .45 [=] | 4.55 |

ALERT

Be careful: the *subtraction* (minus) key looks like [−], whereas the *negative* key looks like (−) or +/−.

EXAMPLE 1.10

$$5 - 0.45 = ?$$

Write the numbers in a column with the decimal points lined up. Include *trailing zeros* to give each number the same amount of decimal places.

$$
\begin{array}{r}
5.00 \\
- 0.45 \\
\hline
4.55
\end{array}
$$

So, the difference between 5 and 0.45 is 4.55.

Multiplying Decimal Numbers

To multiply two decimal numbers, first multiply ignoring the decimal points. Then count the total number of decimal places (digits to the right of the decimal point) in the original two numbers. That sum equals the number of decimal places in the answer.

Keystroke Sequence for Example 1.11:

304.2 [×] .16 [=]

| 48.672 |

You need not press the leading zero when entering 0.16

EXAMPLE 1.11

$$304.2 \times 0.16 = ?$$

$$
\begin{array}{r}
304.2 \\
\times\ 0.16 \\
\hline
18252 \\
3042 \\
\hline
48.672
\end{array}
$$

← 1 decimal place ⎫ Total of 3
← 2 decimal places ⎬ decimal places

There are 3 decimal places in the answer.

Place the decimal point here.

So, 304.2 × 0.16 = 48.672.

Keystroke Sequence for Example 1.12:

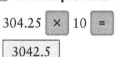

304.25 [×] 10 [=]

| 3042.5 |

EXAMPLE 1.12

$$304.25 \times 10 = ?$$

$$
\begin{array}{r}
304.25 \\
\times\ \ \ \ 10 \\
\hline
3\,042.50
\end{array}
$$

← 2 decimal places ⎫ Total of 2
← 0 decimal places ⎬ decimal places

There are 2 decimal places in the answer.

Place the decimal point here.

So, 304.25 × 10 = 3,042.50 or 3,042.5.

There is a quicker way to do Example 1.12. To *multiply any decimal number by 10, move* the decimal point in the number being multiplied *one place to the right*. Notice that there is one zero in 10.

$$304.25 \times 10 = 304.25 \quad \text{or} \quad 3{,}042.5$$

To *multiply a number by 100, move* the decimal point in the number *two places to the right* because there are two zeros in 100. So, the quick way to multiply by 10; 100; 1,000; and so on is to count the zeros and then move the decimal point to the right the same number of places. The answer should always be a *larger* number than the original. Check your answer to be sure.

EXAMPLE 1.13

$$23.597 \times 1{,}000 = ?$$

There are three zeros in 1,000, so move the decimal point in 23.597 three places to the right.

$$23.597 \times 1{,}000 = 2\,3\,.5\,9\,7 \quad \text{or} \quad 23{,}597$$

So, $23.597 \times 1{,}000 = 23{,}597$.

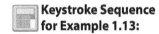

Keystroke Sequence for Example 1.13:

23.597 ⨯ 1000 =
23597

Dividing Decimal Numbers

When dividing with decimal numbers, be sure that you are careful where you place the decimal point in the answer.

EXAMPLE 1.14

Write the fraction $\frac{106.8}{15}$ as a decimal number rounded off to the nearest tenth; that is, round off the answer to one decimal place.

Treat this fraction as a division problem.

$$\frac{106.8}{15} \quad \text{means} \quad 15\overline{)106.8}$$

Step 1 $15\overline{)106.8}$

Step 2   Because you want the answer to the nearest tenth (one decimal place), do the division to two decimal places and then round off the answer.

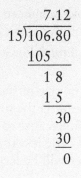

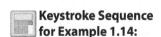

Keystroke Sequence for Example 1.14:

106.8 ÷ 15 = 7.12

≈ 7.1 after rounding off. The symbol ≈ means "is approximately equal to."

Because the hundredths place digit in the answer is *less than 5*, leave the tenths place digit alone. Finally, drop the digit in the hundredths place. So, $\frac{106.8}{15}$ is approximated by the decimal number 7.1 to the nearest tenth.

Keystroke Sequence for Example 1.15:

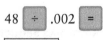

24000

EXAMPLE 1.15

Simplify $\dfrac{48}{0.002}$

Think of this fraction as a division problem. Because there are three decimal places in 0.002, move the decimal points in both numbers three places to the right.

$$\frac{48}{0.002} \quad \text{means} \quad 0.002\overline{)48.} \quad \text{or} \quad 0.002\overline{)48.000}$$

$$\begin{array}{r} 24{,}000. \\ 2\overline{)48{,}000.} \\ \underline{4} \\ 08 \\ \underline{8} \\ 0 \end{array}$$

So, $\dfrac{48}{0.002} = 24{,}000.$

Example 1.15 could also have been done by eliminating the decimal point from the given fraction by multiplying by $\frac{1000}{1000}$ as follows:

$$\frac{48}{0.002} \times \frac{1000}{1000} = \frac{48000}{2} = 24{,}000$$

Estimating Answers

When you use a calculator, errors in the keystroke sequence may lead to dangerously high or dangerously low dosages. To help avoid such mistakes:

1. *Carefully* enter the keystroke sequence. A calculator that simultaneously shows both your entries and the answer in the display is desirable.
2. Think: *Is the answer reasonable?* For example, an oral dosage of 50 tablets is not reasonable!
3. Use rounding to *estimate* the size of the answer. The product of 498 and 49 can be estimated by rounding the numbers off to 500 and 50, respectively. $500 \times 50 = 25{,}000$. Because each factor was made larger, the product of 498 and 49 is a little less than 25,000. Sometimes it is useful to know whether an answer will be larger or smaller than a given number.

EXAMPLE 1.16

Which is larger, 0.4 or 0.23?

Write the numbers in a column with the decimal points lined up, and include trailing zeros to give each number the same amount of decimal places.

$$0.40$$
$$0.23$$

Because 40 hundredths is larger than 23 hundredths, 0.4 is larger than 0.23.

For positive numbers, when one number is divided by a second number, if the answer is larger than 1, the first number is the larger. If the answer is less than 1, the second number is larger.

EXAMPLE 1.17

Is $\frac{0.9}{0.45}$ smaller or larger than 1?

Because the value in the numerator 0.9 is larger than the value in the denominator 0.45, the fraction represents a quantity larger than 1.

EXAMPLE 1.18

Estimate the value of $\frac{200}{2.2}$

Because the denominator is approximately equal to 2, the given fraction will be close in value to $\frac{200}{2}$ or 100. In this case, by making the denominator smaller (2 instead of 2.2), you made the value of the entire fraction larger. Therefore, 100 is too large (an overestimate). So, the actual value of $\frac{200}{2.2}$ is a number somewhat less than 100.

Multiplying Fractions

To *multiply fractions*, multiply the numerators to get the new numerator and multiply the denominators to get the new denominator.

EXAMPLE 1.19

$$\frac{3}{5} \times 6 \times \frac{1}{5} = ?$$

A whole number can be written as a fraction with 1 in the denominator. So, in this example, write 6 as $\frac{6}{1}$ to make all the numbers fractions.

$$\frac{3}{5} \times \frac{6}{1} \times \frac{1}{5} = \frac{3 \times 6 \times 1}{5 \times 1 \times 5} = \frac{18}{25}$$

Keystroke Sequence for Example 1.16:

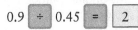

Because 1.7 is larger than 1, the first number entered (0.4) is larger than the second (0.23).

Keystroke Sequence for Example 1.17:

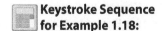

Keystroke Sequence for Example 1.18:

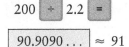

Three Different Keystroke Sequences for Example 1.19:

- Use parentheses:

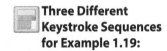

- Multiply the numerators, and then divide by each of the denominators:

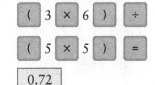

- Use the fraction key:

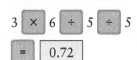
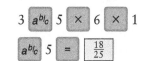

Keystroke Sequence for Example 1.20:

Multiply the numerators and divide by each of the denominators:

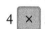

Do not verify the answer to Example 1.20 on the calculator by using the cancelled numbers 4

because the calculator will not uncover previous cancellation errors. Therefore, use the original numbers as shown in the keystroke sequences.

 Keystroke Sequence for Example 1.21:

 45

It is often convenient to cancel before you multiply.

EXAMPLE 1.20

$$\frac{4}{5} \times \frac{3}{10} \times \frac{20}{7} = ?$$

$$\frac{4}{5} \times \frac{3}{\overset{}{\underset{1}{10}}} \times \frac{\overset{2}{20}}{7} = \frac{24}{35}$$

EXAMPLE 1.21

Simplify $\frac{21 \times 15}{7}$

Method 1: Multiply the numbers in the numerator, which yields $\frac{315}{7}$, and then divide 315 by 7, which yields 45

Method 2: First cancel by 7, and then multiply

$$\frac{\overset{3}{21} \times 15}{\underset{1}{7}} = \frac{3 \times 15}{1} = \frac{45}{1} = 45$$

So, $\frac{21 \times 15}{7} = 45$.

Dividing Fractions

To *divide fractions*, change the division problem to an equivalent multiplication problem by inverting the second fraction.

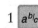 **Keystroke Sequence for Example 1.22:**

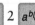

EXAMPLE 1.22

$$1\frac{2}{5} \div \frac{7}{9} = ?$$

Write $1\frac{2}{5}$ as the improper fraction $\frac{7}{5}$.

The *division* problem

$$\frac{7}{5} \div \frac{7}{9}$$

becomes the *multiplication* problem by inverting the second fraction.

$$\frac{7}{5} \times \frac{9}{7}$$

$$\frac{\overset{1}{7}}{5} \times \frac{9}{\underset{1}{7}} = \frac{9}{5} = 1\frac{4}{5}$$

In the next three examples you must deal with whole numbers, fractions, and decimal numbers in the same multiplication problem.

EXAMPLE 1.23

Give the answer to the following problem in simplified fractional form.

$$\frac{1}{300} \times 60 \times \frac{1}{0.4} = ?$$

Write 60 as a fraction and cancel.

$$\frac{1}{\cancel{300}_{5}} \times \frac{\cancel{60}^{1}}{1} \times \frac{1}{0.4} = \frac{1}{5 \times 0.4} = \frac{1}{2}$$

NOTE

Avoid cancelling decimal numbers. It is a possible source of error.

Keystroke Sequence for Example 1.23:

60 ÷ 300 ÷ .4

= 0.5

EXAMPLE 1.24

Give the answer to the following problem in simplified fractional form.

$$0.35 \times \frac{1}{60} = ?$$

Write 0.35 as the fraction $\frac{0.35}{1}$.

$$\frac{0.35}{1} \times \frac{1}{60} = \frac{0.35}{60}$$

The numerator of this fraction is 0.35, a decimal number. You can write an equivalent form of the fraction by multiplying the numerator and denominator by 100.

$$\frac{0.35}{60} \times \frac{100}{100} = \frac{0.35}{60.00} = \frac{35}{6,000} = \frac{7}{1,200}$$

Two Different Keystroke Sequences for Example 1.24:

● .35 ÷ 60 =

0.0058...

● If you think of 0.35 as $\frac{35}{100}$, then use the fraction key:

35 $a^{b}/_{c}$ 100 × 1 $a^{b}/_{c}$

60 = $\frac{7}{1,200}$

EXAMPLE 1.25

Give the answer to the following problem in simplified fractional form.

$$0.88 \times \frac{1}{2.22} = ?$$

$$\frac{0.88}{1} \times \frac{1}{2.2} = \frac{0.88}{2.2}$$

Multiply the numerator and the denominator of this fraction by 100 to eliminate both decimal numbers.

$$\frac{0.88}{2.2} \times \frac{100}{100} = \frac{0.88}{2.2} = \frac{88}{220} = \frac{2}{5}$$

You can simplify $\frac{0.88}{2.2}$ a different way by dividing 0.88 by 2.2

$$2.2\overline{)0.88} = 0.4 \quad \text{and} \quad 0.4 = \frac{4}{10} \quad \text{or} \quad \frac{2}{5}$$

Keystroke Sequence for Example 1.25:

.88 ÷ 2.2 = 0.4

To change 0.4 to a fraction in lowest terms:

4 $a^{b}/_{c}$ 10 = $\frac{2}{5}$

Complex Fractions

Fractions that have numerators or denominators that are themselves fractions are called **complex fractions.**

The longest line in the complex fraction separates the numerator from the denominator of the complex fraction. As with any fraction, you can write the complex fraction as a division problem: *Top ÷ Bottom*.

In the complex fraction $\dfrac{1}{\frac{2}{5}}$, the numerator is 1 and the denominator is $\frac{2}{5}$.

You can simplify this complex fraction as follows:

$$\frac{1}{\frac{2}{5}} \quad \text{means} \quad 1 \div \frac{2}{5} \quad \text{or} \quad 1 \times \frac{5}{2}, \quad \text{which is} \quad \frac{5}{2}$$

In the complex fraction $\dfrac{\frac{1}{2}}{5}$, the numerator is $\frac{1}{2}$ and the denominator is 5.

You can simplify this complex fraction as follows:

$$\frac{\frac{1}{2}}{5} \quad \text{means} \quad \frac{1}{2} \div 5 \quad \text{or} \quad \frac{1}{2} \times \frac{1}{5}, \quad \text{which is} \quad \frac{1}{10}$$

In the complex fraction $\dfrac{\frac{3}{5}}{\frac{2}{5}}$, the numerator is $\frac{3}{5}$ and the denominator is $\frac{2}{5}$.

You can simplify this complex fraction as follows:

$$\frac{\frac{3}{5}}{\frac{2}{5}} \quad \text{means} \quad \frac{3}{5} \div \frac{2}{5} \quad \text{or} \quad \frac{3}{\overset{}{\underset{1}{5}}} \times \frac{\overset{1}{5}}{2}, \quad \text{which is} \quad \frac{3}{2}$$

Keystroke Sequence for Example 1.26:

- For a fractional answer:

  (16 $a^{b/}c$ 3) ÷

  (36 $a^{b/}c$ 5) =

  $\dfrac{20}{27}$

- For a decimal number answer:

  (16 ÷ 3) ÷

  (36 ÷ 5) =

  0.7407...

Two Different Keystroke Sequences for Example 1.27:

- (2 ÷ 3) ×

  (1 ÷ (3 ÷ 4

)) =   0.8888...

- To obtain the fractional form:

  2 $a^{b/}c$ 3 × (1 $a^{b/}c$

  (3 $a^{b/}c$ 4))

  = $\dfrac{8}{9}$

EXAMPLE 1.26

Simplify $\dfrac{\frac{16}{3}}{\frac{36}{5}}$ as a decimal number rounded off to the nearest tenth.

Divide the numerator $\dfrac{16}{3}$ by the denominator $\dfrac{36}{5}$.

$$\frac{16}{3} \div \frac{36}{5}$$

$$\frac{16}{3} \times \frac{5}{36} = \frac{20}{27} = 0.740 \ldots \approx 0.7$$

EXAMPLE 1.27

$$\frac{\frac{2}{3} \times \frac{1}{3}}{4} = ?$$

You can multiply the numerators to get the new numerator and multiply the denominators to get the new denominator, as follows:

$$\frac{2}{3} \times \frac{1}{\frac{3}{4}} = \frac{2 \times 1}{3 \times \frac{3}{4}} = \frac{2}{\frac{9}{4}}$$

Now, the numerator is 2 and the denominator is $\frac{9}{4}$, so you get

$$\frac{2}{1} \div \frac{9}{4}$$

which becomes $\quad \frac{2}{1} \times \frac{4}{9} = \frac{8}{9}$

This problem could have been done another way by simplifying $\frac{1}{\frac{3}{4}}$ first.

You can write $\frac{1}{\frac{3}{4}}$ as $\quad 1 \div \frac{3}{4}\quad$ as $\quad 1 \times \frac{4}{3}\quad$ or $\quad \frac{4}{3}$

Then

$$\frac{2}{3} \times \frac{4}{3} = \frac{8}{9}$$

Addition and Subtraction of Fractions

Addition and subtraction of fractions in this textbook generally involves fractions with denominators of 2, 4, or 8.

Same Denominators

When adding or subtracting fractions that have the *same denominators, add or subtract the numerators and keep the common denominator.*

Add $\frac{1}{2}$ and $\frac{1}{2}$

$$\frac{1}{2} + \frac{1}{2} = \frac{1+1}{2} = \frac{2}{2}, \text{ which equals } 1$$

From $\frac{11}{4}$ subtract $\frac{5}{4}$

$$\frac{11}{4} - \frac{5}{4} = \frac{11-5}{4} = \frac{6}{4}, \text{ which can be reduced to } \frac{3}{2} \text{ or } 1\frac{1}{2}$$

For *mixed numbers* add (or subtract) the whole number and fraction parts separately.

Add $3\frac{1}{4}$ and $2\frac{1}{4}$

$$
\begin{array}{r}
3 \quad \frac{1}{4} \\
+\,2 \quad \frac{1}{4} \\
\hline
5 \quad \frac{1+1}{4} = 5\frac{2}{4}, \text{ which equals } 5\frac{1}{2}
\end{array}
$$

From $10\frac{3}{4}$ *subtract* $6\frac{1}{4}$

$$
\begin{array}{r}
10 \quad \dfrac{3}{4} \\[2mm]
-\ 6 \quad \dfrac{1}{4} \\[2mm]
\hline
4 \quad \dfrac{3-1}{4} = 4\dfrac{2}{4},\ \text{which equals } 4\dfrac{1}{2}
\end{array}
$$

Different Denominators

When adding or subtracting fractions that have *different denominators*, build the fraction(s) so that the denominators are the same (have a common denominator), and proceed as before.

Add $\frac{1}{2}$ and $\frac{1}{4}$

This problem has fractions with different denominators. Recall that $\frac{1}{2} = \frac{2}{4}$. Then the problem becomes

$$
\frac{2}{4} + \frac{1}{4} = \frac{2+1}{4} = \frac{3}{4}
$$

From $\frac{3}{4}$ subtract $\frac{1}{2}$

Recall that $\frac{1}{2} = \frac{2}{4}$. Then the problem becomes

$$
\frac{3}{4} - \frac{2}{4} = \frac{3-2}{4} = \frac{1}{4}
$$

For *mixed numbers* add (or subtract) the whole number and fraction parts separately.

Add $9\frac{3}{4}$ and $6\frac{1}{2}$

To make the denominators the same, use $\frac{1}{2} = \frac{2}{4}$

$$
\begin{array}{r}
9 \quad \dfrac{3}{4} \quad = \quad 9 \quad \dfrac{3}{4} \\[2mm]
+\ 6 \quad \dfrac{1}{2} \quad = \quad 6 \quad \dfrac{2}{4} \\[2mm]
\hline
15 \quad \dfrac{3+2}{4} = 15\dfrac{5}{4},\ \text{which equals } 16\dfrac{1}{4}
\end{array}
$$

From $9\frac{3}{4}$ subtract $6\frac{3}{8}$

To make the denominators the same, use $\frac{3}{4} = \frac{6}{8}$

$$
\begin{array}{r}
9 \quad \dfrac{3}{4} \quad = \quad 9 \quad \dfrac{6}{8} \\[2mm]
-\ 6 \quad \dfrac{3}{8} \quad = \quad 6 \quad \dfrac{3}{8} \\[2mm]
\hline
3 \quad \dfrac{6-3}{8} = 3\dfrac{3}{8}
\end{array}
$$

From $6\frac{1}{4}$ subtract $4\frac{3}{4}$

Method 1: Use borrowing (renaming).

Because $\frac{3}{4}$ is larger than $\frac{1}{4}$, subtraction of the fractions is not possible. Therefore, you may rename $6\frac{1}{4}$ as follows: Borrow 1 from the whole number part (6), and add the 1 to the fractional part ($\frac{1}{4}$). This results in $6\frac{1}{4} = (6 - 1) + (1 + \frac{1}{4})$ or $5\frac{5}{4}$.

$$
\begin{array}{rcl}
6 \ \frac{1}{4} &=& 5 \ \frac{5}{4} \\[2mm]
-6 \ \frac{3}{4} &=& 4 \ \frac{3}{4} \\[2mm]
\hline
1 \ \dfrac{5-3}{4} &=& 1\frac{2}{4} \ \text{or} \ 1\frac{1}{2}
\end{array}
$$

Method 2: Change the mixed numbers to improper fractions.

$$
\begin{array}{rcl}
6\frac{1}{4} &=& \dfrac{25}{4} \\[3mm]
-4\frac{3}{4} &=& \dfrac{19}{4} \\[2mm]
\hline
& & \dfrac{25-19}{4} = \dfrac{6}{4} \ \text{which also equals} \ 1\frac{1}{2}
\end{array}
$$

EXAMPLE 1.28

Add $4\frac{1}{2} + 5\frac{1}{2}$.

$$
\begin{array}{rl}
4 & \dfrac{1}{2} \\[3mm]
+5 & \dfrac{1}{2} \\[2mm]
\hline
9 & \dfrac{1+1}{2} = 9\frac{2}{2}, \text{ which equals } 9 + 1 \text{ or } 10
\end{array}
$$

Keystroke Sequence for Example 1.28:

4 $a^{b}\!/_{c}$ 1 $a^{b}\!/_{c}$ 2 $+$ 5

$a^{b}\!/_{c}$ 1 $a^{b}\!/_{c}$ 2 $=$ 10

Percentages

Percent (%) means *parts per 100* or *divided by 100.* Thus 50% means *50 parts per hundred* or *50 divided by 100,* which can also be written as the fraction $\frac{50}{100}$. The fraction $\frac{50}{100}$ can be changed to the decimal numbers 0.50 and 0.5 or reduced to the fraction $\frac{1}{2}$.

13%   means $\dfrac{13}{100}$ or   0.13

100%   means $\dfrac{100}{100}$ or   1

12.3%   means $\dfrac{12.3}{100}$ or   0.123

$6\frac{1}{2}$ %   means   6.5%   or $\dfrac{6.5}{100}$ or   0.065

ALERT

Calculating with numbers in percent form can be difficult, so percentages should be converted to either fractional or decimal form before performing any calculations.

EXAMPLE 1.29

Write 0.5% as a fraction in lowest terms and as a decimal number.

$$0.5\% = \frac{0.5}{100} = \frac{5}{1,000} = \frac{1}{200}$$

There is another way to get the answer. Because you understand that $0.5 = \frac{1}{2}$, then

$$0.5\% = \frac{1}{2}\% = \frac{1}{2} \div 100 = \frac{1}{2} \div \frac{100}{1} = \frac{1}{2} \times \frac{1}{100} = \frac{1}{200}$$

To obtain a decimal number, write

$$0.5\% = \frac{0.5}{100} = 0.5 = 0.005$$

EXAMPLE 1.30

Write $\frac{3}{4}$ as a decimal number and as a percent.

$$\frac{3}{4} = 3 \div 4 = 0.75$$

To change the decimal number 0.75 to a percent, move the decimal point two places to the right and add the percent sign.

$$0.75 = 75\%$$

To find a *percent of a number* or a *fraction of a number*, translate the word "of" as "multiplication," as illustrated in Examples 1.31 and 1.32.

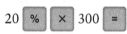

Keystroke Sequence for Example 1.31:

20 % × 300 =

60

EXAMPLE 1.31

What is 20% of 300?

To find a percent of a number, translate the "of" as multiplication.

$$20\% \text{ of } 300 \quad \text{means} \quad 20\% \times 300 \text{ or}$$
$$0.20 \times 300 = 60$$

So, 20% of 300 is 60.

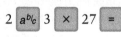

Keystroke Sequence for Example 1.32:

2 a^b/c 3 × 27 =

18

EXAMPLE 1.32

What is two-thirds of 27?

To find a fraction of a number, translate the "of" as multiplication.

$$\frac{2}{3} \text{ of } 27 \quad \text{means} \quad \frac{2}{3} \times 27 = 18$$

So, two-thirds of 27 is 18.

Percent of Change

It is often useful to determine a *percent of change* (increase or decrease). For example, you might want to know if a 20-pound weight loss for a patient is significant. For an adult patient who was 200 pounds, a 20-pound loss would be a decrease in weight of 10%. However, for a child who was 50 pounds, a 20-pound loss would be a decrease in weight of 40%, which is far more significant than a 10% loss.

To obtain the fraction of change, you may use the formula:

$$\text{Fraction of Change} = \frac{Change}{Original}$$

Change the above fraction to a percent to obtain the *percent of change*.

EXAMPLE 1.33

A daily dosage increases from 4 tablets to 5 tablets. What is the fraction of change and percent of change in daily dosage?

$$\text{Fraction of Change} = \frac{Change}{Original}$$

Because the original (old) dosage is 4 tablets, and the new dosage is 5 tablets, then the change in dosage is

$$\text{Change} = 5 \text{ tablets} - 4 \text{ tablets} = 1 \text{ tablet}$$

$$\text{Fraction of Change} = \frac{Change}{Original} = \frac{1}{4} \text{ or } 25\%$$

So, the dosage has increased by $\frac{1}{4}$ or 25%.

EXAMPLE 1.34

A person was drinking 40 ounces of fluid per day, but this was reduced to 10 ounces of fluid per day. What is the percent of change in fluid intake?

$$\text{Fraction of Change} = \frac{Change}{Original}$$

Because the original (old) amount is 40 ounces, and the new amount is 10 ounces, the change is

$$\text{Change} = 40 - 10 = 30 \text{ ounces}$$

$$\text{Fraction of Change} = \frac{Change}{Original} = \frac{30}{40} = \frac{3}{4} \text{ or } 75\%$$

So, this is a 75% decrease in fluid intake.

Summary

In this chapter, all the essential mathematical skills that are needed for dosage calculation were reviewed.

When working with fractions:
- Proper fractions have smaller numbers in the numerator than in the denominator.
- Improper fractions have numerators that are larger than or equal to their denominators.
- Improper fractions can be changed to mixed numbers, and vice versa.
- Any number can be changed into a fraction by writing the number over 1.
- Cancel first when you multiply fractions.
- Change a fraction to a decimal number by dividing the numerator by the denominator.
- A ratio may be written as a fraction.
- Simplify complex fractions by dividing the numerator by the denominator.

When working with decimals:
- Line up the decimal points when adding or subtracting.
- Move the decimal point three places to the right when multiplying a decimal number by 1,000.
- Move the decimal point three places to the left when dividing a decimal number by 1,000.
- Count the total number of places in the numbers you are multiplying to determine the number of decimal places in the answer.
- Avoid cancelling with decimal numbers.

When working with percentages:
- Change to fractions or decimal numbers before doing any calculations.
- "Of" means multiply when calculating a percent of a number.
- Fraction of Change $= \dfrac{Change}{Original}$

Practice Sets

Workspace

The answers to *Try These for Practice* and *Exercises* are found in Appendix A. Ask your instructor for the answers to the *Additional Exercises*.

Try These for Practice

Test your comprehension after reading the chapter.

1. Write $\frac{7}{16}$ as a decimal number rounded off to the hundredths place.

2. Find 23% of 59 and round down the answer to the tenths place.

3. Fill in the missing numbers in this chart.

Fraction	Decimal	Percent
½	0.5	50%
⅗		
	0.45	
		3%

4. Perform the multiplication: $\frac{6}{35} \times \frac{55}{6} \times 14$

5. Write the value of this expression as an ordinary fraction: $\dfrac{\frac{21}{80}}{\frac{7}{8}}$

Exercises

Reinforce your understanding in class or at home.

Convert to whole numbers, proper fractions, or mixed numbers (Questions 1–7).

1. $0.55 = $ _____

2. $4\frac{1}{4} + 3\frac{3}{4} = $ _____

3. $15 \times \frac{3}{5} \times \frac{4}{27} = $ _____

4. $2\frac{3}{4} \div 7 = $ _____

5. $36 \div \frac{9}{10} = $ _____

6. $0.72 \div \frac{9}{20} = $ _____

7. $20,000 \times \frac{7}{15,000} \times \frac{1}{56} = $ _____

Convert to decimal numbers (Questions 8–19).

8. $\frac{3}{8} = $ _____ (round down to the hundredths place)

9. $\frac{16}{25} = $ _____

10. $6\frac{7}{10} = $ _____

11. $\frac{3}{200} = $ _____

12. $\frac{5}{24} = $ _____ (round off to the hundredths place)

13. $\frac{457}{1,000} = $ _____

14. $\frac{6.55}{500}$

15. $\frac{11}{13}$ (round down to the hundredths place)

16. $\frac{0.48}{0.8}$

17. $\frac{0.054}{0.06}$

18. $16\frac{2}{3}\%$ (round off to two decimal places)

19. 0.9%

Simplify and write the answer in decimal form (Questions 20–24).

20. 5.437×0.05 (round off to the nearest hundredth)

21. $0.0657 \times 1,000$

22. $4.7 \div 100$

23. $9 \div 0.17$ (round off to the hundredths place)

24. 0.45×0.03 (round up to two decimal places)

Simplify and write the answer in fractional and in decimal form rounded off to the nearest tenth (Questions 25–30).

25. $\frac{6}{35} \times \frac{55}{18} \times 14$

26. $\frac{\frac{3}{4}}{\frac{3}{7}}$

Workspace

27. $\dfrac{\frac{5}{7}}{100} \times \dfrac{200}{7} = $ _____

28. $\dfrac{15 \times \frac{3}{8}}{\frac{7}{8}} = $ _____

29. $12.5\% = $ _____

30. $37\frac{1}{2}\% = $ _____

31. Express the ratio 25:50 as a fraction in lowest terms.

    _____

32. Express the ratio 24 to 36 as a fraction in lowest terms.

    _____

33. Find the numerator of the equivalent fraction with the given denominator.
    $\dfrac{3}{5} = \dfrac{?}{100}$ _____

34. Find the numerator of the equivalent fraction with the given denominator.
    $\dfrac{3}{4} = \dfrac{?}{8}$ _____

35. Simplify $0.4 + 7 + 2.55$ _____

36. Simplify $2.06 - 1.222$ _____

37. Which is larger, 0.7 or 0.24? _____

38. What is 20% of 80? _____

39. The number of patients in the hospital has increased from 160 to 200. What is the percent of change? _____

40. A patient weighed 400 pounds before a diet program. After the program she weighed 280 pounds. What was the percent of change in the patient's weight? _____

Additional Exercises

Now, test yourself!

Convert to proper fractions or mixed numbers (Questions 1–7).

1. $0.65 = $ _____

2. $3\frac{1}{4} + 4\frac{1}{4} = $ _____

3. $50 \times \dfrac{3}{5} \times \dfrac{1}{30} = $ _____

4. $6\frac{3}{5} \div 11 = $ _____

5. $60 \div \dfrac{13}{5} = $ _____

6. $6.3 \div \dfrac{3}{4} = $ _____

7. $52 \times \dfrac{5}{8,400} \times \dfrac{21}{0.13} = $ _____

Convert to decimal numbers (Questions 8–19).

8. $\dfrac{1}{8} = $ _____ (round down to the hundredths place)

9. $\dfrac{14}{25} = $ _____

10. $5\dfrac{3}{10} = $ _____

11. $\dfrac{1}{200} = $ _____

12. $\dfrac{1}{75}$ = _____ (round off to the nearest hundredth)

13. $\dfrac{870}{1,000}$ = _____

14. $\dfrac{4.56}{200}$ = _____

15. $\dfrac{20}{7}$ = _____ (round down to the tenths place)

16. $\dfrac{0.72}{0.9}$ = _____

17. $\dfrac{0.072}{0.08}$ = _____

18. $6\dfrac{1}{4}\%$ = _____

19. 0.9% = _____

Simplify and write the answer in decimal form (Questions 20–24).

20. 0.24×6.23 = _____ (round off to the nearest hundredth)

21. 0.0047×100 = _____

22. $0.0047 \times 1,000$ = _____

23. $0.77 \div 0.3$ = _____ (round off to the nearest tenth)

24. $7 \div 0.13$ = _____ (round down to the hundredths place)

Simplify and write the answer in fractional form and in decimal form rounded off to the nearest tenth (Questions 25–30).

25. $0.56 \div \dfrac{1}{0.9}$ = _____

26. $\dfrac{13}{\frac{3}{4}}$ = _____

27. $\dfrac{\frac{2}{5}}{100} \times \dfrac{500}{6}$ = _____

28. $\dfrac{26 \times \frac{5}{13}}{\frac{9}{100}}$ = _____

29. 10.3% = _____

30. 99.5% = _____

31. Express the ratio 25:40 as a fraction in lowest terms. _____

32. Express the ratio 60 to 90 as a fraction in lowest terms. _____

33. Find the numerator of the equivalent fraction with the given denominator. $\dfrac{3}{7} = \dfrac{?}{21}$ _____

34. Find the numerator of the equivalent fraction with the given denominator. $\dfrac{6}{11} = \dfrac{?}{55}$ _____

35. Simplify $0.3 + 2 + 2.55$ _____

36. Simplify $2.56 - 1.93$ _____

37. Which is larger, 0.37 or 0.244? _____

38. What is 30% of 500? _____

39. The number of nurses on the night shift has increased from 4 to 5. What is the percent of change? _____

40. A patient was 300 pounds before a diet program. Now he is 240 pounds. What is the percent of change in the patient's weight? _____

Chapter

2

Safe and Accurate Medication Administration

Learning Outcomes

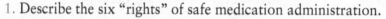

After completing this chapter, you will be able to

1. Describe the six "rights" of safe medication administration.
2. Explain the legal implications of medication administration.
3. Describe the routes of medication administration.
4. Identify common abbreviations used in medication administration.
5. Compare the trade name and generic name of drugs.
6. Describe the forms in which medications are supplied.
7. Identify and interpret the components of a Drug Prescription, Physician's Order, and Medication Administration Record.
8. Interpret information found on drug labels and in prescribing information.

This chapter introduces the process of safe and accurate medication administration. Patient safety is an ongoing critical issue and a primary goal for all healthcare providers. Safety in medication administration involves more than merely calculating accurate dosages. Patient rights, knowledge of potential sources of error, critical thinking, and attention to detail are all important in ensuring patient safety. The responsibilities of the people involved in the administration of medication are described.

The various forms and routes of drugs are presented, as well as abbreviations used in prescribing and documenting the administration of medications. You will learn how to interpret information found in drug labels, Web site "prescribing information," the *Physician's Desk Reference (PDR)*, package inserts, and drug guide books.

The Medication Administration Process

Medication administration is a process involving a chain of healthcare professionals. It includes five stages: (a) ordering/prescribing, (b) transcribing and verifying, (c) dispensing and delivering, (d) administering, and (e) monitoring and reporting.

Physicians, medical doctors (MD), osteopathic doctors (DO), podiatrists (DPM), and *dentists (DDS)* can legally prescribe medications. In many states, *physician's assistants, certified nurse midwives*, and *nurse practitioners* can also prescribe a range of medications related to their areas of practice.

Nurses and pharmacists are involved in transcribing, verifying, dispensing, and delivering medications.

The **prescriber writes** the order, the **pharmacist fills** the order, and the **nurse administers** the medication to the patient; each is responsible for the accuracy of the order.

Although prescribers may administer drugs to patients, the *registered professional nurse (RN), licensed practical nurse (LPN), licensed vocational nurse (LVN)*, and in some states, the *medication technician* may be responsible for administering drugs ordered by the prescriber.

To ensure patient safety, all healthcare professionals must understand how a patient's medications act and interact. Drugs can be life-saving or life-threatening. Every year, thousands of deaths occur because of medication errors. Errors can occur at any point in the medication process.

Preventing Medication Errors

Medication errors may occur anywhere in the medication administration process. When an error occurs it may be caused by failure to comply with the required policies or procedures errors in calculating dosages failure to follow the "six rights of medication administration" and miscommunication of orders. Miscommunication of orders can include illegible handwriting, incorrect use of zeros and decimal points, confusion of metric and other dosing units, as well as inappropriate abbreviations.

Other causes of medication errors include confusing drug names (look-alike or sound-alike); unclear or absent drug labels and packages; and lack of information about the drug or the patient (e.g., allergies, other medications the patient is taking). *High-alert* medications are those that have the highest risk of causing injury when misused. The top high-alert medications are insulin, heparin, injectable potassium chloride, opiates and narcotics, neuromuscular drugs, and chemotherapy drugs.

The **Institute for Safe Medication Practices (ISMP)**, the **United States Pharmacopeia (USP)**, and **The Joint Commission (TJC)** are organizations that are actively involved in preventing medication errors and monitoring medication error reports. Personnel who administer medications must be familiar with and follow applicable laws, policies, and procedures relative to the administration of medications, and they have a legal and ethical responsibility to report medication errors. When an error occurs, it must be reported immediately, the patient assessed for any *adverse drug events (ADEs)*, and an incident report prepared. The reason for the error must be determined, and corrective policies or procedures must be instituted. Best practices for

NOTE

The National Coordinating Council for Medication Error Reporting and Prevention is operated by the ISMP. The Council defines a medication error as "any preventable event that may cause or lead to inappropriate medication use or patient harm while the medication is in the control of the health care professional, patient, or consumer. Such events may be related to professional practice, health care products, procedures, and systems, including prescribing; order communication; product labeling, packaging, and nomenclature; compounding; dispensing; distribution; administration; education; monitoring; and use." When a medication error is identified, the National Alert Network (NAN) issues alerts.

NOTE

For additional information about preventing medication errors and about Medication Reconciliation, refer to The Joint Commission's National Patient Safety Goals (www.jointcommission.org), the Institute for Healthcare Improvement (www.ihi.org), and the Institute for Safe Medication Practices (www.ismp.org).

ALERT

The person who administers the drug has the last opportunity to identify an error before a patient might be injured.

NOTE

A generic drug may be manufactured by different companies under different trade names. For example, the generic drug ibuprofen is manufactured by McNeil PPC under the trade name Motrin, and by Pfizer Consumer Healthcare under the trade name Advil. The active ingredients in Motrin and Advil are the same, but the size, shape, color, or fillers may be different. Be aware that patients may become confused and worried about receiving a medication that has a different name or appears to be dissimilar from their usual medication. State and federal governments now permit, encourage, and, in some states, mandate that the consumer be given the generic form when buying prescription drugs.

preventing ADEs begin with a review of the patient's current drug regimen, allergies, and diagnosis. The healthcare professional must be knowledgeable of the drug's expected benefits, actions, adverse reactions, interactions, and appropriateness for the patient's diagnosis.

TJC requires healthcare facilities to "maintain and communicate accurate patient medication information" (National Patient Safety Goal 03.06.01, 2013). *Medication Reconciliation* is a process that includes developing a list of all current medications that a patient is taking, making a list of medications to be prescribed, comparing the lists, making clinical decisions based on the comparison, and communicating the new list to appropriate caregivers and to the patient. This procedure must be performed at every transition of care, including changes in setting, service, practitioner, and level of care. Medication Reconciliation helps to prevent medication errors such as omissions, duplications, dosing errors, or drug interactions.

Six Rights of Medication Administration

To prepare and administer drugs safely, it is imperative that you understand and follow the **Six Rights of Medication Administration:**

- Right drug
- Right dose
- Right route and form
- Right time
- Right patient
- Right documentation

These six "rights" should be checked before administering any medications. Failure to achieve any of these rights constitutes a medication error.

Some institutions recognize additional rights, such as the *right to know* and the *right to refuse*. Patients need to be educated about their medications, and if a patient refuses a medication, the reason must be documented and reported.

The Right Drug

A drug is a chemical substance that acts on the physiological processes in the human body. For example, the drug insulin is given to patients whose bodies do not manufacture sufficient insulin. Some drugs have more than one action. Aspirin, for example, is an antipyretic (fever-reducing), analgesic (pain-relieving), and anti-inflammatory drug that also has anticoagulant properties (keeps the blood from clotting). A drug may be taken for one, some, or all its therapeutic properties.

The **generic** name is the official accepted name of a drug, as listed in the United States Pharmacopeia (USP). The designation of USP after a drug name indicates that the drug meets government standards. A drug has only one generic name, but can have many trade names. By law, generic names must be identified on all drug labels.

Many companies may manufacture the same drug using different **trade** (patented, brand, or proprietary) names. The drug's trade name is prominently displayed and followed by the trademark symbol (™) or the registration symbol (®). For example, ZyPREXA is the trade name and olanzapine is the generic name for the drug shown in • **Figure 2.1**.

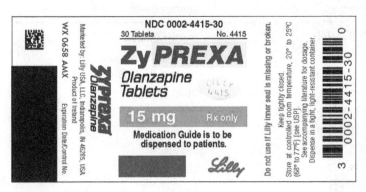

• **Figure 2.1**
Drug label for ZyPREXA.

Dosage strength indicates the amount of drug in a specific unit of measurement. The dosage strength of ZyPREXA is 15 *mg* per tablet.

Each drug has a unique identification number. This number is called the **National Drug Code (NDC) number**. The NDC number for ZyPREXA is 0002-4415-30. It is printed in two places on the label and is also encoded in the bar code. The *Food and Drug Administration (FDA)* regulates the manufacturing, sale, and effectiveness of all medications sold in the United States. Legislatures and other governmental agencies also regulate the administration of medications. The FDA estimates that the bar coding of prescription drugs reduces medication errors by as much as 50 *percent*.

To help avoid errors, drugs should be prescribed with only the generic name or with both the generic and trade names. Many drugs have names that sound alike, or have names or packaging that look alike. To avoid medication errors, the *FDA, Institute for Safe Medication Practice (ISMP), Joint Commission,* and *National Board of Pharmacy* recommend the use of TALL MAN Lettering in drug names. TALL MAN letters are uppercase letters used in a drug name to highlight the primary dissimilarities with look-alike drug names (ISMP Nov, 2010). For example, in Figure 2.1, the drug name ZyPREXA uses tall man lettering to help distinguish it from the drug ZyrTEC.

To meet the National Patient Safety Goals of The Joint Commission, a healthcare organization must develop its own list of look-alike/sound-alike drugs that it stores, dispenses, or administers. Table 2.1 includes a sample list of drugs whose names may be confused. See Appendix B for more complete FDA and ISMP Lists of Look-Alike Drug Names with Recommended Tall Man letters. See www.ismp.org for the ISMP's List of *Confused Drug Names*.

The Right Dose

A person prescribing or administering medications has the *legal responsibility* of knowing the correct dose. Calculations may be necessary, and appropriate equipment must be used to measure the dose. Because no two people are exactly alike, and no drug affects every human body in exactly the same way, drug doses must be individualized. Responses to drug actions may differ according to the gender, race, genetics, nutritional and health status, age, and weight of the patient (especially children and the elderly), as well as the route and time of administration.

Table 2.1	Look-Alike/Sound-Alike Drugs with Tall Man Lettering

Drug Name	Confused with
acetaZOLAMIDE	acetoHEXAMIDE
buPROPion	busPIRone
chloproMAZINE	chloproPAMIDE
DAUNOrubicin	DOXOrubicin
DOBUTamine	DOPamine
EPINEPHrine	ePHEDrine
fentaNYL	SUFentanil
glipiZIDE	glyBURIDE
hydrALAZINE	hydrOXYzine
HumaLOG	HumuLIN
niCARdipine	NIFEdipine
prednisoLONE	prednisone
TOLAZamide	TOLBUTamide
vinBLAStine	vinCRIStine

The **standard adult dosage** for each drug is determined by its manufacturer. A standard adult dosage is recommended based on the requirements of an average-weight adult and may be stated either as a *set dose* (20 *mg*) or as a *range* (150–300 *mg*). In the latter case, the minimum and maximum recommended dosages given are referred to as the **safe dosage range**. Recommended dosage may be found in many sources, including the package insert, the Hospital Formulary, and the prescribing information on the manufacturer's Web site.

Body surface area (BSA) is an estimate of the total skin area of a person measured in meters squared (m²). BSA is determined by formulas based on height and weight (see Chapter 6). Many drug doses administered to children or used for cancer therapy are calculated based on BSA.

Carefully read the drug label to determine the *dosage strength*. Perform and *check calculations*, and pay special attention to decimal points. When giving an intravenous drug to a pediatric patient or giving a high-alert drug, always *double check the dosage and pump settings*, and confirm these with a colleague. Be sure to check for the recommended *safe dosage range* based on the patient's age, BSA, or weight. After you have calculated the dose, be certain to use a standard measuring device such as a calibrated medicine dropper, syringe, or cup to administer the drug.

Medications may be prepared by the pharmacist or drug manufacturer in unit-dose packaging or multiple-dose packaging. **Unit-dose** medications may be in the forms of single tablets, capsules, or a liquid dosage sealed in an individual package. Unit-dose medications may be packaged in vials, bottles, prefilled syringes, or ampules, each of which contains only one dosage of a medication. When more than one dose is contained in a package, this is referred to as **multidose** packaging. See • **Figures 2.2** and **2.3**.

The Right Route and Form

Medications must be administered *in the form* and *via the route specified by the prescriber*. Medications are manufactured in the **form** of tablets, capsules, liquids, suppositories, creams, patches, and injectable medications (which are

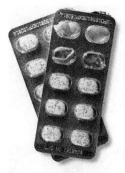 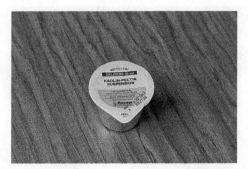

● **Figure 2.2**
Unit-dose packages.

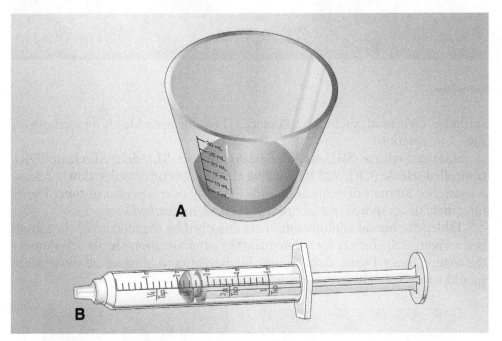

● **Figure 2.3**
Liquid medication in a
a. medication cup
b. oral syringe

supplied in solution or in a powdered form to be reconstituted). The form (preparation) of a drug affects its speed of onset, intensity of action, and route of administration. The **route** indicates the site of the body and method of drug delivery.

Oral Medications

Oral medications are administered **by mouth** (PO) and are supplied in both solid and liquid form. The most common solid forms are *tablets* (tab), *capsules* (cap), and *caplets* (● **Figure 2.4**).

Scored tablets have a groove down the center so that the tablet can be easily broken in half. To avoid an incorrect dose, unscored tablets should never be broken.

Enteric-coated tablets are meant to dissolve in the intestine rather than in the stomach. Therefore, they should be swallowed whole and neither chewed nor crushed. A **capsule** is a gelatin case containing a powder, a liquid, or granules (pulverized fragments of solid medication). When a patient cannot swallow, certain capsules may be opened and their contents mixed in a liquid or

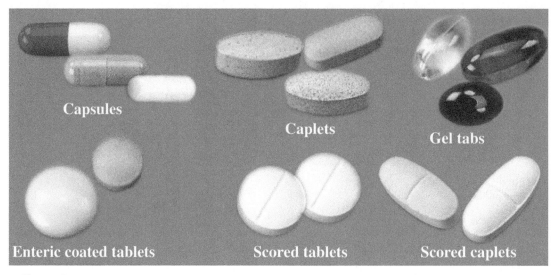

● **Figure 2.4**
Forms of oral medications.

sprinkled on a food, such as applesauce. Theo-dur Sprinkles is an example of such a medication.

Sustained-release (SR), **extended-release (ER** or **XL)**, **delayed-release (DR)**, **controlled-release (CR)**, and **long-acting (LA)** tablets or capsules slowly release a controlled amount of medication into the body over a period of time. Therefore, these drugs *should not be opened, chewed, or crushed.*

Tablets for **buccal** administration are absorbed by the mucosa of the mouth (see ● **Figure 2.5**). Tablets for **sublingual (SL)** administration are absorbed under the tongue (see ● **Figure 2.6**). Tablets for buccal or sublingual administration should never be swallowed.

ALERT

DO NOT substitute a different route for the prescribed route because a serious overdose or underdose may occur. Giving medication by the wrong route is a medication error.

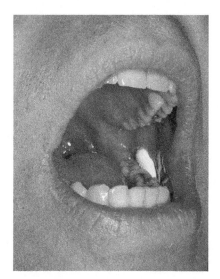

● **Figure 2.5**
Buccal route: Tablet between cheek and teeth.

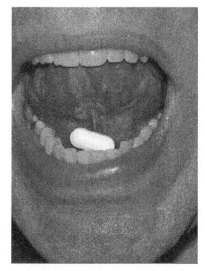

● **Figure 2.6**
Sublingual route: Tablet under tongue.

Oral drugs also come in liquid forms: *elixirs, syrups,* and *suspensions.* An **elixir** is an alcohol solution, a **syrup** is a medication dissolved in a sugar-and-water solution, and a **suspension** consists of an insoluble drug in a liquid base. Liquid medications may also be administered **enterally** into the gastrointestinal tract via a specially placed tube, such as a *nasogastric (NG)*, *gastrostomy (GT)*, or *percutaneous endoscopic gastrostomy (PEG) tube* (see Chapter 10).

Parenteral Medications. Parenteral medications are those that are injected (via needle) into the body by various routes. They are absorbed faster and more completely than drugs given by other routes. Drug forms for parenteral use are sterile and must be administered using aseptic (sterile) technique. See Chapters 7 and 9.

The most common parenteral sites are the following:

- **Epidural:** into the epidural space (in the lumbar region of the spine)
- **Intramuscular (IM):** into the muscle
- **Subcutaneous (subcut):** into the subcutaneous tissue
- **Intravenous (IV):** into the vein
- **Intradermal (ID):** beneath the skin
- **Intracardiac (IC):** into the cardiac muscle
- **Intrathecal:** into the spinal column or in the space under the arachnoid membrane of the brain or spinal cord

Cutaneous Medications. Cutaneous medications are those that are administered through the skin or mucous membrane. Cutaneous routes include the following:

- **Topical:** administered *on the skin surface* and may provide either a *local* or a *systemic* effect. Those drugs applied for a **local** effect are absorbed slowly, and amounts reaching the general circulation are minimal. Those administered for a **systemic** effect provide a slow release and absorption in the general circulation.
- **Transdermal:** contained *in a patch or disk and applied to the skin*. These are administered for their *systemic* effect. Patches allow constant, controlled amounts of drug to be released over 24 *hours* or more. Examples include nitroglycerin for angina or chest pain, nicotine to control the urge to smoke, and fentanyl for chronic pain. See • **Figure 2.7.**

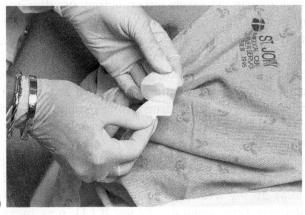
(a)

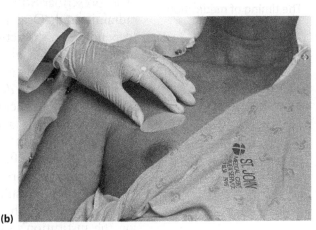
(b)

• **Figure 2.7**
Transdermal patch: (a) protective coating removed; (b) patch immediately applied to clean, dry, hairless skin and labeled with date, time, and initials.

- **Inhalation:** breathed into the respiratory tract through the nose or mouth. *Nebulizers, dry powder inhalers (DPI)*, and *metered dose inhalers (MDI)* are types of devices used to administer drugs via inhalation. A **nebulizer** vaporizes a liquid medication into a fine mist that can then be inhaled using a face mask or handheld device. A **DPI** is a small device used for solid drugs. The device is activated by the process of inhalation, and a fine powder is inhaled. An **MDI** uses a propellant to deliver a measured dose of medication with each inhalation. See • **Figure 2.8**.

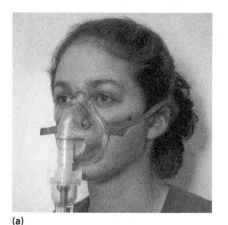
(a)

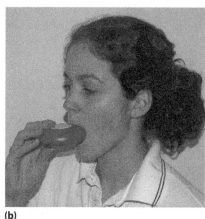
(b)

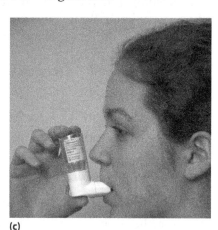
(c)

• **Figure 2.8**
Inhalation devices: (a) nebulizer with face mask; (b) dry powder inhaler; (c) metered dose inhaler.

- **Solutions and ointments:** applied to the mucosa of the eyes (optic), nose (nasal), ears (otic), or mouth
- **Suppositories:** are shaped for insertion into a body cavity (vagina, rectum, or urethra) and dissolve at body temperature

Some drugs are supplied in multiple forms and therefore can be administered by a variety of routes. For example, Tigan (trimethobenzamide HCl) is supplied as a capsule, suppository, or solution for injection.

The Right Time

The prescriber will indicate when and how often a medication should be administered. Oral medications can be given either before or after meals, depending on the action of the drug. Factors such as the purpose of the drug, drug interactions, absorption of the drug, and side effects must be considered when medication times are scheduled. Medications can be ordered *once a day* (daily), *twice a day* (b.i.d.), *three times a day* (t.i.d.), and *four times a day* (q.i.d). Most healthcare facilities designate specific times for these administrations. To maintain a more stable level of the drug in the patient, the period between administrations of the drug should be prescribed at regular intervals, such as q4h (every four hours), q6h, q8h, or q12h.

Incorrect interpretation of abbreviations related to medication administration times could result in drug errors. For example, *30 mg B.I.D.* (twice a day) is not necessarily the same as *30 mg q12h* (every twelve hours). Depending on the institution's drug delivery time schedule, *30 mg B.I.D.* may mean to administer 30 *mg* at 10:00 A.M. and 30 *mg* at 6:00 P.M., whereas *30 mg q12h* may mean to administer 30 *mg* at 10:00 A.M. and 30 *mg* at 10:00 P.M.

B.I.D. should also not be confused with "daily in two divided doses." For example, *30 mg B.I.D.* requires administering two doses of 30 *mg* each for a total daily dose of 60 *mg*. In contrast, *30 mg daily in two divided doses* requires administering two doses of 15 *mg* each for a total daily dose of 30 *mg*.

In 2011, the **Centers for Medicare and Medicaid Services (CMS)** revised the so-called "30-minute rule" on the administration of medication, which had established a uniform 30-minute-window before or after the scheduled time for all scheduled medication administration. Hospitals now must establish policies and procedures for the timing of medication administration that take into account the nature of the prescribed medication, specific clinical applications, and patient needs.

"Hospitals are expected to identify those medications which require exact or precise timing of administration, and which are not, therefore, eligible for scheduled dosing times." Some examples are: stat doses, loading doses, one-time doses (doses specifically timed for procedures), and time-sequenced doses (doses timed for serum drug levels).

"For medications that are eligible for scheduled dosing times, hospitals are expected to distinguish between those that are time-critical and those that are not, and to establish policies governing timing of medication administration accordingly. **Time-critical** scheduled medications are those for which an early or late administration of greater than thirty minutes might cause harm." Some examples are: antibiotics, insulin, anticoagulants, anticonvulsants, and pain medication.

"**Non-time-critical** scheduled medications are those for which a longer or shorter interval of time since the prior dose does not significantly change the medication's therapeutic effect or otherwise cause harm." Therefore, the hospital may establish, as appropriate, either a 1- or 2-hour window for administration.

The Right Patient

Before administering any medication, it is essential to determine the identity of the recipient. Administering a medication to a patient other than the one for whom it was ordered is one example of a medication error. The Joint Commission continues to include proper patient identification in its National Patient Safety Goals, and it requires the use of at least two forms of patient identification. Suggested identifiers include: the patient identification bracelet information, verbalization of the patient's name by the patient or parent, the patient's home telephone number, and the patient's hospital number.

After identifying the patient, match the drug order, patient's name, and age to the Medication Administration Record (MAR). To help reduce errors, many agencies now use computers at the bedside or use handheld devices (scanners) to read the bar code on a patient's identification bracelet and on the medication packages. See • **Figure 2.9.**

> **NOTE**
>
> Because regulations are evolving, healthcare providers should refer to the CMS Web site (www.cms.gov) for current regulations.

> **ALERT**
>
> The patient's bed number or room number is *not* to be used for patient identification. Know and use the identifiers recognized and required by your agency. Administering a medication to the wrong patient is one of the most common medication errors.

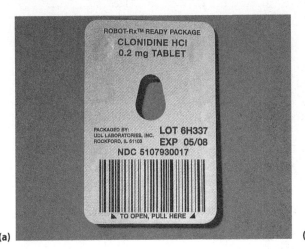
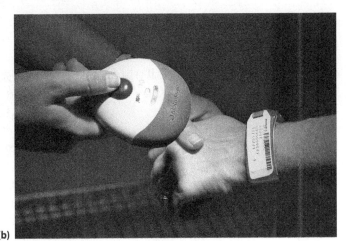

(a) (b)

• **Figure 2.9**
Bar codes: (a) unit-dose drug; (b) scanner reading a patient's identification band.

The Right Documentation

Always document the name and dosage of the drug, as well as the route and time of administration on the MAR. Sign your initials *immediately after, but never before*, the dose is given. It is important to include any relevant information. For example, document patient allergies to medications, patient pain level, heart rate (when giving digoxin), and blood pressure (when giving antihypertensive drugs). All documentation must be legible. Remember the axiom "If it's not documented, it's not done."

Anticipate side effects! A **side effect** is an undesired physiologic response to a drug. For example, codeine relieves pain, but its side effects include constipation, nausea, drowsiness, and itching. Be sure to record any observed side effects and discuss them with the prescriber.

Safe drug administration requires a knowledge of common abbreviations. For instance, when the prescriber writes "*Demerol 75 mg IM q4h prn pain*," the person administering the drug reads this as "Administer the drug Demerol;

Table 2.2 **Common Abbreviations Used for Medication Administration**

Abbreviation	Meaning	Abbreviation	Meaning
Route:		Q.I.D. or q.i.d.	four times per day
GT	gastrostomy tube	Stat	immediately
ID	intradermal	T.I.D. or t.i.d.	three times per day
IM	intramuscular	**General:**	
IV	intravenous	c	with
IVP	intravenous push	CR	controlled release
IVPB	intravenous piggyback	cap	capsule
NGT	nasogastric tube	d.a.w.	dispense as written
PEG	percutaneous endoscopicgastrostomy	DR	delayed release
		ER	extended release
PO	by mouth	g	gram
PR	by rectum	gr	grain
SL	sublingual	gtt	drop
subcut	subcutaneously	kg	kilogram
Supp	suppository	L	liter
Frequency:		LA	long acting
ac	before meals	mcg	microgram
ad lib	as desired	mg	milligram
B.I.D. or b.i.d.	two times a day	mL	milliliter
h, hr	hour	NKDA	no known drug allergies
hs	at bedtime	NPO	nothing by mouth
pc	after meals	s	without
prn	whenever needed or necessary	Sig	directions to patient
q	every	Susp	suspension
q2h	every two hours	SR	sustained release
q4h	every four hours	t or tsp	teaspoon
q6h	every six hours	T or tbs	tablespoon
q8h	every eight hours	tab	tablet
q12h	every twelve hours	XL or XR	extended release

the dose is seventy-five milligrams, the route is intramuscular, the time is every four hours, and it is to be given when the patient has pain." Be cautious with abbreviations because they can be a source of medication error. Only approved abbreviations should be used (Table 2.2).

The Joint Commission requires healthcare organizations to follow its official "*Do Not Use List*" that applies to all medication orders and all medication documentation. See Table 2.3.

Table 2.3   JCAHO Official "Do Not Use List"[1]

Do Not Use	Potential Problem	Use Instead
U (for unit)	Mistaken for "0" (zero), the number "4" (four) or "cc"	Write "unit"
IU (International Unit)	Mistaken for IV (intravenous) or the number 10 (ten)	Write "International Unit"
Q.D., QD, q.d., qd (daily)	Mistaken for each other	Write "daily"
Q.O.D., QOD, q.o.d, qod (every other day)	Period after the Q mistaken for "I" and the "O" mistaken for "I"	Write "every other day"
Trailing zero (X.0 mg)[2]	Decimal point is missed	Write X mg
Lack of leading zero (.X mg)		Write 0.X mg
MS	Can mean morphine sulfate or magnesium sulfate	Write "morphine sulfate" Write "magnesium sulfate"
MSO_4 and $MgSO_4$	Confused for one another	

[1] Applies to all orders and all medication-related documentation that is handwritten (including free-text computer entry) or on preprinted forms.

[2] **Exception:** A "trailing zero" may be used only where required to demonstrate the level of precision of the value being reported, such as for laboratory results, imaging studies that report size of lesions, or catheter/tube sizes. It may not be used in medication orders or other medication-related documentation.

Additional Abbreviations, Acronyms, and Symbols
(For *possible* future inclusion in the Official "Do Not Use" List)

Do Not Use	Potential Problem	Use Instead
> (greater than)	Misinterpreted as the number	Write "greater than"
< (less than)	"7" (seven) or the letter "L" Confused for one another	Write "less than"
Abbreviations for drug names	Misinterpreted due to similar abbreviations for multiple drugs	Write drug names in full
Apothecary units	Unfamiliar to many practitioners Confused with metric units	Use metric units
@	Mistaken for the number "2" (two)	Write "at"
cc	Mistaken for U (units) when poorly written	Write "mL" or "milliliters"
μg	Mistaken for mg (milligrams) resulting in one thousand-fold overdose	Write "mcg" or "micrograms"

Drug Prescriptions

Before anyone can administer any medication, there must be a legal order or prescription for the medication.

A **drug prescription** is a directive to the pharmacist for a drug to be given to a patient who is being seen in a medical office or clinic or is being discharged from a healthcare facility. A prescription may be written, or it can be faxed, phoned, or emailed from a secure, encrypted computer system to a pharmacist. There are many varieties of prescription forms. All prescriptions should contain the following:

- Prescriber's full name, address, telephone number, and (when the prescription is given for a controlled substance) the Drug Enforcement Administration (DEA) number
- Date the prescription is written
- Patient's full name, address, and age or date of birth
- Drug name (generic name should be included), dosage, route, frequency, and amount to be dispensed
- Indication whether it is acceptable to substitute a generic form (when only the trade name is given)
- Directions to the patient that must appear on the drug container
- Number of refills permitted

If any of this information is missing or unclear, the prescription is considered incomplete and is therefore *not* a legal order. Every state has a drug substitution law that either mandates or may permit a less-expensive generic drug substitution by the pharmacist. If the prescriber has an objection to a generic drug substitute, the prescriber will write "do not substitute," "dispense as written," "no generic substitution," or "medically necessary" (• **Figure 2.10**). Some states require bar codes on prescription forms.

Adam Smith, M.D.
100 Main Street
Utopia, New York 10000
Phone (212) 345-6789

DEA # 56777   License # 123456

Name: _Joan Soto_   Date: _November 24, 2016_

Address: _4205 Main Street_   Age/DOB: _04/20/48_
Utopia, NY 10000

Rx   _Zocor 10 mg tablets_
Sig: _1 tablet PO, daily in the evening_

Dispense: _90_
Refills: _0_

THIS PRESCRIPTION WILL BE FILLED GENERICALLY UNLESS THE PRESCRIBER WRITES "d a w" IN THE BOX BELOW.

| _d a w_ | |

Adam Smith MD

• **Figure 2.10**
Drug prescription for Zocor.

This prescription is interpreted as follows:

- Prescriber: Adam Smith, M.D.
- Prescriber address: 100 Main Street, Utopia, NY 10000
- Prescriber phone number: (212) 345-6789
- Date prescription written: November 24, 2016
- Patient's full name: Joan Soto
- Patient address: 4205 Main Street, Utopia NY 10000
- Patient date of birth: April 20, 1948
- Drug name: Zocor (trade name)
- Dosage: 10 *mg*
- Route: by mouth (PO)
- Frequency: once a day
- Amount to be dispensed: 90 *tablets*
- Acceptable to substitute   no, the prescriber has written "d a w"
  a generic form?
- Directions to the patient: take 1 *tablet* by mouth daily in evening
- Refill instructions: no refills permitted

EXAMPLE 2.1

Read the prescription in • Figure 2.11 and complete the following information.

```
              OFFICIAL STATE PRESCRIPTION
              Primary Care Associates
           1234 Spring Street, Manhattan, Kansas 10001
                      (913) 999-5678

   CERT#: Fxxxxxx                    DEA#: xxxxxx
   [ ][ ][ ][ ][ ][ ][ ]  [ ][ ][ ][ ][ ][ ][ ]   [ ][ ][ ]


   Patient Name  Steven James
   Address  124 Winding Lane          Date  10/22/16
                                                    Sex
   City  Manhattan    State  KS  Zip  10001  Age  64   [M] F

   Rx
         Dilantin (phenytoin sodium) 100 mg
         1 cap po t.i.d.
         # 90

   Refills: 2                              | 300 mg |

   Prescriber Signature   Alicia Rodriguez NP


              |   no substitution   |

                 Substitution is mandatory
         unless the words "no substitution" appear in the box above.
```

• Figure 2.11
Drug prescription for Dilantin (phenytoin sodium).

- Date prescription written: _____
- Patient full name: _____
- Patient address: _____
- Patient age: _____
- Generic drug name: _____
- Dosage: _____
- Route: _____
- Frequency: _____
- Amount to be dispensed: _____
- Acceptable to substitute a generic form? _____
- Directions to the patient: _____
- Refill instructions: _____

This is what you should have found:

- Date prescription written: 10/22/2016
- Patient full name: Steven James
- Patient address: 124 Winding Lane
  Manhattan, Kansas 10001
- Patient age: 64
- Generic drug name: phenytoin sodium
- Dosage: 100 *mg*
- Route: by mouth
- Frequency: three times a day
- Amount to be dispensed: 90 *capsules*
- Acceptable to substitute a
  generic form? No
- Directions to the patient: take one capsule three times a day
- Refill instructions: may be refilled two times

Medication Orders

Medication orders are directives to the pharmacist for the drugs prescribed in a hospital or other healthcare facility. The terms *medication orders, drug orders,* and *physician's orders* are used interchangeably, and the forms used will vary from agency to agency. No medication should be given without a medication order. Medication orders can be *written* or *verbal*. Each medication order should follow a specific sequence: drug name, dose, route, and frequency.

Written medication orders are documented in a special book for doctors' orders, on a physician's order sheet in the patient's chart, or in a computer.

A **verbal** order must contain the same components as a written order—otherwise, it is invalid. The Joint Commission requires that an *authorized person* write the order in the patient's chart and then read it back to the prescriber. The prescriber must confirm that the order is correct. Hospitals must have policies stating when the order must be signed by the prescriber—for example, within 24 *hours*. To provide for the safety of the patient, generally verbal orders may be taken only in an emergency.

Types of Medication Orders

The most common type of medication order is the **routine order**, which indicates that the ordered drug is administered until a discontinuation order is written or until a specified date is reached.

A **standing order** is prescribed in anticipation of sudden changes in a patient's condition. Standing orders are used frequently in critical care units, where a patient's condition may change rapidly and immediate action would be required. Standing orders may also be used in long-term care facilities where a physician may not be readily available; for example, "*Tylenol (acetaminophen) 650 mg PO q4h for temperature of 101° F or higher.*" This is interpreted as "Administer the drug Tylenol (acetaminophen), a dose of six hundred fifty milligrams; the route is by mouth, the time is every four hours, and it is to be given whenever the patient's temperature is one hundred one degrees Fahrenheit or more."

A **prn order** is written by the prescriber for a drug to be given when a patient needs it; for example, "*morphine sulfate 5 mg subcut q4h prn mild-moderate pain.*" This is interpreted as "Administer the drug morphine sulfate, a dose of five milligrams; the route is subcutaneous, the time is every four hours, and it is to be given as needed when the patient has mild or moderate pain."

A **stat order** is an order that is to be administered immediately. Stat orders are usually written for emergencies or when a patient's condition suddenly changes; for example, "*Lasix (furosemide) 80 mg IV stat.*" This is interpreted as "Administer the drug Lasix (furosemide), a dose of eighty milligrams; the route is intravenous, and the drug is to be given immediately."

Components of a Medication Order

The essential components of a medication order are the following:

- **Patient's full name and date of birth:** Often this information is stamped or imprinted on the medication order form. Additional information may include the patient's admission number, religion, type of insurance, and physician's name.

- **Date and time the order was written:** This includes the month, day, year, and time of day. Many institutions use military time, which is based on a "24-hour clock" that does not use A.M. or P.M. (• **Figure 2.12**). Military times are written as four-digit numbers followed by the word *hours*.

Thus, 2:00 A.M. in military time is 0200 *h* (pronounced *Oh two hundred hours*), 12 noon is 1200 *h* (pronounced *twelve hundred hours*), 2:00 P.M. is 1400 *h* (pronounced *fourteen hundred hours*), and midnight is 2400 *h*.

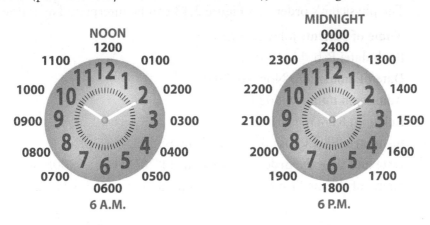

• **Figure 2.12**
Clocks showing 10:10 A.M. (1010 *h*) and 10:10 P.M. (2210 *h*).

There is confusion between the meanings of 12 A.M. and 12 P.M. Twelve noon, for example, is literally neither A.M. (ante meridiem: before midday), nor is it P.M. (post meridiem: after midday). Noon *is* midday! Therefore, to avoid confusion when administering medications, for noon and midnight use *12 noon* and *12 midnight*, or use military time (*1200h* and *2400h*). The FDA recomends the use of military time.

- **Name of the medication:** The generic name is recommended. If a prescriber desires to prescribe a trade name drug, "no generic substitution" must be specified.
- **Dosage of the medication:** The amount of the drug.
- **Route of administration:** Only approved abbreviations may be used.
- **Time and frequency of administration:** When and how often the drug is to be given.
- **Signature of the prescriber:** The medication order is not legal without the signature of the prescriber.
- **Signature of the person transcribing the order:** This may be the responsibility of a nurse or others identified by agency policy.

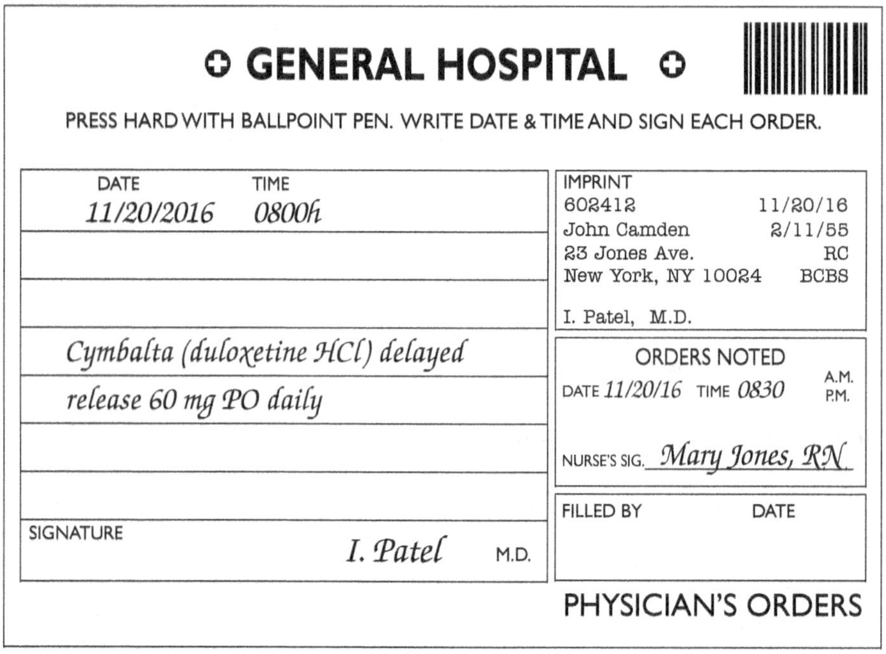

● **Figure 2.13**
Physician's order for Cymbalta (duloxetine HCl).

The physician's order in ● **Figure 2.13** can be interpreted as follows:

Name of patient: John Camden

Birth date: Feb. 11, 1955

Date of admission: Nov. 20, 2016

Admission number: 602412

Religion: Roman Catholic (RC)

Insurance: Blue Cross Blue Shield (BCBS)

Date and time the order was written: 11/20/2016 at 0800h or 8:00 A.M.

Name of the medication: Cymbalta (duloxetine HCl delayed release)

Dosage: 60 *mg*
Route of administration: PO (by mouth)
Frequency of administration: once a day
Signature of person writing the order: I. Patel, MD
Person who transcribed the order: Mary Jones, RN

EXAMPLE 2.2

Interpret the physician's order sheet shown in • Figure 2.14 and record the following information:

⊕ GENERAL HOSPITAL ⊕

PRESS HARD WITH BALLPOINT PEN. WRITE DATE & TIME AND SIGN EACH ORDER.

DATE	TIME
11/22/2016	1800h

IMPRINT
422934   11/22/16
Catherine Rodriguez 12/01/62
40 Addison Avenue
Rutlans, VT 06701   Prot

M. Ling, M.D.   GHI-CBP

Timoptic (timolol maleate) 0.5% opthalmic solution 1 drop B.I.D. to right eye

ORDERS NOTED   A.M.
DATE 11/22/16 TIME 1830h   P.M.

NURSE'S SIG. *Sara Gordon RN*

SIGNATURE   *Mae Ling* M.D.

FILLED BY   DATE

PHYSICIAN'S ORDERS

• **Figure 2.14**
Physician's order for Timoptic.

Date order written: _____
Time order written: _____
Name of drug: _____
Dosage: _____
Route of administration: _____
Frequency of administration: _____
Name of prescriber: _____
Name of patient: _____
Birth date: _____
Religion: _____
Type of insurance: _____
Person who transcribed the order: _____

This is what you should have found:

- **Date order written:**   11/22/2016
- **Time order written:**   1800 *h* or 6:00 P.M.

- **Name of drug:** Timoptic (timolol maleate) 0.5% ophthalmic solution
- **Dosage:** 1 *drop*
- **Route:** topical to right eye
- **Frequency of administration:** 2 times a day
- **Name of prescriber:** Mae Ling, M.D.
- **Name of patient:** Catherine Rodriguez
- **Birth date:** December 1, 1962
- **Religion:** Protestant
- **Type of insurance:** GHI-CBP
- **Person who transcribed the order:** Sara Gordon, RN

ALERT

Before administering any medication, always compare the label on the medication with the information on the MAR. If there is a discrepancy, you must check the prescriber's original order.

Medication Administration Records

A **Medication Administration Record (MAR)** is a form used by healthcare facilities to document all drugs administered to a patient. It is a legal document, part of the patient's medical record, and the format varies from agency to agency. Patient confidentiality must be maintained, and photocopying of any part of the medical record requires patient permission. Every agency develops policies related to using the MAR, including: how to add new medications, discontinue medications, how to document one-time or stat medications, the process to follow if a medication is not administered or a patient refuses a medication, and how to correct an error on the MAR.

Routine, PRN, and STAT medications all may be written in separate locations on the MAR. PRN and STAT medications may also have a separate form. If a medication is to be given regularly, a complete schedule is written for all administration times. Each time a dose is administered, the healthcare worker initials the time of administration. The full name, title, and initials of the person who gave the medication must be recorded on the MAR.

After a prescriber's order has been verified, a nurse or other healthcare provider transcribes the order to the MAR. This record is used to check the medication order; prepare the correct medication dose; and record the date, time, and route of administration.

The essential components of the MAR include the following:

- **Patient information:** a stamp or printed label with patient identification (name, date of birth, medical record number).
- **Dates:** when the order was written, when to start the medication, and when to discontinue it.
- **Medication information:** full name of the drug, dose, route, and frequency of administration.
- **Time of administration:** frequency as stated in the prescriber's order—for example, t.i.d. Times for PRN and one-time doses are recorded *precisely* at the time they are administered.
- **Initials:** the initials and the signature of the person who administered the medication are recorded.
- **Special instructions:** instructions relating to the medication—for example, "Hold if systolic BP is less than 100."

EXAMPLE 2.3

Study the MAR in • Figure 2.15, and then complete the following chart and answer the questions.

	UNIVERSITY HOSPITAL	789652 Wendy Kim 44 Chester Avenue New York, NY 10003	9/11/2016 12/20/60 RC Medicaid
	DAILY MEDICATION ADMINISTRATION RECORD	Dr. Juan Rodriguez, M.D.	

PATIENT NAME ___*Wendy Kim*___

ROOM # ___*422*___   IF ANOTHER RECORD IS IN USE ☐

ALLERGIC TO (RECORD IN RED): ___*tomato, codeine*___

DATES GIVEN ⬇   DATE DISCHARGED:

RED CHECK INITIAL	ORDER DATE	INITIAL	EXP DATE	MEDICATION, DOSAGE, FREQUENCY AND ROUTE	HOURS	12	13	14	15							
	9/12	JY	9/19	Rocephin (ceftriaxone) 1 g	0600	/	MC	MC								
				IVPB q12h for 7 days begin at 1800h	1800	MJ	SG	SG								
	9/12	JY	9/18	digoxin 0.125 mg PO daily	0900	JY	JY	JY								
	9/12	JY	9/18	Vasotec (enalapril maleate)	0900	JY	JY	JY								
				20 mg PO q12h	2100	MJ	SG	SG								
	9/12	JY	9/18	Plavix (clopidogrel bisulfate)	0900	JY	JY	JY								
				75 mg PO daily												
	9/12	JY	9/18	Ditropan XL (oxybutynin chloride)	2100	MJ	SG	SG								
				10 mg PO HS												

INT.	NURSES' FULL SIGNATURE AND TITLE	INT.	CODES FOR INJECTION SITES	
JY	Jim Young, RN		A- left anterior thigh	H- right anterior thigh
MC	Marie Colon, RN		B- left deltoid	I- right deltoid
MJ	Mary Jones, LPN		C- left gluteus medius	J- right gluteus medius
SG	Sara Gordon, RN		D- left lateral thigh	K- right lateral thigh
			E- left ventral gluteus	L- right ventral gluteus
			F- left lower quadrant	M- right lower quadrant
			G- left upper quadrant	N- right upper quadrant

• **Figure 2.15**
MAR for Wendy Kim.

Name of Drug	Dose	Route of Administration	Time of Administration

1. Identify the drugs and their doses administered at 9:00 A.M.

   _____

2. Identify the drugs and their doses administered at 9:00 P.M.

   _____

3. Who administered the clopidogrel bisulfate on 9/14?

   _____

4. What is the route of administration for ceftriaxone?

   _____

5. What is the time of administration for enalapril maleate?

   _____

This is what you should have found:

Name of Drug	Dose	Route of Administration	Time of Administration
ceftriaxone	1 *g*	IVPB	0600 *h* (6 A.M.) &1800 *h* (6 P.M.)
digoxin	0.125 *mg*	PO	0900 *h* (9 A.M.)
Vasotec (enalapril maleate)	20 *mg*	PO	0900 *h* (9 A.M.) & 2100 *h* (9 P.M.)
Plavix (clopidogrel bisulfate)	75 *mg*	PO	0900 *h* (9 A.M.)
Ditropan XL (oxybutynin chloride)	10 *mg*	PO	2100 *h* (9 P.M.)

1. digoxin 0.125 *mg*; Vasotec (enalapril maleate) 20 *mg*; Plavix (clopidogrel bisulfate) 75 *mg*
2. Vasotec (enalapril maleate) 20 *mg*, and Ditropan XL (oxybutynin chloride) 10 *mg*
3. Jim Young, RN
4. Intravenous
5. 0900 *h* (9:00 A.M.) and 2100 *h* (9:00 P.M.)

EXAMPLE 2.4

Study the MAR in • Figures 2.16a and 2.16b, and then fill in the following chart and answer the questions.

UNIVERSITY HOSPITAL

659204   11/20/2016
Mohammad Kamal   10/2/52
4103 Ely Avenue   Musl
Bronx, NY 10466   GHI-CBP

DAILY MEDICATION ADMINISTRATION RECORD

Dr. Indu Patel, M.D.

PATIENT NAME ___Mohammad Kamal___

ROOM # ___302___   IF ANOTHER RECORD IS IN USE ☐

ALLERGIC TO (RECORD IN RED): ___sulfa, fish___

DATES GIVEN ⬇ MONTH/DAY   YEAR: _2016_

RED CHECK INITIAL	ORDER DATE	INITIAL	EXP DATE	MEDICATION, DOSAGE, FREQUENCY AND ROUTE	TIME	11/20	11/21	11/22	11/23	11/24	11/25	11/26
	11/20	MC	11/26	Protonix (pantoprazole sodium) DR 40 mg	10 AM	—	MC	MC	MC	MJ	MJ	JY
				PO daily								
	11/20	MC	11/26	captopril 25 mg	10 AM	—	MC	MC	MC	MJ	MJ	JY
				PO B.I.D.	BP		160/110	150/70	160/110	138/86	130/80	130/80
					6 PM	MC	MC	MC	MC	MJ	MJ	JY
					BP	160/100	150/90	160/100	140/80	130/80	128/80	128/80
	11/20	MC	11/26	Lasix (furosemide) 20 mg PO daily	10 AM	—	MC	MC	MC	MJ	MJ	JY
	11/20	SG	11/27	cefotaxime	10 AM	—	MC	MC	MC	MJ	MJ	JY
				1g IVPB q12hr for 7 days	10 PM		SG	SG	SG	SG	SG	SG
	11/21	MC	11/27	Procrit (epoetin alfa) 3,000 units	10 AM		MC		MC		MJ	
				subcutaneous, three times per week,								
				start on 11/21								
	11/21	MC	11/27	digoxin, 0.125 mg PO daily	10 AM		MC	MC	MC	MJ	MJ	JY
					HR		72	70	96	76	80	80

INT.	NURSES' FULL SIGNATURE AND TITLE	INT.	NURSES' FULL SIGNATURE AND TITLE
MC	Marie Colon, RN		
SG	Sara Gordon, RN		
MJ	Mary Jones, LPN		
JY	Jim Young, RN		

• **Figure 2.16a**
MAR for Mohammad Kamal.

UNIVERSITY HOSPITAL

659204
Mohammad Kamal
4103 Ely Avenue
Bronx, NY 10466

11/20/2016
10/2/52
Musl
GHI-CBP

DAILY MEDICATION ADMINISTRATION RECORD

Dr. Indu Patel, M.D.

PATIENT NAME ___Mohammad Kamal___

ROOM # ___302___

ALLERGIC TO (RECORD IN RED): ___sulfa, fish___

IF ANOTHER RECORD IS IN USE ☐

DATES GIVEN ↧ MONTH/DAY   YEAR: ___2016___

PRN MEDICATION

ORDER DATE	EXPIRATION DATE/TIME	MEDICATION, DOSAGE, FREQUENCY AND ROUTE		DOSES GIVEN						
11/20	11/27	Tylenol (acetaminophen) 650 mg PO q6h prn mild pain	DATE	11/20	11/21	11/22				
			TIME	6 PM	10 AM	6 PM				
			INIT	MJ	MC	6 PM				
11/20	11/27	Robitussin DM 10 ml PO q12h prn	DATE	11/20	11/21					
			TIME	10 AM	10 PM					
			INIT	MJ	SG					

STAT-ONE DOSE-PRE-OPERATIVE MEDICATIONS   ◯ Check here if additional sheet in use.

ORDER DATE	MEDICATION-DOSAGE ROUTE	DATE	TIME	INIT	ORDER DATE	MEDICATION-DOSAGE ROUTE	DATE	TIME	INIT
11/23	labetalol 20 mg IVP over 2 min stat	11/23	10 AM	MC					

INT.	NURSES' FULL SIGNATURE AND TITLE	INT.	NURSES' FULL SIGNATURE AND TITLE
MJ	Mary Jones, RN		
MC	Marie Colon, RN		
SG	Sara Gordon, RN		

• **Figure 2.16b**
MAR for Mohammad Kamal.

Name of Routine Drug	Dose	Route of Administration	Time of Administration

1. Which drugs were administered at 10:00 A.M. on 11/23?

___

2. Which drug was given stat, and what was the route? Date and time?

___

3. Who administered the captopril at 6:00 P.M. on 11/21?

_____

4. What is the route of administration for Procrit?

_____

5. How many doses of captopril did the patient receive by 7:00 P.M. on 11/24?

_____

Here is what you should have found:

Name of Routine Drug	Dose	Route of Administration	Time of Administration
Protonix (pantoprazole sodium)	40 _mg_	PO	10:00 A.M.
captopril	25 _mg_	PO	10:00 A.M. & 6:00 P.M.
Lasix (furosemide)	20 _mg_	PO	10:00 A.M.
cefotaxime	1 _g_	IVPB	10:00 A.M. & 10:00 P.M.
Procrit (epoetin alfa)	3,000 _units_	subcutaneously	three times a week at 10:00 A.M.
digoxin	0.125 _mg_	PO	10:00 A.M.

1. Protonix 40 _mg_, captopril 25 _mg_; Lasix 20 _mg_; cefotaxime 1 g, Procrit 3,000 _units_, digoxin 0.125 _mg_, labetalol 20 _mg_.
2. labetalol IV on 11/23 at 10:00 A.M.
3. Marie Colon, RN
4. subcutaneous
5. 9

Technology in the Medication Administration Process

Many healthcare agencies have computerized the medication process. Those who prescribe or administer medications must use security codes and passwords to access the computer system. Prescribers input orders and all other essential patient information directly into a computer terminal. This system may be referred to as **Computerized Physician Order Entry (CPOE)**. The order is received in the pharmacy, where a patient's drug profile (list of drugs) is maintained. The nurse verifies the order on the computer and inputs his or her digital ID on the **eMAR (electronic Medication Administration Record)** after the medication is administered. A computer printout replaces the handwritten MAR.

One advantage of a computerized system is that handwritten orders do not need to be deciphered or transcribed. The computer program can also identify possible interactions among the patient's medications and automatically alert the pharmacist and persons administering the drugs. However, though technology can reduce medication errors and enhance patient safety, it also has the potential to cause new types of unintended errors.

Some institutions use _Automated Dispensing Cabinets (ADCs)_ to dispense medications. See • **Figure 2.17**. The healthcare provider must still be vigilant when

NOTE

Healthcare facilities must provide employees with adequate training regarding medication administration devices and routinely verify that users are competent with the equipment.

using such technology and must be sure to follow the "Six Rights of Medication Administration"; refer to the ISMP guidelines for the safe use of ADCs.

• **Figure 2.18** is a portion of a *computerized MAR* for a 24-hour period stated in military time. This MAR divides the day into three shifts. Note that

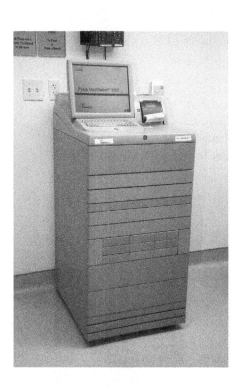

• Figure 2.17
Automated Dispensing Cabinet (ADC).

SCHEDULED	12/06/16–12/07/16 2301–0700	12/07/16 0701–1500	12/07/16 1501–2300
℞ Cefepime (Maxipime)		0840 **2 g IVPB** MAB	2015
℞ Emoxaparin Na (Lovenox)		1026 **40 mg subcutaneous** MAB	
℞ Furosemide (Lasix)	0611 **20 mg IVP** DJS		
℞ Hetastarch (he SPAN)		0920 **250 mL IVPB** MAB	
℞ KCl (Potassium chloride)		1026 **20 mEq ER tab PO** MAB	
℞ Metoprolol XL (Toprol XL)		1000 **CANCEL** MAB	2200
℞ Metronidazole (Flagyl)	0611 **500 mg IVPB** DJS	1324 **500 mg IVPB** MAB	2200
℞ NTG (Nitroglycerin)	0110 **15 mg oint topical** DJS 0611 **15 mg oint topical** DJS	1231 **15 mg oint topical** MAB	1800
℞ Pantoprazole (Protonix) 40 mg IVPB		1026 **40 mg IVPB** MAB	
PRN	12/06/16–12/07/16 2301–0700	12/07/16 0701–1500	12/07/16 1501–2300
℞ Saline flush	0110 **2 mL IV flush** DJS	0829 **2 mL IV flush** MAB	1600
℞ Morphine	0115 **4 mg IVP** DJS 0439 **4 mg IVP** DJS	1306 **2 mg IVP** MAB	
IV	12/06/16–12/07/16 2301–0700	12/07/16 0701–1500	12/07/16 1501–2300
℞ NS (NaCl, 0.9%, 1 L)		0810	2130
PRN ORDERS			
Hydrocodone 5 mg and Acetaminophen 500 mg	x 1–2 tab PO q4h prn process if pain		
Saline flush	2 mL IV flush q8 at 0000/0800/1600 and prn		
Insulin, human regular sliding scale {Novolin R SS}	See scale prn if BS 200–249 mg/dL give 4 Units of Reg insulin subcut		

• Figure 2.18
A portion of an eMAR.

no medications have yet been recorded for the 3:01 P.M.–11:00 P.M. shift (1501 *h*–2300 *h*).

Scheduled (routine), IV, and PRN orders are shown. For each order administered, the MAR indicates the time, order, and the nurse's digital identification. Currently there is a variety of computerized medication systems in use. The healthcare provider has a responsibility to be both knowledgeable of the facility's policies and proficient in using its system.

EXAMPLE 2.5

Use the MAR in Figure 2.18 to answer the following questions:

1. Which drug was ordered in milliequivalents?

   _____

2. What drugs were administered at 6:11 A.M. on 12/07/2016?

   _____

3. Identify the dosage, route, and time that Flagyl was administered after noon on 12/07/2016.

   _____

4. Identify the name, dosage, route, and time of administration of the PRN drugs administered after noon on 12/07/2016.

   _____

5. What is the form and route of administration for nitroglycerin on 12/07/2016?

   _____

This is what you should have found:

1. KCl (potassium chloride)
2. furosemide (Lasix), metronidazole (Flagyl), and NTG (nitroglycerin)
3. 500 *mg*, IVPB at 1324 *h* (1:24 P.M.)
4. morphine 2 *mg* IVP was given at 1306 *h* (1:06 P.M.)
5. Ointment, topical

Drug Labels

You will need to understand the information found on drug labels to calculate drug dosages. The important features of a drug label are identified in • **Figure 2.19**.

1. **Name of drug:** Bosulif is the trade name. In this case, the name begins with an uppercase letter, is in large type, and is boldly visible on the label. The generic name is bosutinib, written in lowercase letters.
2. **Form of drug:** The drug is in the form of a tablet.
3. **National Drug Code (NDC) number:** 0069-0136-01.
4. **Bar code:** Has the NDC number encoded in it.

Always read the expiration date! After the expiration date, the drug may lose its potency or act differently in a patient's body. Follow the healthcare facility's policy regarding disposal of expired drugs. Never give expired drugs to patients!

• **Figure 2.19**
Drug label for Bosulif.

(Reg. Trademark of Pfizer Inc. Reproduced with permission.)

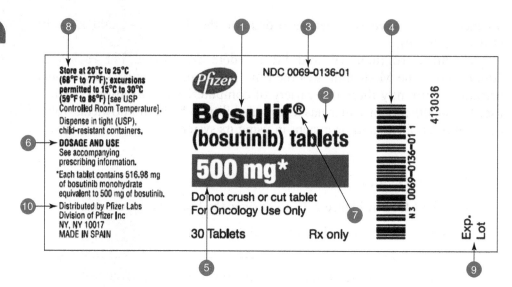

5. **Dosage strength:** *500 mg* of the drug are contained in one tablet.

6. **Dosage recommendations: Note that the manufacturer informs you to see accompanying prescribing information.**

7. Bosulif® is the registered trade name for the drug.

8. **Storage directions:** Some drugs have to be stored under controlled conditions if they are to retain their effectiveness. This drug should be stored at 20°C to 25°C (68°F to 77°F).

9. **Expiration date:** The expiration date specifies when the drug should be discarded. For the sake of simplicity, not every drug label in this textbook will have an expiration date.

10. **Manufacturer:** Pfizer Inc.

The label in Figure 2.20 expresses the strength as 5 *mg*/5 *mL*. The ISMP recommends that the slash mark (/) not be used to indicate *per* or to separate two doses because it might be mistaken for the number *1*.

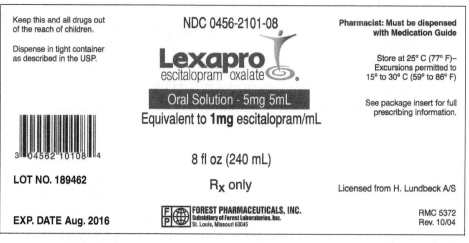

• **Figure 2.20**
Drug label for Lexapro.

The label in • **Figure 2.20** indicates the following information:

1. **Trade name:** Lexapro

2. **Generic name:** escitalopram oxalate

3. **Form:** oral solution

4. **Dosage strength:** *5 mg/5 mL*, equivalent to 1 *mg* of escitalopram per *mL*

5. **Dosage recommendations:** See package insert for full prescribing information

6. **NDC number:** 0456-2101-08

7. **Expiration date:** August 2016

8. **Total volume in container:** 8 *fl oz* (240 *mL*)

9. **Manufacturer:** Forest Pharmaceuticals, Inc.

10. **Lot number** or **control number:** The lot number of this drug is 189462. This number identifies where and when a drug was manufactured. When there is a problem with particular batches of a drug and these batches must be recalled, lot numbers are useful for identifying which items are to be taken off the market.

EXAMPLE 2.6

Read the label in • Figure 2.21 and find the following:

1. Trade name: _____

2. Generic name: _____

3. Form: _____

4. Dosage strength: _____

5. NDC number: _____

6. Dosage and use: _____

7. Instructions for dispensing: _____

Store at 20-25°C (68-77°F) [See USP Controlled Room Temperature]. Preserve in tight, light-resistant containers. Protect from moisture.

Dispense in tight (USP), light-resistant, child-resistant containers.

NOTE TO PHARMACISTS - Do not dispense capsules which are discolored.

DOSAGE AND USE: See accompanying prescribing information.

Each capsule contains 100 mg phenytoin sodium, USP.

Distributed by Parke-Davis Division of Pfizer Inc, NY, NY 10017

ALWAYS DISPENSE WITH ACCOMPANYING MEDICATION GUIDE

NDC 0071-0369-24

Pfizer

Dilantin®

(extended phenytoin sodium capsules, USP)

100 mg

100 Capsules   Rx only

FPO (80% x 5.5mm)
N3 0071-0369-24 5
11137802

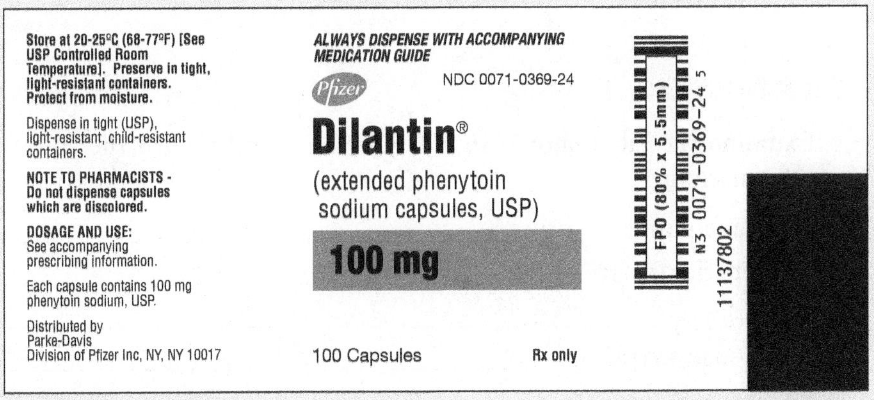

• **Figure 2.21**
Drug label for Dilantin.

(Reg. Trademark of Pfizer Inc. Reproduced with permission.)

The label for the antiseizure drug Dilantin in Figure 2.21 indicates the following:

1. **Trade name:** Dilantin

2. **Generic name:** extended phenytoin sodium

3. **Form:** capsules

4. **Dosage strength:** 100 *mg* per capsule

5. **NDC number:** 0071-0369-24

6. **Dosage and use:** See accompanying information

7. **Instructions for dispensing:** Do not dispense capsules which are discolored

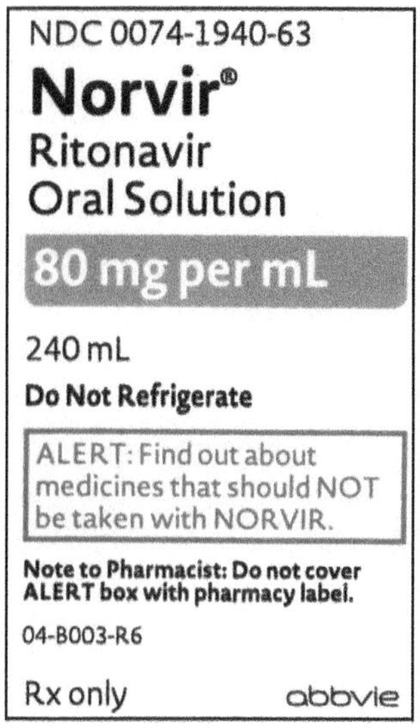

NDC 0074-1940-63

Norvir®

Ritonavir
Oral Solution

80 mg per mL

240 mL

Do Not Refrigerate

ALERT: Find out about
medicines that should NOT
be taken with NORVIR.

**Note to Pharmacist: Do not cover
ALERT box with pharmacy label.**

04-B003-R6

Rx only   abbvie

● **Figure 2.22**
Drug label for Norvir.

EXAMPLE 2.7

Examine the label shown in ● Figure 2.22 and record the following information:

1. Trade name: _____
2. Generic name: _____
3. Form: _____
4. Dosage strength: _____
5. Amount of drug in container: _____
6. Storage temperature: _____
7. Special instructions: _____

This is what you should have found:

1. **Trade name:** Norvir
2. **Generic name:** ritonavir
3. **Form:** Oral solution
4. **Dosage strength:** 80 mg per mL
5. **Amount of drug in container:** 240 mL
6. **Storage temperature:** Do not refrigerate
7. **Special instructions:** ALERT: Find out about medicines that should NOT be taken with Norvir.

EXAMPLE 2.8

Examine the label shown in ● Figure 2.23 and record the following information:

1. Trade name: _____
2. Generic name: _____
3. Form: _____
4. Dosage strength: _____

NDC 0009-3359-01

Prepidil® Gel
dinoprostone cervical gel

0.5 mg*

For endocervical administration
Sterile
DOSAGE AND USE: See accompanying prescribing
information.
* Each 3 gram syringe applicator contains 0.5 mg
dinoprostone. Also contains 240 mg colloidal silicon
dioxide NF, 2760 mg triacetin USP.
Store in a refrigerator 2° to 8°C (36° to 46°F).
MADE IN USA (includes foreign content)

Distributed by
Pharmacia & Upjohn Co
Division of Pfizer Inc, NY, NY 10017

Rx only

8Q3906

LOT/EXP.:

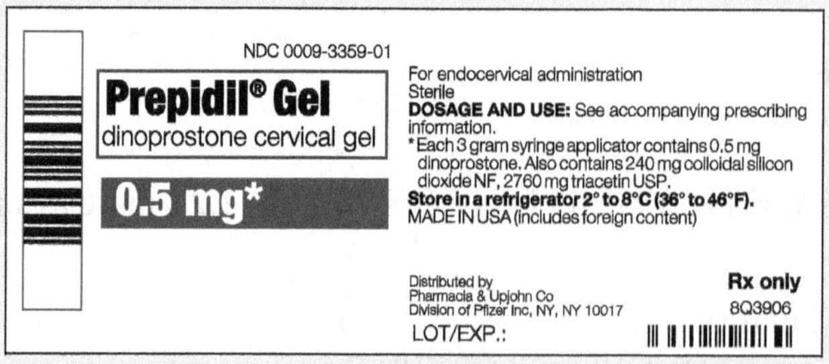

● **Figure 2.23**
**Drug label for
Prepidil Gel.**

This is what you should have found:

1. **Trade name:** Prepidil Gel
2. **Generic name:** dinoprostone cervical gel
3. **Form:** topical gel
4. **Dosage strength:** 0.5 mg

Combination Drugs

Combination drugs contain two or more generic drugs in one form. Both names and strengths of each drug are on the label. Two such medication labels follow.

Examine the label shown in • **Figure 2.24.** The label for this antihypertensive and cholesterol-lowering combination drug indicates that each tablet contains 2.5 *mg* of amlodopine besylate and 20 *mg* of atorvaststin calcium. A combination drug is sometimes prescribed indicating both the dose and the number of tablets or milliliters to be administered. For example, *Caduet (amlodopine beyslate/atorvastatin calcium) 2.5 mg/20 mg 1 tab PO daily.*

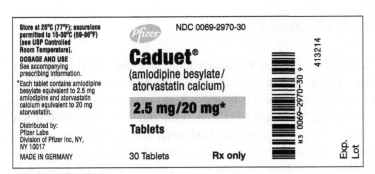

• **Figure 2.24**
Drug label for Caduet.

EXAMPLE 2.9

Examine the label shown in • Figure 2.25 and answer the following questions:

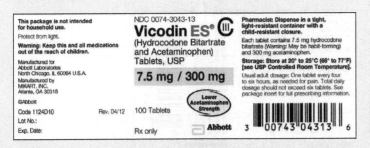

• Figure 2.25
Drug label for
Vicodin ES.

1. What is the trade name and dosage strength of the drug?

2. What is the dosage strength of acetaminophen?

3. What is the route of administration?

4. What is the amount of drug in the container?

5. What is the usual adult dose?

This is what you should have found:

1. Vicodin ES is the trade name, and the dosage strength is 7.5 *mg*/300 *mg* per tablet
2. 300 *mg* of acetaminophen per tablet
3. By mouth
4. 100 *tablets*
5. 1 *tablet* q4-6h prn pain, not to exceed 6 *tab/d*

Controlled Substances

Certain drugs that can lead to abuse or dependence are classified by law as **controlled substances**. These drugs are divided into five categories, called schedules. Schedule I drugs are those with the highest potential for abuse (e.g., heroin, marijuana). Schedule V drugs are those with the lowest potential for abuse (e.g., cough medications containing codeine). Controlled substances must be stored, handled, disposed of, and administered according to regulations established by the *U.S. Drug Enforcement Agency (DEA)*. Hospitals and pharmacies must register with the DEA and use their assigned numbers to purchase scheduled drugs. Those who prescribe medications must have a DEA number to prescribe controlled substances.

The controlled substance OxyContin (oxycodone hydrochloride) is a Schedule II drug, as indicated by the CII on the label. (See the arrow in • **Figure 2.26**.)

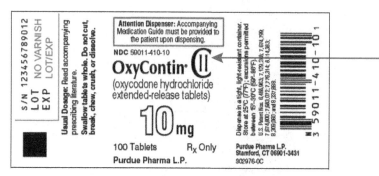

• Figure 2.26

Drug Information

In an effort to manage the risks of medications and reduce medical errors and adverse drug events, the U.S. Food and Drug Administration (FDA) mandates the format in which information about drugs is provided.

Drug information can be obtained online. Prescription drug information is also found on the package insert, whereas information on over-the-counter (OTC) drugs is found on the packaging itself.

Prescription Drug Package Inserts

The FDA has mandated that a new format for package inserts be phased in by 2016. The new categories for the format are:

- **Highlights of Prescribing Information:** provides immediate access to the most important facts.
- **Proprietary name, dosage form, route of administration, and initial U.S. approval (year):** gives the date of initial product approvals, thereby making it easier to determine how long a product has been on the market.
- **Boxed Warning:** identifies the dangers of the medication.
- **Recent Major Changes:** notes the changes made within the past year to ensure the most up-to-date information.
- **Indications and Usage:** includes conditions for which the product is effective.
- **Dosage and Administration:** describes the recommended dose and routes of administration.
- **Dosage Forms and Strengths:** indicates how the product is supplied and its strength (e.g., 10 *mg/tab*).
- **Contraindications:** gives reasons for which it is inadvisable to use the product.
- **Warnings and Precautions:** provides notice of things that may cause harm.
- **Adverse Reactions:** The following statement must be included in this section: "To report SUSPECTED ADVERSE REACTIONS, contact (manufacturer) at (phone # and Web address) or FDA at 1-800-FDA-1088 or www.fda.gov/medwatch.
- **Drug Interactions:** lists other drugs that, when taken in combination, may cause concern.
- **Use in Specific Populations:** indicates target populations (e.g., pregnancy, nursing mothers, pediatric, and geriatric patients).

Over-the-Counter (OTC) Labels

Over-the-counter (OTC) medicines are drugs that can be obtained without a prescription. In the United States, the FDA decides which drugs are safe enough to sell over the counter. Taking OTC drugs still has risks. Some interact with other drugs, supplements, foods, or drinks, whereas others may cause problems for people with certain medical conditions. The FDA format for OTC drug labels is much simpler than that for prescription drugs. The categories are as follows:

- **Drug Facts:** includes the name of the drug and its purpose.
- **Uses:** indicates the conditions for which the drug is effective.

> **NOTE**
>
> Prescription drug information is accessible on "Daily Med," an interagency online health information clearing house created cooperatively by the FDA and the National Library of Medicine (NLM) at http://dailymed.nlm.nih.gov.

- **Warnings:** indicates the effects of the medication of which to be aware.
- **Directions:** specifies the quantity of the drug to take and how often to take it—for example, 2 *tablets* every 8 *hours* with water.
- **Other Information:** provides miscellaneous information—for example, expiration date and storage directions.
- **Inactive ingredients:** lists other substances in the drug that are not active ingredients.
- **Questions or comments:** provides a contact number for consumer questions.

● Figure 2.27 shows an excerpt from the prescribing information for the drug Bosulif (bosutinib).

HIGHLIGHTS OF PRESCRIBING INFORMATION
These highlights do not include all the information needed to use BOSULIF safely and effectively. See full prescribing information for BOSULIF.
BOSULIF® (bosutinib) tablets, for oral use
Initial U.S. Approval: 2012

----------- **INDICATIONS AND USAGE** -----------

- BOSULIF is a kinase inhibitor indicated for the treatment of adult patients with chronic, accelerated, or blast phase Ph+ chronic myelogenous leukemia (CML) with resistance or intolerance to prior therapy.

-------- **DOSAGE AND ADMINISTRATION** --------

- Recommended Dose: 500 *mg* orally once daily with food.
- Consider dose escalation to 600 *mg* daily in patients who do not reach complete hematologic response by week 8 or complete cytogenetic response by week 12 and do not have Grade 3 or greater adverse reactions.
- Adjust dosage for hematologic and non-hematologic toxicity.
- Hepatic impairment (at baseline): reduce BOSULIF dose to 200 *mg* daily.

------- **DOSAGE FORMS AND STRENGTHS** -------

Tablets: 100 *mg* and 500 *mg*.

------------- **CONTRAINDICATIONS** -------------

Hypersensitivity to BOSULIF.

-------- **WARNINGS AND PRECAUTIONS** ---------

- Gastrointestinal toxicity: Monitor and manage as necessary. Withhold, dose reduce, or discontinue BOSULIF.

- Myelosuppression: Monitor blood counts and manage as necessary.
- Hepatic toxicity: Monitor liver enzymes at least monthly for the first three months and as needed. Withhold, dose reduce, or discontinue BOSULIF.
- Fluid retention: Monitor patients and manage using standard of care treatment. Withhold, dose reduce, or discontinue BOSULIF.
- Embryofetal toxicity: May cause fetal harm. Females of reproductive potential should avoid becoming pregnant while being treated with BOSULIF.

------------- **ADVERSE REACTIONS** --------------

Most common adverse reactions (incidence greater than 20%) are diarrhea, nausea, thrombocytopenia, vomiting, abdominal pain, rash, anemia, pyrexia, and fatigue.

To report SUSPECTED ADVERSE REACTIONS, contact Pfizer Inc. at 1-800-438-1985 or FDA at 1-800-FDA-1088 or www.fda.gov/medwatch.

------------- **DRUG INTERACTIONS** --------------

- CYP3A Inhibitors and Inducers: Avoid concurrent use of BOSULIF with strong or moderate CYP3A inhibitors and inducers.
- Proton Pump Inhibitors: May decrease bosutinib drug levels. Consider short-acting antacids in place of proton pump inhibitors.

See 17 for PATIENT COUNSELING INFORMATION and FDA-approved patient labeling.
Revised: 09/2012

● **Figure 2.27**
Excerpts of package insert for Bosulif.

EXAMPLE 2.10

Read the excerpts of the package insert in Figure 2.27 and fill in the requested information.

1. What is the generic name of the drug?

   _____

2. For what condition is this drug used?

   _____

3. What are the most common adverse reactions of this drug?

   _____

4. What is the recommended dose?

   _____

5. What should the prescriber do if a person taking Bosulif develops fluid retention?

   _____

   _____

This is what you should have found:

1. bosutinib
2. Treatment of adult patients who have chronic, accelerated, or blast phase Ph+ chronic myelogenous leukemia
3. Diarrhea, nausea, thrombocytopenia, vomiting, abdominal pain, rash, anemia, pyrexia, and fatigue
4. 500 *mg* once daily by mouth with food
5. Withhold dose, reduce or discontinue Bosulif

EXAMPLE 2.11

Read the drug information in • Figures 2.28 and 2.29 and answer the following questions.

1. What is the generic name of the drug?

   _____

2. What is the purpose of this drug?

   _____

3. Who should not use this drug?

   _____

4. What does this product contain that may cause severe stomach bleeding?

   _____

5. What should you do if you experience sustained stomach pain after using this drug?

   _____

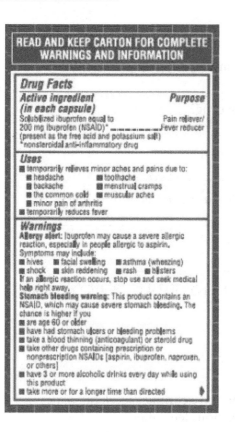

READ AND KEEP CARTON FOR COMPLETE WARNINGS AND INFORMATION

Drug Facts

Active ingredient (in each capsule)	Purpose
Solubilized ibuprofen equal to 200 mg ibuprofen (NSAID)* (present as the free acid and potassium salt) *nonsteroidal anti-inflammatory drug	Pain reliever/ Fever reducer

Uses
- temporarily relieves minor aches and pains due to:
  - headache
  - toothache
  - backache
  - menstrual cramps
  - the common cold
  - muscular aches
  - minor pain of arthritis
- temporarily reduces fever

Warnings

Allergy alert: Ibuprofen may cause a severe allergic reaction, especially in people allergic to aspirin. Symptoms may include:
- hives
- facial swelling
- asthma (wheezing)
- shock
- skin reddening
- rash
- blisters

If an allergic reaction occurs, stop use and seek medical help right away.

Stomach bleeding warning: This product contains an NSAID, which may cause severe stomach bleeding. The chance is higher if you
- are age 60 or older
- have had stomach ulcers or bleeding problems
- take a blood thinning (anticoagulant) or steroid drug
- take other drugs containing prescription or nonprescription NSAIDs [aspirin, ibuprofen, naproxen, or others]
- have 3 or more alcoholic drinks every day while using this product
- take more or for a longer time than directed

Drug Facts (continued)

Do not use
- if you have ever had an allergic reaction to any other pain reliever/fever reducer
- right before or after heart surgery

Ask a doctor before use if
- stomach bleeding warning applies to you
- you have problems or serious side effects from taking pain relievers or fever reducers
- you have a history of stomach problems, such as heartburn
- you have high blood pressure, heart disease, liver cirrhosis, kidney disease, or asthma
- you are taking a diuretic

Ask a doctor or pharmacist before use if you are
- under a doctor's care for any serious condition
- taking aspirin for heart attack or stroke, because ibuprofen may decrease this benefit of aspirin
- taking any other drug

When using this product
- take with food or milk if stomach upset occurs
- the risk of heart attack or stroke may increase if you use more than directed or for longer than directed

Stop use and ask a doctor if
- you experience any of the following signs of stomach bleeding:
  - feel faint
  - vomit blood
  - have bloody or black stools
  - have stomach pain that does not get better
- pain gets worse or lasts more than 10 days
- fever gets worse or lasts more than 3 days
- redness or swelling is present in the painful area
- any new symptoms appear

If pregnant or breast-feeding, ask a health professional before use. It is especially important not to use ibuprofen during the last 3 months of pregnancy unless definitely directed to do so by a doctor because it may cause problems in the unborn child or complications during delivery.

Drug Facts (continued)

Keep out of reach of children. In case of overdose, get medical help or contact a Poison Control Center right away.

Directions
- do not take more than directed
- the smallest effective dose should be used
- adults and children 12 years and over: take 1 capsule every 4 to 6 hours while symptoms persist
- if pain or fever does not respond to 1 capsule, 2 capsules may be used
- do not exceed 6 capsules in 24 hours, unless directed by a doctor
- children under 12 years: ask a doctor

Other Information
- each capsule contains: potassium 20 mg
- read all warnings and directions before use. Keep carton.
- store at 20-25°C (68-77°F)
- avoid excessive heat above 40°C (104°F)

Inactive Ingredients
FD&C green no. 3, gelatin, light mineral oil, pharmaceutical ink, polyethylene glycol, potassium hydroxide, purified water, sorbitan, sorbitol

Questions or comments?
call toll free 1-800-88-ADVIL

• **Figure 2.28**
Information found on Advil packaging.

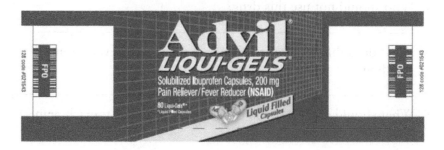

• **Figure 2.29**
Advil packaging.

This is what you should have found:

1. ibuprofen
2. Pain reliever/fever reducer
3. People who have ever had an allergic reaction to any other pain reliever/fever reducer or right before or after heart surgery
4. An NSAID
5. Stop taking the drug and consult a doctor

Summary

In this chapter, the medication administration process was discussed, including the people who may administer drugs; the "six rights" and "three checks" of medication administration; and how to interpret prescriptions, medication orders, Medication Administration Records, drug labels, and drug package inserts.

- The six rights of medication administration serve as a guide for *safe* administration of medications to patients.
- Failure to achieve any of the six rights constitutes a medication error.
- A person administering medications has a legal and ethical responsibility to report medication errors.
- Medication errors can occur at any point in the medication process.
- A drug should be prescribed using its generic name.
- Understanding drug orders requires the interpretation of common abbreviations.
- Never use any abbreviations on The Joint Commission "Official Do Not Use" list.
- Read drug labels carefully; many drugs have look-alike/sound-alike names.
- Carefully read the label to determine dosage strength and check calculations, paying special attention to decimal points.
- Medications must be administered in the form and via the route specified by the prescriber.
- The form of a drug affects its speed of onset, intensity of action, and route of administration.

- The *oral (PO)* route is the one most commonly used.
- *Buccal* and *sublingual* medications must be kept in the mouth until they are completely dissolved.
- *Topical* medications may have local and systemic effects. *Transdermal patches* are applied for their systemic effect.
- *Inhalation* medications may be administered with various devices, such as *nebulizers, dry powder*, and *metered dose inhalers*.
- *Parenteral* medications are injected into the body. To prevent infection, sterile technique must be used for their administration.
- Before administering any medication, it is essential to identify the patient.
- Medications should be documented immediately after, but never before, they are administered.
- No medication should be given without a legal order.
- If persons administering medications have difficulty understanding or interpreting the order, they must clarify the order with the prescriber.
- The medication administration process is rapidly becoming computerized.
- Drug package inserts contain detailed information about the drug indications and usage, dosage and administration, forms and strengths, contraindications, warnings and precautions, adverse reactions, drug interactions, use in special populations, and contact information to report suspected adverse reactions.
- Information for prescription drugs is found in package inserts, whereas information for OTC drugs is found on the packaging itself.

Practice Sets

The answers to *Try These for Practice* and *Exercises* are found in Appendix A. Ask your instructor for the answers to the *Additional Exercises*.

Try These for Practice

Test your comprehension after reading the chapter.

Study the labels in • **Figures 2.30** to **2.34** and answer the following questions.

1. What is the trade name for alprazolam?

   _____

2. What is the route of administration for clindamycin?

   _____

3. What is the generic name for Crixivan?

   _____

4. Which drug is a combination drug?

   _____

5. What is the dosage strength for paricalcitol?

   _____

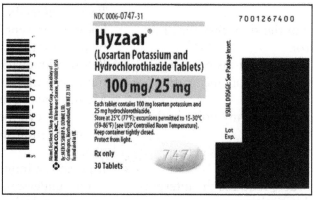

• **Figure 2.30**
Drug label for Hyzaar.

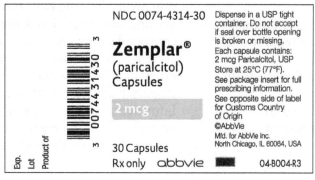
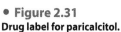
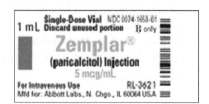

• **Figure 2.31**
Drug label for paricalcitol.

Workspace

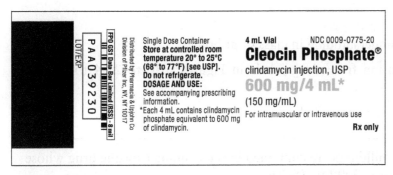

● Figure 2.32
Drug label for Cleocin.

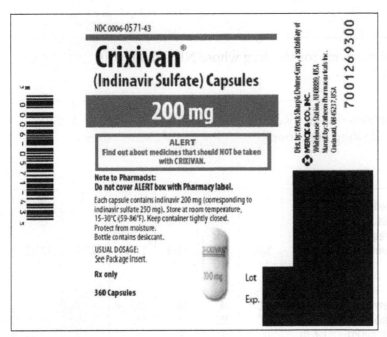

● Figure 2.33
Drug label for Crixivan.

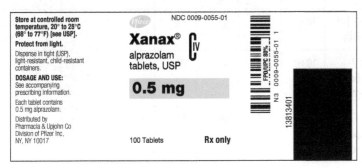

● Figure 2.34
Drug label for Xanax.

Workspace

Exercises

Reinforce your understanding in class or at home.

Use the information from drug labels in Figures 2.30 to 2.34 to complete Exercises 1 to 5.

1. Which drug is a controlled substance?

   _____

2. How many milliliters are contained in the container for the drug whose NDC number is 0009-0775-20?

   _____

3. What is the dosage strength of Crixivan?

   _____

4. How many milligrams of hydrochlorothiazide are contained in one tablet of Hyzaar?

   _____

5. Write the generic name for the drug whose NDC number is 0006-0571-43.

   _____

6. Study the portions of a MAR in • **Figures 2.35a, 2.35b,** and **2.35c** to answer the following questions.

Order Date	Exp Date	Medication Dosage Frequency & Route	Time	12/7	12/8	12/9	12/10	12/11	12/12
12/7	12/13	Neurontin (gabapentin) 100 mg PO t.i.d.	10 AM 2 PM 6 PM	MC MC JY	MC MC JY	MC MC JY	MC MC JY		
12/7	12/16	Vantin (cefpodoxime) 200 mg PO q12h for 10 days	8 AM 8 PM	SG JY	SG JY	SG JY	SG JY		
12/7	12/13	digoxin 0.125 mg PO daily	10 AM	MC	MC	MC	MC		
12/7	12/13	Levemir 7 units subcut at bedtime	10 PM	JY	JY	JY	JY		
12/7	12/13	Norvasc (amlodipine) 5 mg PO daily	10 AM	MC	MC	MC	MC		

• **Figure 2.35a**
Portion of a MAR.

PRN Medication		Medication Dosage Route & Time	Doses Given						
Order Date	Expiration Date		Date	12/10					
12/10	12/13	Tylenol with codeine #3 (300 mg /30 mg) tab 1 PO q4h prn mild-moderate pain	Time	10 PM					
			Init	JY					

• **Figure 2.35b**
Portion of a MAR.

Initial	Nurse's Signature	Initial	Nurse's Signature
SG	Sara Gordon RN		
MC	Marie Colon RN		
JY	Jim Young LPN		

• **Figure 2.35c**
Portion of a MAR.

(a) Which drugs were administered at 10 P.M. on 12/10?

_____

(b) Using military time, designate the time(s) of day when the patient received gabapentin.

_____

(c) How many doses of cefpodoxime were administered by nurse Gordon?

_____

(d) What is the route of administration for Levemir?

_____

(e) Which drugs were administered by nurse Colon on 12/8?

_____

Workspace

Workspace

7. Study the portion of a physician's order sheet in • **Figure 2.36** to answer the following questions.

(a) Which drug(s) is/are given four times a day?

_____

(b) Which drug(s) is/are given once a day?

_____

(c) How many times a day should the patient receive Vibramycin?

_____

(d) What is the route of administration for Dilaudid?

_____

(e) How many times a day can the patient receive hydromorphone HCl?

_____

PHYSICIAN'S ORDERS

Order Date	Date Disc	
4/20/2016	4/30/2016	Vibramycin (doxycycline hydrochloride) 100 mg PO q12h
4/20/2016	4/27/2016	digoxin 0.125 mg PO daily
4/20/2016	4/27/2016	Mevacor (lovastatin) 20 mg PO with the evening meal
4/20/2016	4/27/2016	metoclopramide HCl 10 mg PO ac and hs. Give 30 minutes before meals and at bedtime.
4/20/2016	4/23/2016	Dilaudid (hydromorphone hydrochloride) 1 mg IVP (over 2-3 min) q3h prn moderate pain
4/20/2016	4/27/2016	Cozaar (losartan potassium) 25 mg PO daily

• **Figure 2.36**
Portion of a physician's order sheet.

8. Use the package insert shown in • **Figure 2.37** to answer the following questions.

(a) What is the generic name and form of the drug?

_____

(b) For what condition is the intramuscular form of ZyPREXA used?

_____

(c) What may occur if the drug is taken with diazepam?

_____

(d) What is the recommended beginning oral dose for adults with schizophrenia?

_____

(e) Should women who are breastfeeding use this drug?

_____

HIGHLIGHTS OF PRESCRIBING INFORMATION

These highlights do not include all the information needed to use ZYPREXA safely and effectively. See full prescribing information for ZYPREXA.

ZYPREXA (olanzapine) Tablet for Oral use
ZYPREXA ZYDIS (olanzapine) Tablet, Orally Disintegrating for Oral use
ZYPREXA IntraMuscular (olanzapine) Injection, Powder, For Solution for Intramuscular use

Initial U.S. Approval: 1996

WARNING: INCREASED MORTALITY IN ELDERLY PATIENTS WITH DEMENTIA-RELATED PSYCHOSIS

See full prescribing information for complete boxed warning.
- **Elderly patients with dementia-related psychosis treated with antipsychotic drugs are at an increased risk of death. ZYPREXA is not approved for the treatment of patients with dementia-related psychosis. (5.1, 5.14, 17.2)**

When using ZYPREXA and fluoxetine in combination, also refer to the Boxed Warning section of the package insert for Symbyax.

--------------------------- RECENT MAJOR CHANGES ---------------------------

Indications and Usage:

Schizophrenia (1.1)	12/2009
Bipolar I Disorder (Manic or Mixed Episodes) (1.2)	12/2009
Special Considerations in Treating Pediatric Schizophrenia and Bipolar I Disorder (1.3)	12/2009
ZYPREXA IntraMuscular: Agitation Associated with Schizophrenia and Bipolar I Mania (1.4)	12/2009

Dosage and Administration:

Schizophrenia (2.1)	12/2009
Bipolar I Disorder (Manic or Mixed Episodes) (2.2)	12/2009

Warnings and Precautions:

Orthostatic Hypotension (5.8)	05/2010
Leukopenia, Neutropenia, and Agranulocytosis (5.9)	08/2009
Hyperprolactinemia (5.15)	01/2010

--------------------------- INDICATIONS AND USAGE ---------------------------

ZYPREXA® (olanzapine) is an atypical antipsychotic indicated:

As oral formulation for the:
- Treatment of schizophrenia. (1.1)
  - Adults: Efficacy was established in three clinical trials in patients with schizophrenia: two 6-week trials and one maintenance trial. (14.1)
  - Adolescents (ages 13-17): Efficacy was established in one 6-week trial in patients with schizophrenia (14.1). The increased potential (in adolescents compared with adults) for weight gain and hyperlipidemia may lead clinicians to consider prescribing other drugs first in adolescents. (1.1)
- Acute treatment of manic or mixed episodes associated with bipolar I disorder and maintenance treatment of bipolar I disorder. (1.2)
  - Adults: Efficacy was established in three clinical trials in patients with manic or mixed episodes of bipolar I disorder: two 3- to 4-week trials and one maintenance trial. (14.2)
  - Adolescents (ages 13-17): Efficacy was established in one 3-week trial in patients with manic or mixed episodes associated with bipolar I disorder (14.2). The increased potential (in adolescents compared with adults) for weight gain and hyperlipidemia may lead clinicians to consider prescribing other drugs first in adolescents. (1.2)
- Medication therapy for pediatric patients with schizophrenia or bipolar I disorder should be undertaken only after a thorough diagnostic evaluation and with careful consideration of the potential risks. (1.3)
- Adjunct to valproate or lithium in the treatment of manic or mixed episodes associated with bipolar I disorder. (1.2)
  - Efficacy was established in two 6-week clinical trials in adults (14.2). Maintenance efficacy has not been systematically evaluated.

As ZYPREXA IntraMuscular for the:
- Treatment of acute agitation associated with schizophrenia and bipolar I mania. (1.4)

- Efficacy was established in three 1-day trials in adults. (14.3)

As ZYPREXA and Fluoxetine in Combination for the:
- Treatment of depressive episodes associated with bipolar I disorder. (1.5)
  - Efficacy was established with Symbyax (olanzapine and fluoxetine in combination) in adults; refer to the product label for Symbyax.
- Treatment of treatment resistant depression (major depressive disorder in patients who do not respond to 2 separate trials of different antidepressants of adequate dose and duration in the current episode). (1.6)
  - Efficacy was established with Symbyax (olanzapine and fluoxetine in combination) in adults; refer to the product label for Symbyax.

--------------------- DOSAGE AND ADMINISTRATION ---------------------

Schizophrenia in adults (2.1)	Oral: Start at 5-10 mg once daily; Target: 10 mg/day within several days
Schizophrenia in adolescents (2.1)	Oral: Start at 2.5-5 mg once daily; Target: 10 mg/day
Bipolar I Disorder (manic or mixed episodes) in adults (2.2)	Oral: Start at 10 or 15 mg once daily
Bipolar I Disorder (manic or mixed episodes) in adolescents (2.2)	Oral: Start at 2.5-5 mg once daily; Target: 10 mg/day
Bipolar I Disorder (manic or mixed episodes) with lithium or valproate in adults (2.2)	Oral: Start at 10 mg once daily
Agitation associated with Schizophrenia and Bipolar I Mania in adults (2.4)	IM: 10 mg (5 mg or 7.5 mg when clinically warranted) Assess for orthostatic hypotension prior to subsequent dosing (max. 3 doses 2-4 hrs apart)
Depressive Episodes associated with Bipolar I Disorder in adults (2.5)	Oral in combination with fluoxetine: Start at 5 mg of oral olanzapine and 20 mg of fluoxetine once daily
Treatment Resistant Depression in adults (2.6)	Oral in combination with fluoxetine: Start at 5 mg of oral olanzapine and 20 mg of fluoxetine once daily

- Lower starting dose recommended in debilitated or pharmacodynamically sensitive patients or patients with predisposition to hypotensive reactions, or with potential for slowed metabolism. (2.1)
- Olanzapine may be given without regard to meals. (2.1)

ZYPREXA and Fluoxetine in Combination:
- Dosage adjustments, if indicated, should be made with the individual components according to efficacy and tolerability. (2.5, 2.6)
- Olanzapine monotherapy is not indicated for the treatment of depressive episodes associated with bipolar I disorder or treatment resistant depression. (2.5, 2.6)
- Safety of co-administration of doses above 18 mg olanzapine with 75 mg fluoxetine has not been evaluated. (2.5, 2.6)

-------------------- DOSAGE FORMS AND STRENGTHS --------------------
- Tablets (not scored): 2.5, 5, 7.5, 10, 15, 20 mg (3)
- Orally Disintegrating Tablets (not scored): 5, 10, 15, 20 mg (3)
- Intramuscular Injection: 10 mg vial (3)

----------------------------- CONTRAINDICATIONS -----------------------------
- None with ZYPREXA monotherapy.
- When using ZYPREXA and fluoxetine in combination, also refer to the Contraindications section of the package insert for Symbyax®. (4)
- When using ZYPREXA in combination with lithium or valproate, refer to the Contraindications section of the package inserts for those products. (4)

---------------------- WARNINGS AND PRECAUTIONS ----------------------
- *Elderly Patients with Dementia-Related Psychosis:* Increased risk of death and increased incidence of cerebrovascular adverse events (e.g., stroke, transient ischemic attack). (5.1)
- *Suicide:* The possibility of a suicide attempt is inherent in schizophrenia and in bipolar I disorder, and close supervision of high-risk patients should accompany drug therapy; when using in combination with fluoxetine, also refer to the Boxed Warning and Warnings and Precautions sections of the package insert for Symbyax. (5.2)
- *Neuroleptic Malignant Syndrome:* Manage with immediate discontinuation and close monitoring. (5.3)

● **Figure 2.37**
Excerpt from package insert for ZyPREXA.

- *Hyperglycemia:* In some cases extreme and associated with ketoacidosis or hyperosmolar coma or death, has been reported in patients taking olanzapine. Patients taking olanzapine should be monitored for symptoms of hyperglycemia and undergo fasting blood glucose testing at the beginning of, and periodically during, treatment. (5.4)
- *Hyperlipidemia:* Undesirable alterations in lipids have been observed. Appropriate clinical monitoring is recommended, including fasting blood lipid testing at the beginning of, and periodically during, treatment. (5.5)
- *Weight Gain:* Potential consequences of weight gain should be considered. Patients should receive regular monitoring of weight. (5.6)
- *Tardive Dyskinesia:* Discontinue if clinically appropriate. (5.7)
- *Orthostatic Hypotension:* Orthostatic hypotension associated with dizziness, tachycardia, bradycardia and, in some patients, syncope, may occur especially during initial dose titration. Use caution in patients with cardiovascular disease, cerebrovascular disease, and those conditions that could affect hemodynamic responses. (5.8)
- *Leukopenia, Neutropenia, and Agranulocytosis:* Has been reported with antipsychotics, including ZYPREXA. Patients with a history of a clinically significant low white blood cell count (WBC) or drug induced leukopenia/neutropenia should have their complete blood count (CBC) monitored frequently during the first few months of therapy and discontinuation of ZYPREXA should be considered at the first sign of a clinically significant decline in WBC in the absence of other causative factors. (5.9)
- *Seizures:* Use cautiously in patients with a history of seizures or with conditions that potentially lower the seizure threshold. (5.11)
- *Potential for Cognitive and Motor Impairment:* Has potential to impair judgment, thinking, and motor skills. Use caution when operating machinery. (5.12)
- *Hyperprolactinemia:* May elevate prolactin levels. (5.15)
- *Use in Combination with Fluoxetine, Lithium or Valproate:* Also refer to the package inserts for Symbyax, lithium, or valproate. (5.16)
- *Laboratory Tests:* Monitor fasting blood glucose and lipid profiles at the beginning of, and periodically during, treatment. (5.17)

------------------------------ ADVERSE REACTIONS ------------------------------

Most common adverse reactions (≥5% and at least twice that for placebo) associated with:

Oral Olanzapine Monotherapy:
- Schizophrenia (Adults) – postural hypotension, constipation, weight gain, dizziness, personality disorder, akathisia (6.1)
- Schizophrenia (Adolescents) – sedation, weight increased, headache, increased appetite, dizziness, abdominal pain, pain in extremity, fatigue, dry mouth (6.1)
- Manic or Mixed Episodes, Bipolar I Disorder (Adults) – asthenia, dry mouth, constipation, increased appetite, somnolence, dizziness, tremor (6.1)

- Manic or Mixed Episodes, Bipolar I Disorder (Adolescents) – sedation, weight increased, increased appetite, headache, fatigue, dizziness, dry mouth, abdominal pain, pain in extremity (6.1)

Combination of ZYPREXA and Lithium or Valproate:
- Manic or Mixed Episodes, Bipolar I Disorder (Adults) – dry mouth, weight gain, increased appetite, dizziness, back pain, constipation, speech disorder, increased salivation, amnesia, paresthesia (6.1)

ZYPREXA and Fluoxetine in Combination: Also refer to the Adverse Reactions section of the package insert for Symbyax. (6)

ZYPREXA IntraMuscular for Injection:
- Agitation with Schizophrenia and Bipolar I Mania (Adults) – somnolence (6.1)

To report SUSPECTED ADVERSE REACTIONS, contact Eli Lilly and Company at 1-800-LillyRx (1-800-545-5979) or FDA at 1-800-FDA-1088 or www.fda.gov/medwatch

---------------------------- DRUG INTERACTIONS ----------------------------
- *Diazepam:* May potentiate orthostatic hypotension. (7.1, 7.2)
- *Alcohol:* May potentiate orthostatic hypotension. (7.1)
- *Carbamazepine:* Increased clearance of olanzapine. (7.1)
- *Fluvoxamine:* May increase olanzapine levels. (7.1)
- *ZYPREXA and Fluoxetine in Combination:* Also refer to the Drug Interactions section of the package insert for Symbyax. (7.1)
- *CNS Acting Drugs:* Caution should be used when taken in combination with other centrally acting drugs and alcohol. (7.2)
- *Antihypertensive Agents:* Enhanced antihypertensive effect. (7.2)
- *Levodopa and Dopamine Agonists:* May antagonize levodopa/dopamine agonists. (7.2)
- *Lorazepam (IM):* Increased somnolence with IM olanzapine. (7.2)
- *Other Concomitant Drug Therapy:* When using olanzapine in combination with lithium or valproate, refer to the Drug Interactions sections of the package insert for those products. (7.2)

----------------------- USE IN SPECIFIC POPULATIONS -----------------------
- *Pregnancy:* ZYPREXA should be used during pregnancy only if the potential benefit justifies the potential risk to the fetus. (8.1)
- *Nursing Mothers:* Breast-feeding is not recommended. (8.3)
- *Pediatric Use:* Safety and effectiveness of ZYPREXA in children <13 years of age have not been established. (8.4)

See 17 for PATIENT COUNSELING INFORMATION and FDA-approved Medication Guide

Revised: 05/2010

● **Figure 2.37**
(*Continued*)

---

9. Fill in the following table with the equivalent times.

Workspace

Standard Time	Military Time
9:30 A.M.	_____
_____	1443 *h*
_____	2400 *h*
11:20 P.M.	_____
_____	0948 *h*
11:40 P.M.	_____
_____	2042 *h*
2:15 A.M.	_____
_____	0002 *h*
7:15 A.M.	_____

10. Interpret the following medication orders:

    (a) Glucophage (metformin) 500 *mg* PO B.I.D.

    (b) heparin 10,000 *units* subcut q8h

    (c) NITRO-BID 2% (nitroglycerin ointment) one-half inch q6h to chest wall

    (d) Accupril (quinapril hydrochloride) 5 *mg* PO daily

    (e) Tylenol (acetaminophen) 650 *mg* PO q4h prn fever over 101°

11. Determine the missing component(s) for each of the following medication orders:

    (a) Wellbutrin XL® (bupropion hydrochloride) PO

    (b) Glucotrol (glipizide) 1 *tab* before breakfast

    (c) Ambien® (zolpidem tartrate) 10 *mg*

    (d) ibuprofen stat

    (e) Timoptic (timolol maleate) 1 *drop* B.I.D.

12. (a) A drug is ordered 10 *mg* daily. How many milligrams will you administer?

    (b) A drug is ordered 10 *mg* B.I.D. How many milligrams will you administer?

    (c) A drug is ordered 10 *mg* q12h. How many milligrams will you administer?

    (d) A drug is ordered 10 *mg* daily in two divided doses. How many milligrams will you administer?

Additional Exercises

Now, test yourself!

Use the information from drug labels in • **Figures 2.38** to **2.42** to complete Exercises 1 to 5.

1. Write the generic name for Singulair.

2. Write the trade name for the drug whose NDC number is 0006-0749-54.

3. What is the total amount of solution in the bottle of clarithromycin?

4. What is the dosage strength of E.E.S. granules?

5. What is the dosage strength of the drug whose NDC number is 0074-3956-46?

Workspace

Workspace

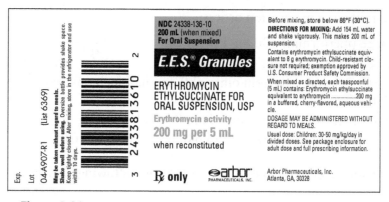

● **Figure 2.38**
Drug label for E.E.S. granules.

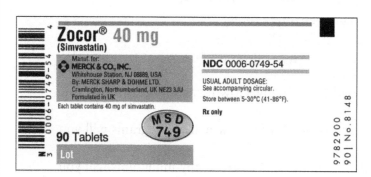

● **Figure 2.39**
Drug label for Zocor.

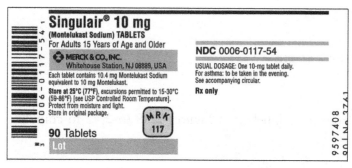

● **Figure 2.40**
Drug label for Singulair.

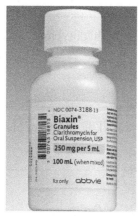

● **Figure 2.41**
Drug label for Biaxin.

NDC 0074-3956-46

Kaletra®
Lopinavir/Ritonavir
Oral Solution

80 mg/20 mg per mL

160 mL

ALERT: Find out about medicines
that should NOT be taken with
KALETRA

**Attention Pharmacist: Do not cover
ALERT box with pharmacy label.**

**Dispense the enclosed Medication
Guide to each patient.**
04-B092-R5

Rx only   abbvie

● **Figure 2.42**
Drug label for Kaletra.

6. Study the MAR in • **Figures 2.43a** and **2.43b** and answer the questions.

(a) Which drugs were administered at 10 P.M. on 12/10/2016?

_____

(b) Designate the time of the day the patient received ibandronate sodium.

_____

(c) How many doses of Dilantin were administered to the patient by nurse Young?

_____

(d) What drugs must be taken before breakfast?

_____

(e) What is the last date on which the patient will receive Bactrim?

_____

‖‖‖‖‖‖	**UNIVERSITY HOSPITAL**	324689 Jane Ambery 2336 17th Avenue Brooklyn, NY 10001	12/7/2016 5/01/47 Protestant HIP
	DAILY MEDICATION ADMINISTRATION RECORD	Dr. Mae Ling	

PATIENT NAME ___Jane Ambery___

ROOM # ___112___   IF ANOTHER RECORD IS IN USE ☐

ALLERGIC TO (RECORD IN RED): ___sulfa, fish___

DATES GIVEN ↓ MONTH/DAY   YEAR: ___2016___

RED CHECK INITIAL	ORDER DATE	INITIAL	EXP DATE	MEDICATION, DOSAGE, FREQUENCY AND ROUTE	TIME	12/7	12/8	12/9	12/10	12/11	12/12	12/13
	12/7	MC	12/13	Dilantin (phenytoin) 100 mg	10AM	MC	MC	MC	MC			
				PO t.i.d.	2PM	MC	MC	MC	MC			
					6PM	JY	JY	JY	JY			
	12/7	SG	12/16	Bactrim DS 2tabs PO q12h	8AM	SG	SG	SG	SG			
				for 10 days	8PM	JY	JY	JY	JY			
	12/7	SG	12/13	Bonivar (ibandronate sodium)	6AM	SG	SG	SG	SG			
				2.5 mg PO daily. Take 60 minutes								
				before first food or drink of day								
				(except plain water)								
	12/7	SG	12/13	Humulin N insulin 15 units subcut	7:30AM	SG	SG	SG	SG			
				every morning								
				30 minutes before breakfast								
	12/7	SG	12/13	Humulin R insulin 8 units subcut	7:30AM	SG	SG	SG	SG			
				every morning								
				30 minutes before breakfast								

INT.	NURSES' FULL SIGNATURE AND TITLE	INT.	NURSES' FULL SIGNATURE AND TITLE
SG	Sara Gordon, RN		
MC	Marie Colon, RN		
JY	Jim Young, RN		

• **Figure 2.43a**
Medication Administration Record for Jane Ambery.

Workspace

<table>
<tr>
<td colspan="3" align="center">UNIVERSITY
HOSPITAL</td>
<td>324689
Jane Ambery
2336 17th Avenue
Brooklyn, NY</td>
<td>12/7/2016
5/01/47
Protestant
HIP</td>
</tr>
<tr>
<td colspan="3" align="center">DAILY MEDICATION
ADMINISTRATION RECORD</td>
<td colspan="2">Dr. Mae Ling, M.D.</td>
</tr>
</table>

PATIENT NAME ___ *Jane Ambery* ___

ROOM # ___ *112* ___   IF ANOTHER RECORD IS IN USE ☐

ALLERGIC TO (RECORD IN RED): ___ *sulfa, fish* ___

DATES GIVEN ↓ MONTH/DAY   YEAR: *2016* ___

PRN MEDICATION

ORDER DATE	EXPIRATION DATE/TIME	MEDICATION, DOSAGE, FREQUENCY AND ROUTE		DOSES GIVEN						
12/10	12/17	*Anusol supp 1 PR q4–6h prn*	DATE	12/10						
			TIME	10 PM						
			INIT	JY						
			DATE							
			TIME							
			INIT							

STAT-ONE DOSE-PRE-OPERATIVE MEDICATIONS   ◯ Check here if additional sheet in use.

ORDER DATE	MEDICATION–DOSAGE ROUTE	DATE	TIME	INIT	ORDER DATE	MEDICATION–DOSAGE ROUTE	DATE	TIME	INIT

INT.	NURSES' FULL SIGNATURE AND TITLE	INT.	NURSES' FULL SIGNATURE AND TITLE
JY	*Jim Young, RN*		

● **Figure 2.43b**
Medication Administration Record for Jane Ambery.

7. Study the physician's order sheet in ● **Figure 2.44** and then answer the following questions.

(a) Which drugs are ordered to be given two times a day?

_____

(b) How many doses of metoclopramide will the patient receive each day?

_____

PHYSICIAN'S ORDERS

ORDER DATE	DATE DISC		
4/20/16	4/30/16	*Omnicef (cefdinir) 300 mg PO q12h for 10 days*	2/28/52 Episcopal Aetna / 4/20/2016
4/20/16	4/27/16	*digoxin 0.125 mg PO daily*	
4/20/16	4/27/16	*Glucophage (metformin HCl) 850 mg PO b.i.d. with breakfast and dinner*	
4/20/16	4/27/16	*Reglan (metoclopramide) 10 mg PO 30 minutes before meals and at bedtime*	
4/20/16	4/23/16	*Duragesic transdermal film ER 25 mg per hour. Remove in 72 hours.*	Jane Myers 23 College Ave Salt Lake City Utah 46022 / Dr. Juan Rodriguez #212332
4/20/16	4/27/16	*Lasix 40 mg PO daily*	
		PLEASE INDICATE BEEPER # → 222	

● **Figure 2.44**
Physician's order sheet for patient Jane Myers.

(c) What is the dose and route of administration of Duragesic?

_____

(d) What is the route of administration for metformin?

_____

(e) How many doses of cefdinir will the patient receive per day?

_____

Workspace

8. Use the package insert shown in • **Figure 2.45** to answer the following questions.

HIGHLIGHTS OF PRESCRIBING INFORMATION
These highlights do not include all the information needed to use Savella safely and effectively. See full prescribing information for Savella.
Savella® (milnacipran HCl) Tablets
Initial U.S. Approval: 2009

WARNING: SUICIDALITY AND ANTIDEPRESSANT DRUGS
See full prescribing information for complete boxed warning.
• **Increased risk of suicidal ideation, thinking, and behavior in children, adolescents, and young adults taking antidepressants for major depressive disorder (MDD) and other psychiatric disorders. Savella is not approved for use in pediatric patients (5.1)**

-------------- RECENT MAJOR CHANGES--------------------
Warnings and Precautions, Serotonin Syndrome or Neuroleptic Malignant Syndrome (NMS)-like Reactions (5.2)
06/2009

------------------INDICATIONS AND USAGE-----------------
Savella® is a selective serotonin and norepinephrine reuptake inhibitor (SNRI) indicated for the management of fibromyalgia (1)
Savella is not approved for use in pediatric patients (5.1)

-------------DOSAGE AND ADMINISTRATION--------------
• Administer Savella in two divided doses per day (2.1)
• Based on efficacy and tolerability, dosing may be titrated according to the following schedule (2.1):
Day 1: 12.5 mg once
Days 2-3: 25 mg/day (12.5 mg twice daily)
Days 4-7: 50 mg/day (25 mg twice daily)
After Day 7: 100 mg/day (50 mg twice daily)
• Recommended dose is 100 mg/day (2.1)
• May be increased to 200 mg/day based on individual patient response (2.1)
• Dose should be adjusted in patients with severe renal impairment (2.2)

-----------DOSAGE FORMS AND STRENGTHS------------
• Tablets: 12.5 mg, 25 mg, 50 mg, 100 mg (3)

--------------------CONTRAINDICATIONS--------------------
• Use of monoamine oxidase inhibitors concomitantly or in close temporal proximity (4.1)
• Use in patients with uncontrolled narrow-angle glaucoma (4.2)

--------------WARNINGS AND PRECAUTIONS--------------
• Suicidality: Monitor for worsening of depressive symptoms and suicide risk (5.1)
• Serotonin Syndrome or Neuroleptic Malignant Syndrome (NMS)-like Reactions: Serotonin syndrome or NMS-like reactions have been reported with SNRIs and SSRIs. Discontinue Savella and initiate supportive treatment (5.2, 7)

• Elevated blood pressure and heart rate: Cases have been reported with Savella. Monitor blood pressure and heart rate prior to initiating treatment with Savella and periodically throughout treatment (5.3, 5.4)
• Seizures: Cases have been reported with Savella therapy. Prescribe Savella with care in patients with a history of seizure disorder (5.5)
• Hepatotoxicity: More patients treated with Savella than with placebo experienced mild elevations of ALT and AST. Rarely, fulminant hepatitis has been reported in patients treated with Savella. Avoid concomitant use of Savella in patients with substantial alcohol use or chronic liver disease (5.6)
• Discontinuation: Withdrawal symptoms have been reported in patients when discontinuing treatment with Savella. A gradual dose reduction is recommended (5.7)
• Abnormal Bleeding: Savella may increase the risk of bleeding events. Caution patients about the risk of bleeding associated with the concomitant use of Savella and NSAIDs, aspirin, or other drugs that affect coagulation (5.9)
• Male patients with a history of obstructive uropathies may experience higher rates of genitourinary adverse events (5.11)

--------------------ADVERSE REACTIONS--------------------
The most frequently occurring adverse reactions (≥ 5% and greater than placebo) were nausea, headache, constipation, dizziness, insomnia, hot flush, hyperhidrosis, vomiting, palpitations, heart rate increased, dry mouth, and hypertension (6.3)

To report SUSPECTED ADVERSE REACTIONS, contact Forest Pharmaceuticals, Inc., at (800) 678-1605 or FDA at 1-800-FDA-1088 or www.fda.gov/medwatch.

--------------------DRUG INTERACTIONS--------------------
• Savella is unlikely to be involved in clinically significant pharmacokinetic drug interactions (7)
• Pharmacodynamic interactions of Savella with other drugs can occur (7)

--------------USE IN SPECIFIC POPULATIONS--------------
• Pregnancy and nursing mothers: Use only if the potential benefit justifies the potential risk to the fetus or child (8.1, 8.3)
• To enroll in the Savella Pregnancy Registry call 1-877-643-3010 (toll free) or download data forms from the registry website: www.savellapregnancyregistry.com (8.1)

See 17 for PATIENT COUNSELING INFORMATION and Medication Guide.
Revised: May 2010

• **Figure 2.45**
Excerpt from package insert for Savella.

Workspace

(a) What is the generic name and form of the drug?

_____

(b) What condition is the drug used to treat?

_____

(c) What is the initial dose on the first day?

_____

(d) Can the drug be used for children?

_____

(e) What is the maximum daily dose?

_____

9. Fill in the following table with the equivalent times.

Standard Time	Military Time
7:30 A.M.	_____
_____	1743 h
	2400 h
8:20 P.M.	_____
	1257 h
10:30 P.M.	_____
	1532 h
4:15 A.M.	_____
	0004 h
9:12 A.M.	_____

10. Interpret the following drug orders:

    (a) Norvasc (amlodipine) 10 mg PO daily, hold for SBP below 100
    (b) morphine sulfate 5 mg subcut q4h prn moderate-severe pain
    (c) Methergine (methylergonovine maleate) 0.2 mg IM stat, then 0.2 mg PO q6h for six doses
    (d) Ceftin (cefuroxime axetil) 1.5 g IVPB 30 minutes before surgery, then 750 milligrams IVPB q8h for 24h
    (e) heparin 5,000 units subcut q12h

11. Determine which part is missing for each of the following drug orders:

    (a) *cephalexin 500 mg q12h*
    (b) *Ziagen (abacavir sulfate) 300 mg PO*
    (c) *Vasotec (enalapril) via PEG hold for HR less than 60 and SBP less than 100*
    (d) *hydrocortisone sodium succinate 140 mg IVPB*
    (e) *acetaminophen PO*

12. (a) A drug is ordered 60 *mg* daily. How many milligrams will you administer?
    (b) A drug is ordered 60 *mg* T.I.D. How many milligrams will you administer?
    (c) A drug is ordered 60 *mg* q8h. How many milligrams will you administer?
    (d) A drug is ordered 60 *mg* daily in three divided doses. How many milligrams will you administer?

Dimensional Analysis

Learning Outcomes

$$\frac{2\,h}{1} \times \frac{60\,min}{1\,h}$$

After completing this chapter, you will be able to

1. Identify some common units of measurement and their abbreviations.
2. Construct unit fractions from equivalences.
3. Convert a quantity expressed with a single unit of measurement to an equivalent quantity with another single unit of measurement.
4. Solve, using Dimensional Analysis, both simple (one-step) and complex (multi-step) problems involving single units of measurement.
5. Convert a quantity expressed as a rate to another rate.
6. Solve, using Dimensional Analysis, both simple (one-step) and complex (multi-step) problems involving rates.

I n this chapter, you will learn to use *Dimensional Analysis*. Dimensional Analysis is a simple approach to drug calculations that largely frees you from the need to memorize formulas. It is the method most commonly employed in the physical sciences. Once this technique is mastered, you will be able to calculate drug dosages quickly and safely.

Introduction to Dimensional Analysis

In courses such as chemistry and physics, students learn to routinely change a quantity in one unit of measurement to an equivalent quantity in a different unit of measurement by cancelling matching units of measurement. In the first edition of this textbook in 1973, "dimensional analysis" was used for the first time in a medical dosage calculation textbook. The name Dimensional Analysis was chosen because the units of measure (for example, feet and inches) are called *dimensions*, and these dimensions have to be *analyzed* in order to see how to do the problems. Dimensional Analysis has become the most popular method of dosage calculation.

The Mathematical Foundation for Dimensional Analysis

Dimensional Analysis relies on two simple mathematical concepts.

Concept 1   When a nonzero quantity is divided by the same amount, the result is 1.

For example: $7 \div 7 = 1$

Because you can also write a division problem in fractional form, you get

$$\frac{7}{7} = 1$$

Because $\frac{7}{7}$ is a fraction equal to 1, and the word "*unit*" means one, the fraction $\frac{7}{7}$ is called a **unit fraction**.

In the preceding unit fraction, you may *cancel* the 7s on the top and bottom. That is, you can divide both numerator and denominator by 7.

$$\frac{\cancel{7}}{\cancel{7}} = \frac{1}{1} = 1$$

Units of measurement are the "labels"—such as *inches, feet, minutes,* and *hours*—that are sometimes written after a number. They are also referred to as **dimensions**, or simply **units**. For example, in the quantity 7 *days, days* is the unit of measurement.

The equivalent quantities you divide may contain **units of measurement**. For example: $7 \ days \div 7 \ days = 1$

Or in fractional form: $\dfrac{7 \ days}{7 \ days} = 1$

In the preceding unit fraction, you may cancel the number 7 and the unit of measurement *days* on the top and bottom and obtain the following:

$$\frac{\cancel{7 \ days}}{\cancel{7 \ days}} = \frac{1}{1} = 1$$

Going one step further, now consider this *equivalence*: **7 *days* = 1 *week*.**

Because 7 *days* is the same quantity of time as 1 *week*, when you divide these quantities, you must get 1.

So, both $7 \ days \div 1 \ week = 1$ **and** $1 \ week \div 7 \ days = 1$

Table 3.1	**Equivalents for Some Common Units of Measurement**

$$12 \text{ inches (in)} = 1 \text{ foot (ft)}$$
$$2 \text{ pints (pt)} = 1 \text{ quart (qt)}$$
$$16 \text{ ounces (oz)} = 1 \text{ pound (lb)}$$
$$60 \text{ seconds (sec)} = 1 \text{ minute (min)}$$
$$60 \text{ minutes (min)} = 1 \text{ hour (h or hr)}$$
$$24 \text{ hours (h or hr)} = 1 \text{ day (d)}$$
$$7 \text{ days (d)} = 1 \text{ week (wk)}$$
$$12 \text{ months (mon)} = 1 \text{ year (yr)}$$

Or in unit fractional form: $\dfrac{7 \text{ days}}{1 \text{ week}} = 1$ **and** $\dfrac{1 \text{ week}}{7 \text{ days}} = 1$

Other unit fractions can be obtained from the equivalences found in Table 3.1.

Concept 2 When a quantity is multiplied by 1, the quantity is unchanged.

In the following examples, the quantity 2 *weeks* will be multiplied by the number 1 and also by the unit fractions $\dfrac{7}{7}, \dfrac{7 \text{ days}}{7 \text{ days}},$ and $\dfrac{7 \text{ days}}{1 \text{ week}}$

$$2 \text{ weeks} \times 1 = \qquad\qquad 2 \text{ weeks}$$

$$2 \text{ weeks} \times \frac{7}{7} = 2 \text{ weeks} \times 1 = 2 \text{ weeks}$$

$$2 \text{ weeks} \times \frac{7 \text{ days}}{7 \text{ days}} = 2 \text{ weeks} \times 1 = 2 \text{ weeks}$$

$$2 \text{ weeks} \times \frac{7 \text{ days}}{1 \text{ week}} = 2 \text{ weeks} \times 1 = 2 \text{ weeks}$$

Consider the previous line again. This time you cancel the *week(s)*!

$$2 \text{ weeks} = 2 \text{ weeks} \times \frac{7 \text{ days}}{1 \text{ week}} = (2 \times 7) \text{ days} = 14 \text{ days}$$

So, 2 *weeks* = 14 *days*.

This shows how to convert a quantity measured in weeks (2 *weeks*) to an equivalent quantity measured in days (14 *days*). With the Dimensional Analysis method, you will be multiplying quantities by unit fractions in order to convert the units of measure. This procedure demonstrates the basic technique of Dimensional Analysis.

Many of the problems in dosage calculation require changing a quantity with a *single unit of measurement* into an equivalent quantity with a *different single unit of measurement*—for example, changing 2 *weeks* to 14 *days* as was done above.

Changing a Single Unit of Measurement to Another Single Unit of Measurement

Simple (One-Step) Problems with Single Units of Measurement

Suppose you want to express 18 *months* in *years*. That is, you want to convert 18 *months* to an equivalent amount of time in *years*.

This is a **simple** problem. Simple problems have only three elements. The elements in this problem are

The given quantity:	18 *months*
The quantity you want to find:	? *years*
An equivalence between the units in question:	1 *year* = 12 *months*

To begin the Dimensional Analysis process in a logical way, write the quantity you are given (18 *months*) on the left of an equal sign and the unit you want to change it to (*years*) on the right side, as follows:

$$18 \ months = ? \ years$$

It may help to write 18 *months* as the fraction $\dfrac{18 \ months}{1}$

Thus, you now have

$$\frac{18 \ months}{1} = ? \ years$$

Determine the Appropriate Unit Fraction

To change *months* to *years*, you need an equivalence between *months* and *years*. That equivalence is

$$12 \ months = 1 \ year$$

From this equivalence, you can get two possible unit fractions:

$$\frac{12 \ months}{1 \ year} \quad \text{and} \quad \frac{1 \ year}{12 \ months}$$

But which of these fractions should you choose? If you multiply $\dfrac{18 \ months}{1}$ by the first of these fractions, you get

$$\frac{18 \ months}{1} \times \frac{12 \ months}{1 \ year}$$

Notice that both of the *months* units are in the numerators of the fractions.

Because no cancellation of the units is possible in this case, do not select this unit fraction.

If instead you multiply 18 *months* by the second of the unit fractions, you get the following:

$$\frac{18\ months}{1} \times \frac{1\ year}{12\ months} = ?\ years$$

Notice that now *one of the months is in the numerator (top), and the other months is in the denominator (bottom) of a fraction*. Because cancellation of the *months* is now possible, this is the appropriate unit fraction to choose.

Cancel the Units of Measurement

$$\frac{18\ \cancel{months}}{1} \times \frac{1\ year}{12\ \cancel{months}} = ?\ years$$

After you cancel the *months*, notice that *year* (the unit of measurement you want to find) is the only remaining unit on the left side.

$$\frac{18\ \cancel{months}}{1} \times \frac{1\ \cancel{year}}{12\ \cancel{months}} = ?\ years$$

Cancel the Numbers and Finish the Multiplication

After you are sure that you have *only the unit of measurement you want (years) remaining on the left side and that it is on the top of a fraction*, you can complete the cancellation and multiplication of the numbers as follows:

$$\frac{\overset{3}{\cancel{18}}\ \cancel{months}}{1} \times \frac{1\ year}{\underset{2}{\cancel{12}}\ \cancel{months}} = \frac{3\ years}{2} \quad or \quad 1\frac{1}{2}\ years$$

So, 18 *months* is equivalent to $1\frac{1}{2}$ *years*.

EXAMPLE 3.1

Change $2\frac{1}{4}$ *hours* to an equivalent amount of time in *minutes*.

The elements in this problem are

The given quantity:	$2\frac{1}{4}$ *hours*
The quantity you want to find:	? *minutes*
An equivalence between them:	1 *hour* = 60 *minutes*

$$2\frac{1}{4}\ hours = ?\ minutes$$

Avoid doing multiplication with mixed numbers; change them to improper fractions or decimal numbers. In this case, you can write

---

NOTE

The unit you want to find must always appear in the numerator (top) of the fraction.

NOTE

When a unit of measure follows a numeric fraction, write the unit of measure in the numerator (top) of the fraction. For example, write $\frac{1}{2}$ *hour* as $\frac{1\ hour}{2}$.

$2\frac{1}{4}$ *hours* as the improper fraction $\frac{9}{4}$ *hours*. It is better to write the quantity $\frac{9}{4}$ *hours* as $\dfrac{9\ hours}{4}$ in order to make it clear that the unit of measurement (*hours*) is in the numerator of the fraction, not in the denominator.

So, the problem becomes $\dfrac{9\ hours}{4} = ?\ minutes.$

Determine the Appropriate Unit Fraction   You want to change *hours* to *minutes*, so you need an equivalence between *hours* and *minutes*. That equivalence is

$$1\ hour = 60\ minutes$$

From this equivalence, you get two possible fractions, which are both equal to 1:

$$\dfrac{1\ hour}{60\ minutes} \quad \text{and} \quad \dfrac{60\ minutes}{1\ hour}$$

But which of these fractions will lead to cancellation? Because you want to eliminate (cancel) the *hours*, and because *hours* are on the top, as follows:

$$\dfrac{9\ hours}{4} = ?\ minutes$$

you need to multiply by the unit fraction with *hour* on the bottom, as follows:

$$\dfrac{9\ hours}{4} \times \dfrac{60\ minutes}{1\ hour} = ?\ minutes$$

This is what you want because cancellation of the *hour(s)* is now possible.

Cancel the Units $\dfrac{9\ \cancel{hours}}{4} \times \dfrac{60\ minutes}{1\ \cancel{hour}} = ?\ minutes$

After you cancel the *hour(s)*, make sure that *minutes* (the unit you want) is the only remaining unit of measurement on the left side and that it is in a numerator (top) of a fraction.

$$\dfrac{9\ \cancel{hours}}{4} \times \dfrac{60\ \boxed{minutes}}{1\ \cancel{hour}} = ?\ minutes$$

Cancel the Numbers and Finish the Multiplication

$$\dfrac{9\ \cancel{hours}}{\underset{1}{\cancel{4}}} \times \dfrac{\overset{15}{\cancel{60}}\ minutes}{1\ \cancel{hour}} = 135\ minutes$$

So, $2\frac{1}{4}$ *hours* = 135 *minutes*.

> **NOTE**
>
> To eliminate a particular unit of measurement in the numerator, use a unit fraction with that same unit of measurement in the denominator.

EXAMPLE 3.2

Change 4.5 *feet* to an equivalent length measured in *inches*.

Given quantity: 4.5 *feet*

Quantity you want to find: ? *inches*

Equivalence between the two quantities: 1 *foot* = 12 *inches*

$$4.5 \text{ } feet = \text{ ? } inches$$

You want to cancel the *feet* and get the answer in *inches*, so choose a fraction with *feet* (or *foot*) on the bottom and *inches* on top. You need a fraction in the form of $\dfrac{\text{? } inches}{\text{? } feet}$.

Because 1 *foot* = 12 *inches*, the fraction you need is $\dfrac{12 \text{ } inches}{1 \text{ } foot}$

$$\frac{4.5 \text{ } feet}{1} \times \frac{12 \text{ } inches}{1 \text{ } foot} = 54 \text{ } inches$$

So, 4.5 *feet* is equivalent to 54 *inches*.

EXAMPLE 3.3

An infant weighs 6 *pounds* 5 *ounces*. What is the weight of the infant in ounces?

$$6 \text{ } pounds \text{ } 5 \text{ } ounces \quad \text{means} \quad 6 \text{ } pounds + 5 \text{ } ounces$$

First, convert 6 *pounds* to *ounces*.

The given quantity: 6 *pounds*

The quantity you want to find: ? *ounces*

An equivalence between them: 1 *pound* = 16 *ounces*

$$6 \text{ } pounds = \text{ ? } ounces$$

$$\frac{6 \text{ } pounds}{1} = \text{ ? } ounces$$

You want to cancel *pounds* and get the answer in *ounces*. So, choose a fraction with *pounds* on the bottom and *ounces* on top—that is, a fraction that looks like $\dfrac{\text{? } ounces}{\text{? } pounds}$

Because 1 *pound* = 16 *ounces*, the fraction is $\dfrac{16\ ounces}{1\ pound}$

$$\frac{6\ pounds}{1} \times \frac{16\ ounces}{1\ pound} = 96\ ounces$$

So, 6 *pounds* = 96 *ounces*, and the infant weighs 96 *ounces* + 5 *ounces*, or 101 *ounces*.

Dimensional Analysis can be applied to a wide variety of problems, as demonstrated by the next example.

EXAMPLE 3.4

Suppose that the currency exchange rate in Mexico is 0.076 U.S. *dollar* for 1 *Mexican peso*. At this rate how many *Mexican pesos* would be exchanged for 190 U.S. *dollars*?

Given quantity: 190 *dollars*

Quantity you want to find: ? *pesos*

Equivalence between them: 0.076 *dollar* = 1 *peso*

$$190\ dollars = ?\ pesos$$

You want to cancel the *dollars* and get the answer in *pesos*, so choose a fraction with *dollars* on the bottom and *pesos* on top. You need a unit fraction in the form of $\dfrac{?\ pesos}{?\ dollars}$

Because 0.076 *dollar* = 1 *peso*, the fraction you need is $\dfrac{1\ peso}{0.076\ dollar}$

$$\frac{190\ dollars}{1} \times \frac{1\ peso}{0.076\ dollar} = \frac{190}{0.076}\ pesos \quad or \quad 2{,}500\ pesos$$

So, 190 U.S. *dollars* are equivalent to 2,500 Mexican *pesos*.

Complex (Multi-Step) Problems with Single Units of Measurement

Sometimes you will encounter problems that will require the procedures used previously to be repeated one or more times. We call such problems **complex or multi-step**. In a complex problem, multiplication by more than one unit fraction is required. The method is very similar to that used with simple problems.

Here is an example: Suppose you want to change 4 *hours* to an equivalent time in *seconds*.

The given quantity: 4 *hours*

The quantity you want to find: ? *seconds*

An equivalence between them: ?

Most people do not know the direct equivalence between hours and seconds. But you do know the following two equivalences related to the units of measurement in this problem: 1 *hour* = 60 *minutes* and 1 *minute* = 60 *seconds*.

So the problem is

$$4 \; hours = ? \; seconds$$

First, you want to cancel *hours*. To do this, you must use an equivalence containing *hours* and a unit fraction with *hours* on the bottom. Because 1 *hour* = 60 *minutes*, this fraction will be $\dfrac{60 \; minutes}{1 \; hour}$

$$\frac{4 \; \cancel{hours}}{1} \times \frac{60 \; minutes}{1 \; \cancel{hour}} = ? \; seconds$$

After the *hours* are cancelled, as shown previously, only *minutes* remain on the left side. So, what you have done at this point is changed 4 *hours* to (4 × 60 = 240) *minutes*, but you want to obtain the answer in *seconds*. Therefore, the *minutes* must now be cancelled. Because *minutes* is in the numerator, a unit fraction with *minutes* in the denominator is required.

Because 1 *minute* = 60 *seconds*, the fraction is $\dfrac{60 \; seconds}{1 \; minute}$

Now, multiplying by this unit fraction, you get

$$\frac{4 \; \cancel{hours}}{1} \times \frac{60 \; minutes}{1 \; \cancel{hour}} \times \frac{60 \; seconds}{1 \; minute} = ? \; seconds$$

Cancel the *minutes* and notice that the only unit of measurement remaining on the left side is *seconds*, the unit you want to find!

$$\frac{4 \; \cancel{hours}}{1} \times \frac{60 \; \cancel{minutes}}{1 \; \cancel{hour}} \times \frac{60 \; \boxed{seconds}}{1 \; \cancel{minute}} = ? \; seconds$$

Now that you have the unit of measurement you want (*seconds*) on the left side, cancel the numbers (not possible in this example) and finish the multiplication:

$$\frac{4 \; \cancel{hours}}{1} \times \frac{60 \; \cancel{minutes}}{1 \; \cancel{hour}} \times \frac{60 \; seconds}{1 \; \cancel{minute}} = 14,400 \; seconds$$

So, 4 *hours* is equivalent to 14,400 *seconds*.

EXAMPLE 3.5

Convert 50,400 *minutes* to an equivalent time in *days*

The given quantity:	50,400 *minutes*
The quantity you want to find:	? *days*
Equivalences between them:	?

You might not know the direct equivalence between minutes and days. But you do know the following two equivalences related to the units in this problem: 60 *minutes* = 1 *hour* and 24 *hours* = 1 *day*.

$$50,400\ minutes = ?\ days$$

You want to cancel *minutes*. To do this, you must use an equivalence containing *minutes* and make a unit fraction with *minutes* on the bottom.

Because 60 *minutes* = 1 *hour*, this fraction will be $\dfrac{1\ hour}{60\ minutes}$.

$$50,400\ \cancel{minutes} \times \frac{1\ hour}{60\ \cancel{minutes}} = ?\ days$$

After the *minutes* are cancelled as shown above, only *hour* remains on the left side, but you want to obtain the answer in *days*. Therefore, the *hour* must now be cancelled. This will require a unit fraction with *hours* in the denominator. Because 1 *day* = 24 *hours*, this fraction is $\dfrac{1\ day}{24\ hours}$.

After cancelling the *hours*, you now have

$$50,400\ \cancel{minutes} \times \frac{1\ \cancel{hour}}{60\ \cancel{minutes}} \times \frac{1\ day}{24\ \cancel{hours}} = ?\ days$$

Because only *day* (in the numerator) is on the left side, the numbers can be cancelled.

$$\overset{840}{\cancel{50,400}}\ \cancel{minutes} \times \frac{1\ \cancel{hour}}{\underset{1}{\cancel{60}}\ \cancel{minutes}} \times \frac{1\ day}{24\ \cancel{hours}} = \frac{840}{24}\ days = 35\ days$$

So, 50,400 *minutes* = 35 *days*.

EXAMPLE 3.6

Kim is having a party for 24 *people* and is serving *hot dogs*. Each person will eat 2 *hot dogs*. How much will the *hot dogs* for the party cost if a *package* of 8 *hot dogs* costs $2.50?

The given single unit of measurement: 24 *people* (1/1)

The single unit of measurement
you want to find: ? *cost* ($)

You might not know the direct equivalence between people and cost. But you do know the following equivalences supplied in this problem:

2 *hot dogs per person*   2 *hot dogs* = 1 *person*
1 *package* of *hot dogs* is $2.50   1 *package* = $2.50
1 *package* has 8 *hot dogs*   1 *package* = 8 *hot dogs*

But where do you start?

In this problem, there are two single units of measurement—one that is given (*persons*) and one you have to find (*cost*). Cost involves a single unit of measurement, namely *dollars* ($). *Because you are looking for a quantity measured in a single unit of measurement* ($), *you should start with the given single unit of measurement* (*persons*).

$$24 \text{ persons} = ? \$$$

You want to cancel *persons*. To do this, you must use an equivalence containing *person(s)* to make a fraction with *person(s)* on the bottom. From the preceding equivalence, 2 *hot dogs* = 1 *person*, this fraction will be $\dfrac{2 \text{ hot dogs}}{\text{person}}$.

$$24 \text{ \cancel{persons}} \times \frac{2 \text{ hot dogs}}{\text{person}} = ? \$$$

After the *person(s)* are cancelled, only *hot dogs* remains on the left side, and it indicates that 48 *hot dogs* are needed. But you want to obtain the answer in $. Therefore, the *hot dogs* must now be cancelled. This will require a fraction with *hot dogs* in the denominator. From the equivalence 1 *package* = 8 *hot dogs*, the unit fraction is $\dfrac{1 \text{ package}}{8 \text{ hot dogs}}$ Thus, you now have

$$24 \text{ \cancel{persons}} \times \frac{2 \text{ \cancel{hot dogs}}}{\text{person}} \times \frac{1 \text{ package}}{8 \text{ \cancel{hot dogs}}} = ? \$$$

After the *hot dogs* are cancelled, only *package* remains on the left side, and (if you do the mathematics now) it indicates the number of *packages* (6) that are needed. But you want to obtain the answer in $. Therefore, the *package* must now be cancelled. This will require a fraction with *package* in the denominator. From the equivalence 1 *package* = $ 2.50, the unit fraction is $\dfrac{\$ 2.50}{1 \text{ package}}$.

$$24 \text{ \cancel{persons}} \times \frac{2 \text{ \cancel{hot dogs}}}{\text{person}} \times \frac{1 \text{ \cancel{package}}}{8 \text{ \cancel{hot dogs}}} \times \frac{\$2.50}{1 \text{ \cancel{package}}} = ? \$$$

Because you now have only $ (in the numerator) on the left side, the numbers can be cancelled and the multiplication finished.

$$\overset{3}{24} \text{ \cancel{persons}} \times \frac{2 \text{ \cancel{hot dogs}}}{\text{person}} \times \frac{1 \text{ \cancel{package}}}{\underset{1}{8} \text{ \cancel{hot dogs}}} \times \frac{\$ 2.50}{1 \text{ \cancel{package}}} = \$ 15$$

So, the hot dogs for the party will cost $15.00.

NOTE

Don't stop multiplying by unit fractions until the unit of measurement you are looking for is the only remaining unit on the left side. Remember that the unit you are looking for must be in the numerator of a fraction.

Changing One Rate to Another Rate

A **rate** is a fraction with different units of measurement on top and bottom. For example, 50 *miles* per *hour* written as 50 *miles/hour* and 3 *pounds* per *week* written as 3 *pounds/week* are rates. In dosage calculation, the bottom unit of measurement is frequently time (for example, *hours* or *minutes*). We sometimes want to change one rate into another rate. For example, in Chapter 10 you will change flow rates from *drops/minute* to *milliliters/hour*. These problems are done in a manner similar to the method that was used to do the single-unit-to-single-unit problems.

Simple (One-Step) Problems with Rates

EXAMPLE 3.7

Convert *5 feet per hour* to an equivalent rate of speed in *inches per hour*.

The given rate: *5 feet per hour*

The rate you want to find: *? inches per hour*

Because you are looking for a **rate**, you start with the *given* **rate**:

$$5 \text{ feet per hour } = \text{ ? inches per hour}$$

Write these rates as fractions:

$$\frac{5 \text{ feet}}{hour} = \frac{? \text{ inches}}{hour}$$

Notice that you are given a rate with *hour* in the denominator, and the rate you are looking for also has *hour* in the denominator. Therefore, *the denominator does not have to be changed!*

But the given rate has *feet* in the numerator, and the rate you want has a different unit, *inches*, in the numerator. Therefore, *feet* must be changed.

To cancel *feet*, you must use an equivalence containing *feet*—namely, 12 *inches* = 1 *foot*. Because *feet* is in the numerator, you need a unit fraction with *feet* in the denominator. This unit fraction is $\frac{12 \text{ inches}}{1 \text{ foot}}$.

After the *feet* are cancelled, *inches* remains on top, and *hour* remains on the bottom, and those are the units you want. Finally, do the multiplication of the numbers.

$$\frac{5 \text{ feet}}{hour} \times \frac{12 \text{ inches}}{1 \text{ foot}} = \frac{60 \text{ inches}}{hour}$$

So, *5 feet per hour* is equivalent to 60 *inches per hour*.

EXAMPLE 3.8

Convert 90 *feet per hour* to an equivalent rate in *feet per minute*.

The given rate: 90 *ft/h*

The rate you want to find: ? *ft/min*

Because you are looking for a rate, you start with the given rate,

$$90 \text{ ft per } h = \text{ ? } ft/min$$

$$\frac{90 \text{ ft}}{h} = \frac{? \text{ ft}}{min}$$

Notice that you are given a rate with *ft* in the numerator, and the answer you are looking for also has *ft* in the numerator. Therefore, the numerator does not have to be changed!

But the given rate has *h* in the denominator, and the rate you want has a different unit, *min*, in the denominator. Therefore, *h* must be eliminated. Because *h* is in the denominator, you need a fraction with *h* in the numerator.

Use the equivalence 1 *h* = 60 *min*. This unit fraction is $\frac{1 \text{ } h}{60 \text{ } min}$.

$$\frac{90 \cancel{(ft)}}{\cancel{h}} \times \frac{1 \cancel{h}}{60 \cancel{(min)}} = \frac{? \text{ ft}}{min}$$

After the *h* is cancelled, *ft* remains on top and *min* is on the bottom, and those are the units you want. Cancel the numbers and finish the multiplication.

$$\frac{\overset{3}{\cancel{90}} \text{ ft}}{\cancel{h}} \times \frac{1 \cancel{h}}{\underset{2}{\cancel{60}} \text{ min}} = \frac{3 \text{ ft}}{2 \text{ min}} = \frac{1.5 \text{ ft}}{min}$$

So, 90 *feet/hour* is equivalent to a rate of 1.5 *feet/minute*.

EXAMPLE 3.9

Convert 3 *ounces per day* to an equivalent rate in *ounces per week*.

$$\frac{3 \text{ oz}}{1 \text{ d}} = \text{ ? } \frac{oz}{wk}$$

Notice that the given rate and the rate you want both have the same numerator, *ounces*. Therefore, the numerator does not have to be changed.

However, the given rate has *day* in the denominator, and the rate you want has a different unit, *week*, in the denominator. Therefore, the denominator, *day*, needs to be cancelled by using a unit fraction with day in the numerator.

Because $7\,days = 1\,week$, the unit fraction needed is $\dfrac{7\,days}{1\,week}$.

$$\frac{3\,oz}{1\,d} \times \frac{7\,d}{1\,wk} = ?\,\frac{oz}{wk}$$

Cancel the days and multiply.

$$\frac{3\,oz}{1\,\cancel{d}} \times \frac{7\,\cancel{d}}{1\,wk} = ?\,\frac{oz}{wk}$$

$$= \frac{21\,oz}{1\,wk}$$

So, 3 *ounces per day* is equivalent to 21 *ounces per week*.

Complex (Multi-Step) Problems with Rates

EXAMPLE 3.10

Convert $10\frac{1}{2}$ *feet/hour* to an equivalent rate in *inches/minute*.

The given rate: $\qquad\qquad 10\frac{1}{2}$ *feet/hour*

The rate you want to find: $\quad$? *inches/minute*

Because you are looking for a rate, you should start with a rate.

$$10\tfrac{1}{2}\ feet/hour = ?\ inches/minute$$

Write $10\frac{1}{2}$ as the improper fraction $\frac{21}{2}$

$$\frac{21\,ft}{2\,h} = \frac{?\,in}{min}$$

You want to cancel *ft*. To do this, you must use an equivalence containing *ft* on the bottom. Because you want to convert to *inches*, use the equivalence 12 *inches* = 1 *foot*, and the unit fraction will be $\dfrac{12\,in}{1\,ft}$.

$$\frac{21\,\cancel{ft}}{2\,h} \times \frac{12\,in}{1\,\cancel{ft}} = \frac{?\,in}{min}$$

After the *ft* are cancelled, *in* is on top, which is what you want. But *h* is on the bottom and it must be cancelled. This will require a fraction with *h* in the numerator. From the equivalence 1 *hour* = 60 *minutes*, the unit fraction is $\dfrac{1\,h}{60\,min}$.

After cancelling the *hours*, you now have

$$\frac{21\,\cancel{ft}}{2\,\cancel{h}} \times \frac{12\,\textcircled{in}}{1\,\cancel{ft}} \times \frac{1\,\cancel{h}}{60\,\textcircled{min}} = \frac{?\,in}{min}$$

You now have *in* on top and *min* on the bottom, so do the cancelling and multiplications of the numbers.

$$\frac{21\ \cancel{ft}}{2\ \cancel{h}} \times \frac{\overset{1}{\cancel{12}}\ in}{1\ \cancel{ft}} \times \frac{1\ \cancel{h}}{\underset{5}{\cancel{60}}\ min} = \frac{21\ in}{10\ min} \quad or \quad \frac{2.1\ in}{min}$$

So, $10\frac{1}{2}$ *feet/hour* = 2.1 *inches/minute*.

EXAMPLE 3.11

Write 3.2 *inches/second* in *feet/minute*.

The given rate: 3.2 *in/sec*
The rate you want to find: *? ft/min*

Because you are looking for a **rate**, you should start with a **rate**.

$$\frac{3.2\ in}{sec} = \frac{?\ ft}{min}$$

You want to cancel *in*. To do this, you must use an equivalence containing *in* on the bottom. This fraction will be $\dfrac{1\ ft}{12\ in}$

$$\frac{3.2\ \cancel{in}}{sec} \times \frac{1\ ft}{12\ \cancel{in}} = \frac{?\ ft}{min}$$

Now, *ft* is on top, which is what you want. But *sec* is on the bottom and it must be cancelled. This will require a fraction with *sec* in the numerator: $\dfrac{60\ sec}{1\ min}$.

Now cancel and multiply the numbers.

$$\frac{3.2\ \cancel{in}}{\cancel{sec}} \times \frac{1\ \cancel{ft}}{\underset{1}{\cancel{12}}\ \cancel{in}} \times \frac{\overset{5}{\cancel{60}}\ \cancel{sec}}{1\ \cancel{min}} = \frac{16\ ft}{min}$$

So, 3.2 *inches/second* = 16 *feet/minute*.

EXAMPLE 3.12

Water is flowing from a hose at the rate of 1.2 *pints per second*. Convert this to an equivalent flow rate measured in *quarts per minute*.

Given rate: 1.2 *pt/sec*
Rate you want to find: *? qt/min*

You want to change one rate to another rate.

$$\frac{1.2\ pt}{sec} = \frac{?\ qt}{min}$$

Neither the units on the tops (*pt* and *qt*), nor those on the bottoms (*sec* and *min*) match, therefore both the *pt* and the *sec* must be changed (cancelled). You may start with either one. Suppose you start with *pt*. Because *pt* is on the top, you must use an equivalent unit fraction with *pt* on the bottom. This fraction will be $\dfrac{1\,qt}{2\,pt}$

$$\frac{1.2\,pt}{sec} \times \frac{1\,\textcircled{qt}}{2\,pt} = \frac{?\,\textcircled{qt}}{min}$$

Now, *qt* is on the top, which is what you want. But *sec* is on the bottom and it must be cancelled. This will require a unit fraction with *sec* in the numerator. This fraction will be $\dfrac{60\,sec}{1\,min}$

After you cancel all the units, you then cancel and multiply the numbers.

$$\frac{1.2\,pt}{sec} \times \frac{1\,qt}{2\,pt} \times \frac{\overset{30}{60}\,sec}{1\,min} = \frac{36\,qt}{min}$$

So, 1.2 *pints per second* is equivalent to 36 *quarts per minute*.

EXAMPLE 3.13

Convert 96 *ounces per year* to an equivalent rate in *pounds per month*.

$$\frac{96\,oz}{1\,yr} = ?\,\frac{lb}{mon}$$

Notice that the given rate and the rate you want have different units of measurement in both the numerators and denominators. Therefore, both have to be changed.

To cancel the *year* in the denominator, you need a unit fraction with *year* in the numerator. Because 12 *months* = 1 *year*, the unit fraction will be $\dfrac{1\,yr}{12\,mon}$.

$$\frac{96\,oz}{1\,yr} \times \frac{1\,yr}{12\,mon} = ?\,\frac{lb}{mon}$$

After cancelling the *years*, *month* is in the denominator, which is what you want. Now you must cancel the *ounce* in the numerator. Because 16 *ounces* = 1 *pound*, the unit fraction will be $\dfrac{1\,lb}{16\,oz}$.

$$\frac{96\,oz}{1\,yr} \times \frac{1\,yr}{12\,mon} \times \frac{1\,lb}{16\,oz} = ?\,\frac{lb}{mon}$$

After the ounces are cancelled, you have the correct units of measurement on both top and bottom, *lb* and *mon*, respectively. Now cancel and multiply the numbers.

$$\frac{\overset{8}{96}\,oz}{1\,yr} \times \frac{1\,yr}{\underset{1}{12}\,mon} \times \frac{1\,lb}{16\,oz} = \frac{1\,lb}{2\,mon}$$

So, 96 *ounces per year* is equivalent to $\frac{1}{2}$ *pound per month*.

Summary

In this chapter, the techniques of Dimensional Analysis were introduced.

Mathematical concepts were reinforced:
- A nonzero number divided by itself equals 1.
- A fraction equal to 1 is called a unit fraction.
- When a quantity is multiplied (or divided) by 1, the quantity is unchanged.
- Cancellation always involves a quantity in a numerator and another quantity in a denominator.

Simple (one-step) single-unit-to-single-unit problems:
- Start with the **given** single unit of measure on the left side of the = sign.
- Write the single unit of measure you want to **find** on the right side of the = sign.
- Identify an **equivalence** containing the units of measure in the problem.
- Use the equivalence to make a unit fraction with the **given** unit of measure in the **denominator.**
- Multiply the given unit of measurement by the unit fraction.
- Cancel the units of measure. The only unit of measurement remaining on the left side (in a numerator) will match the unit of measure on the right side.
- Cancel the numbers and finish the multiplication.

Simple (one-step) rate-to-rate problems:
- Start with the given rate on the left side of the equal sign.
- Write the rate you want to **find** on the right side of the equal sign.
- Identify a unit of measure that must be cancelled.
- Find an **equivalence** containing the unwanted unit of measure you want to cancel.
- Choose a unit fraction that leads to cancellation of the unwanted unit of measurement.
- Cancel the units of measurement. The only units of measurement remaining on the left side (in a numerator) will match the units of measure on the right side.
- Cancel the numbers and finish the multiplication.
- In medical dosage calculations involving rates of flow, time (in minutes or hours) will always be in the denominator.

Complex (multi-step) problems:
- Repeat the preceding steps until the only unit of measurement(s) remaining on the left side is the same as the unit of measurement(s) on the right side.

Practice Sets

The answers to *Try These for Practice* and *Exercises* are found in Appendix A. Ask your instructor for the answers to the *Additional Exercises*.

Workspace

Try These for Practice

Test your comprehension after reading the chapter.

1. How many seconds are in *6.5 minutes?* _____

2. What is the weight in ounces of an infant who weighs 4 *pounds 6 ounces?* _____

3. How many hours are equivalent to 5,400 *seconds?*

4. A child is gaining weight at the rate of 11 *ounces per week*. Express this rate of weight gain measured in ounces per day. Round off the answer to the nearest tenth of an ounce per day.

5. A ball is rolling at the speed of 2 *feet per minute*. Find this speed in *inches per minute*. _____

Workspace

Exercises

Reinforce your understanding in class or at home.

1. $0.2\ h =$ _____ *min*

2. $1\frac{1}{2}\ yr =$ _____ *mon*

3. $2\frac{3}{4}\ d =$ _____ *h*

4. $5.25\ lb =$ _____ *oz*

5. $\frac{1}{4}\ h =$ _____ *sec*

6. $\dfrac{1\ ft}{min} =$ _____ $\dfrac{in}{min}$

7. $\dfrac{1\ ft}{min} =$ _____ $\dfrac{ft}{h}$

8. How many hours are equivalent to 720 *minutes*?

9. A faucet is running water at the rate of one-half pint every minute. What is this flow rate expressed in pints per hour?

10. A neonate weighs 4 *pounds* and 6 *ounces*. Express the weight of this baby in ounces.

11. What fraction of an hour is 900 *seconds*?

12. Each team in a basketball league has 12 players. There are 8 teams in the league. Each player has 2 uniforms. It costs $5 to dry-clean 2 uniforms. How much will it cost to dry-clean all the uniforms of all the league's players?

13. How many seconds are in 1 *week*?

14. If a person is 70 *inches* tall, express this *height* in *feet* and *inches*.

15. $4\ pt/min = ?\ qt/min$

16. $2\ pt/min = ?\ pt/h$

17. $0.2\ pt/min = ?\ qt/h$

18. $2\ in/min = ?\ ft/h$

19. $2\ oz/d = ?\ lb/wk$

20. 0.02 *inches per second* is equivalent to how many feet per hour?

Additional Exercises

Now, test yourself!

1. 0.25 *hours* = _____ *minutes*

2. $5\frac{1}{4}$ *years* = _____ *months*

3. $2\frac{1}{3}$ *days* = _____ *hours*

4. $2.5\ lb =$ _____ *oz*

5. $\frac{3}{4} h =$ _____ *min*

6. 18 *mon* = _____ *yr*

7. 36 *in* = _____ *ft*

8. 40 *oz* = _____ *lb*

9. An infant weighs 6 *pounds 5 ounces* at birth. What is the weight in ounces? _____

10. There are 12 cans of soda in a case. Each can contains 16 ounces of soda. Every 24 ounces of soda contains 1 cup of sugar. How many cups of sugar are in 3 cases of soda? _____

11. What fraction of an hour is 1,350 *seconds*? _____

12. What is the height in inches of a person who is 6 *feet 2 inches* tall? _____

13. Write 604,800 *seconds* as an equivalent amount of time in weeks. _____

14. If a person measures 54 *inches in height*, what does the person measure in feet? _____

15. What fraction of an hour is 2,700 *seconds*? _____

16. Change $6 \dfrac{pints}{h}$ to an equivalent rate in $\dfrac{quarts}{day}$. _____

17. Change $6 \dfrac{quarts}{day}$ to an equivalent rate in $\dfrac{pints}{hour}$. _____

18. Change 1,680 *hours* to *weeks*. _____

19. Write 1,209,600 *seconds* as an equivalent amount of time in *weeks*. _____

20. There are 24 cans of soda in a case. Each can contains 12 ounces of soda. Every 60 ounces of soda contains 1 cup of sugar. How many cups of sugar are in 5 cases of soda? _____

Workspace

Unit

2

Systems of Measurement

Chapter

The Household and Metric Systems

Learning Outcomes

$0.4\ g = 400\ mg$

After completing this chapter, you will be able to

1. Identify the units of measurement in the household and metric systems.
2. Recognize the abbreviations for the units of measurement in the two systems.
3. State the equivalents for the units of volume.
4. State the equivalents for the units of weight.
5. State the equivalents for the units of length.
6. Convert from one unit to another within each of the two systems.

Historically, the United States has used three different systems to measure drugs: the apothecary, household, and metric systems.

The **apothecary** system is the oldest of the three systems, and it is difficult to use. Because its use led to many medication errors, the Joint Commission, FDA, and ISMP have suggested that it be discontinued. Package inserts and other drug references no longer use the apothecary system for recommended medication dosages. Therefore, the apothecary system is not included in this chapter.

The **household** system is designed so that dosages can be measured at home using ordinary containers found in the kitchen, such as cups and teaspoons. The household system is sometimes referred to as the English system.

The **metric** system is the most logically organized and easiest to use of all the systems of measurement. It was first adopted by France a few years after the French revolution of 1789. It is also referred to as the *International System of Units*. It can be abbreviated as *SI*, which are the first two initials of its French name, *Système International d'Unités*. The metric system will eventually replace all other systems of measurement used in healthcare.

In this chapter you will be introduced to the household and metric systems.

The Household System

Liquid Volume in the Household System

Occasionally, household measurements are used when prescribing liquid medication. Table 4.1 lists equivalent values, with their abbreviations, for units of liquid measurement in the household system.

Table 4.1 Household Equivalents of Liquid Volume

1 quart (qt) =	2 pints (pt)
1 pint (pt) =	2 measuring cups
1 measuring cup =	8 ounces (oz)
1 ounce (oz) =	2 tablespoons (T)
1 tablespoon (T) =	3 teaspoons (t)

You can use Dimensional Analysis to convert from one unit of measurement to an equivalent unit of measurement within the household system the same way you converted units of measurement in Chapter 3. You multiply the given measurement by a unit fraction that is equal to 1; the unit fraction has the *given units of measurement on the bottom* (the denominator) and the *desired units of measurement on top* (the numerator), as the following examples show.

EXAMPLE 4.1

How many cups of water are contained in a 16-*fluid-ounce* bottle of water?

$$\frac{16 \text{ oz}}{1} = ? \text{ cup}$$

You want to cancel the *ounces* and get the answer in *cups*. You need a unit fraction in the form of $\frac{? \text{ cup}}{? \text{ oz}}$.

Because 1 *cup* = 8 *ounces*, the unit fraction is $\frac{1 \text{ cup}}{8 \text{ oz}}$.

$$\frac{\overset{2}{\cancel{16} \text{ oz}}}{1} \times \frac{1 \text{ cup}}{\underset{1}{\cancel{8} \text{ oz}}} = 2 \text{ cups}$$

So, 2 *cups* of water are contained in a 16-*fluid-ounce* bottle of water.

EXAMPLE 4.2

A patient needs to drink $1\frac{1}{2}$ *ounces* of an elixir per day. How many *teaspoons* would be equivalent to this dosage?

$$1\frac{1}{2} \text{ ounces} = ? \text{ teaspoons}$$

ALERT

Using ordinary tableware to measure medications may constitute a safety risk because ordinary tableware does not come in standard sizes. Therefore, patients and their families should be advised to use the measuring device provided with the medication rather than a kitchen tablespoon, for example.

NOTE

The unit *ounce*, which is used to measure liquid volumes, is sometimes referred to as *fluid ounce*.

NOTE

In the household system for quantities less than 1, either decimal numbers or fractions may be used. However, fractions are preferred. For example, $\frac{1}{2}$ *qt* is preferred over 0.5 *qt*.

If you do not know a direct equivalence between *ounces* and *teaspoons*, then this will be a complex (multi-step) problem, which requires first changing *ounces* to *tablespoons* and then changing *tablespoons* to *teaspoons*.

$$1\tfrac{1}{2} \; ounces \rightarrow ? \; tablespoons \rightarrow ? \; teaspoons$$

Because calculating with mixed numbers is difficult, you should write $1\tfrac{1}{2}$ *ounces* as either 1.5 *ounces* or $\dfrac{3 \; ounces}{2}$

Now you want to cancel the *ounces* and get the answer in *tablespoons*, so choose a unit fraction with *ounces* on the bottom and *tablespoons* on top. That is, you need a unit fraction in the form of

$$\frac{? \; tablespoons}{? \; ounces}$$

Because $1 \; ounce = 2 \; tablespoons$, the fraction you need is $\dfrac{2 \; tablespoons}{1 \; ounce}$

Cancel the *ounces*.

$$\frac{3 \; \cancel{ounces}}{2} \times \frac{2 \; \boxed{tablespoons}}{1 \; \cancel{ounce}} = ? \; teaspoons$$

After cancelling the *ounces* as shown above, only *tablespoons* remain in the numerator on the left side. But you want the answer to be in *teaspoons*, so you must cancel the *tablespoons*. This requires a second unit fraction with *tablespoons* in the denominator. The fraction is $\dfrac{3 \; teaspoons}{1 \; tablespoon}$

$$\frac{3 \; \cancel{ounces}}{2} \times \frac{2 \; \cancel{tablespoons}}{1 \; \cancel{ounce}} \times \frac{3 \; \boxed{teaspoons}}{1 \; \cancel{tablespoon}} = ? \; teaspoons$$

After cancelling the *tablespoons* as shown above, only *teaspoons* remain in the numerator on the left side. *Teaspoons* is the unit you want on the left side, so now focus on the numbers. Cancel the twos and multiply:

$$\frac{3 \; \cancel{oz}}{\cancel{2}} \times \frac{\cancel{2} \; \cancel{T}}{1 \; \cancel{oz}} \times \frac{3 \; t}{1 \; \cancel{T}} = 9 \; t$$

So, $1\tfrac{1}{2}$ *ounces* is equivalent to 9 *teaspoons*.

Weight in the Household System

The only units of weight used in the household system of medication administration are *ounces* (*oz*) and *pounds* (*lb*), as shown in Table 4.2.

Table 4.2 **Household Equivalents of Weight**

1 *pound* (*lb*) = 16 *ounces* (*oz*)

EXAMPLE 4.3

An infant weighs 5 *lb* 8 *oz*. What is the weight of the infant in *ounces*?

First change the 5 *lb* to *ounces*.

$$5 \ lb = ? \ oz$$

Cancel the pounds and obtain the equivalent amount in *ounces*.

$$5 \ lb \times \frac{? \ oz}{? \ lb} = ? \ oz$$

Because 16 *oz* = 1 *lb*, the unit fraction is $\dfrac{16 \ oz}{1 \ lb}$

$$5 \ lb \times \frac{16 \ oz}{1 \ lb} = 80 \ oz$$

Now add the extra 8 *oz*.

$$80 \ oz + 8 \ oz = 88 \ oz$$

So, the 5 *lb* 8 *oz* infant weighs 88 *oz*.

Length in the Household System

The only units of length used in the household system for medication administration are *feet* (*ft*) and *inches* (*in*), as shown in Table 4.3.

Table 4.3   Household Equivalents for Length

1 *foot* (*ft*) = 12 *inches* (*in*)

EXAMPLE 4.4

A child is 3 *ft* 2 *in* tall. Find the child's height in *inches*.

First, change the 3 *feet* to *inches*.

$$3 \ feet = ? \ inches$$

You want to cancel the *feet* and get the answer in *inches*, so choose a fraction with *feet* on the bottom and *inches* on top. You need a unit fraction in the form of $\dfrac{? \ inches}{? \ feet}$

Because 1 *foot* = 12 *inches*, the fraction you need is $\dfrac{12 \ inches}{1 \ foot}$

$$\frac{3 \ feet}{1} \times \frac{12 \ inches}{1 \ foot} = 36 \ inches$$

So, 3 *feet* is equivalent to 36 *inches*. Now add the extra 2 *inches*.

$$36 \ in + 2 \ in = 38 \ inches$$

The 3 *feet* 2 *inch* child is 38 *inches* tall.

Decimal-Based Systems

As seen in Chapter 1, our *place-value number system* is a *decimal* system—that is, it is based on the number 10. The *United States monetary system* and the *metric system* are also decimal systems.

The *U.S. monetary system* uses the dollar as its fundamental unit. All other denominations are decimal multiples or fractions of the dollar.

hundred-dollar bill	ten-dollar bill	dollar bill	dime	penny

An amount of money measured in one denomination can be easily converted to another denomination by merely moving the decimal point the appropriate number of places.

For example, to convert *60 dimes* to *pennies*, see in the chart that *dime* to *penny* is one jump to the *right*.

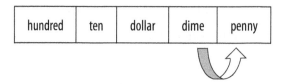

So, move the decimal point in 60 *dimes* one place to the *right* as follows:

60 *dimes* = 60.0 *dimes* = 6 0 0. *pennies*, or 600 *pennies*

To convert *80 dollars* to *ten dollar bills*, see in the chart that *dollar* to *ten* is one jump to the *left*.

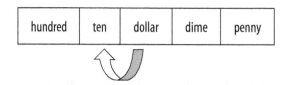

So, move the decimal point in 80 *dollars* one place to the *left*, as follows:

80 *dollars* = 80. *dollars* = 8 . 0 *tens* = 8 *tens*

To convert *4 hundred-dollar bills* to *dimes*, see in the chart that *hundred* to *dime* is a jump of *3 places to the right*.

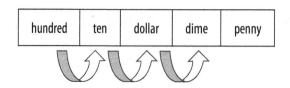

So, move the decimal point in 4 *hundreds* 3 *places to the right*.

4 *hundreds* = 4.000 *hundreds* = 4 0 0 0. *dimes*, or 4,000 *dimes*.

The Metric System

The metric system is the most widely used general system of measurement in the world today, with the United States being the only exception among developed countries. However, in all countries the metric system is the preferred system for prescribing medications.

Because the *metric system* is based on 10, converting quantities in this system can also be accomplished by merely shifting the decimal point. The simplicity of its decimal basis has encouraged the proliferation of the metric system.

At the heart of the metric system are the *fundamental* or *base units*. The **base units** needed for medical dosages are *gram (g)*, *liter (L)*, and *meter (m)*; these base units are used to measure weight, liquid volume, and length, respectively.

Decimal multiples of any of the base units are obtained by appending standard *metric prefixes* to the base unit. Table 4.4 shows both the base units and their **metric prefixes** with their abbreviations. Note that only the prefixes in blue are used in dosage calculation.

Table 4.4 Format of the Metric System

Name	kilo	hecto	deka	BASE UNIT	deci	centi	milli	*	*	micro
Abbreviation	k	h	da	g, L, m	d	c	m	*	*	mc
Multiple of the Base	1,000	100	10	1	0.1	0.01	0.001	*	*	0.000001

In the metric system, the prefixes indicate multiples of 10 times the base unit or the base unit divided by multiples of 10. The meanings of the necessary prefixes are found in Table 4.5.

Table 4.5 Metric Prefixes Used in Dosage Calculation

Metric Prefixes			
kilo	means	one thousand	(1,000 times the base)
centi	means	one hundredth	(0.01 times the base)
milli	means	one thousandth	(0.001 times the base)
micro	means	one millionth	(0.000001 times the base)

NOTE

To help remember the important metric prefixes, various mnemonics may be employed. Two are: <u>K</u>ing <u>H</u>enry <u>D</u>oesn't <u>U</u>sually <u>D</u>rink <u>C</u>old <u>M</u>alted <u>M</u>ilk, or <u>K</u>ids <u>H</u>ate <u>D</u>rudgery <u>U</u>ntil <u>D</u>awn <u>C</u>alculating <u>M</u>any <u>M</u>etrics (<u>k</u>ilo, <u>h</u>ecto, <u>d</u>eka, <u>u</u>nit, <u>d</u>eci, <u>c</u>enti, <u>m</u>illi, <u>m</u>icro).

NOTE

Depending on the country, spellings are *meter/metre*, *liter/litre*, and *deca/deka*.

The metric prefixes are appended to the base units. For example,

$$1 \underline{kilo}gram = 1,000 \; grams$$

and

$$1 \underline{milli}liter = \frac{1}{1,000} \; of \; a \; liter \; or \; 0.001 \; L$$

Fractions, such as $\frac{1}{2}$, are not formally used in the metric system. For example, $3\frac{1}{2}$ *grams* is written as 3.5 *grams*.

Liquid Volume in the Metric System

Drugs in liquid form are measured by volume. The volume of a liquid is the amount of space it occupies. In dosage calculations for liquid volumes only, *liters* and *milliliters* are used (see Table 4.6).

Table 4.6 **Metric Equivalents of Liquid Volume**
1 *cubic centimeter (cc or cm³)* = 1 *milliliter (mL)*
1,000 *milliliters (mL)* = 1 *liter (L)*

Milliliters are used for smaller amounts of fluids. The prefix *milli* means $\frac{1}{1,000}$, so

$$1 \text{ } liter \text{ } (L) = 1,000 \text{ } milliliters \text{ } (mL)$$

Milliliters are equivalent to *cubic centimeters* (cm^3 or *cc*), so

$$1 \text{ } mL = 1 \text{ } cm^3 = 1 \text{ } cc$$

You must be able to convert from one unit of measurement to another within the metric system. With liquids in the metric system, you need to make conversions only between *liters* and *milliliters*. Of course, you could make such conversions by using *Dimensional Analysis*. However, conversions involving metric-system units can be done by merely *moving the decimal point*. In Example 4.5, these methods will be compared.

EXAMPLE 4.5

If the prescriber ordered 0.5 *L* of 5% dextrose in water, how many *milliliters* were ordered?

Method 1: *By Dimensional Analysis*

$$0.5 \text{ } liters = ? \text{ } milliliters$$

You want to cancel the *liters* and get the answer in *milliliters*, so choose a unit fraction with *liters* on the bottom and *milliliters* on top. You need a fraction in the form of $\frac{?\text{ }mL}{?\text{ }L}$

Because 1 *L* = 1,000 *milliliters*, the fraction you need is $\frac{1,000\text{ }mL}{1\text{ }L}$

$$\frac{0.5 \text{ } \cancel{L}}{1} \times \frac{1,000 \text{ } \widehat{mL}}{1 \text{ } \cancel{L}} = 500 \text{ } mL$$

Method 2: *By moving the decimal point*

The metric system for *liters* has the following format, but only the units in blue are used in dosage calculations of liquid volume:

kilo	hecto	deka	Base Unit	deci	centi	milli	*	*	micro
kL	hL	daL	liter (L)	dL	cL	mL			mcL

Because for liquid volume the only units needed for medical dosage calculations are *liter* (L) and *milliliter* (mL), the jump will always be three places.

Base Unit	deci	centi	milli
L	dL	cL	mL

For this example, to convert *liters* to *milliliters* is a jump of *3 places to the right*, so, in the quantity 0.5 L, move the decimal point *3 places to the right*, as follows:

$$0.5 \ L = 0.500 \ L = 0 \ 5 \ 0 \ 0. \ mL = 500. \ mL = 500 \ mL$$

So, the prescriber ordered 500 *milliliters* of 5% dextrose in water.

EXAMPLE 4.6

The patient is to receive *1,750 milliliters of 0.9% NaCl IV q12h.* What is this volume in *liters*?

Method 1:   Dimensional Analysis

$$1,750 \ mL = ? \ L$$

Cancel the *milliliters* and obtain the equivalent amount in *liters*.

$$\frac{1,750 \ mL}{1} \times \frac{? \ L}{? \ mL} = ? \ L$$

Because 1,000 *mL* = 1 *L*, the unit fraction you want is $\dfrac{1 \ L}{1,000 \ mL}$

$$\frac{1,750 \ \cancel{mL}}{1} \times \frac{1 \ \cancel{L}}{1,000 \ \cancel{mL}} = \frac{1,750 \ L}{1,000} = 1.75 \ L$$

Method 2:   *Moving the decimal point*

For this example, to convert *1,750 milliliters* to *liters* is a jump of *3 places to the left*.

liter	deci	centi	milli
L			mL

So, in 1,750 *mL* move the decimal point *3 places to the left* as follows:

$$1{,}750 \, mL = 1{,}750. \, mL = 1 \underset{\curvearrowleft\curvearrowleft\curvearrowleft}{.7\,5\,0} \, L = 1.750 \, L = 1.75 \, L$$

So, 1,750 *mL* of 0.9% NaCl is the same amount as 1.75 *L* of 0.9% NaCl.

Weight in the Metric System

Drugs in dry form are generally measured by weight. In dosage calculations, *kilograms, grams, milligrams,* and *micrograms* (written in order of size) are used to measure weight. *Kilograms* are the largest of these units of measurement, and *micrograms* are the smallest (see Table 4.7).

Table 4.7 **Metric Equivalents of Weight**		
1 kilogram (kg)	=	1,000 grams (g)
1 gram (g)	=	1,000 milligrams (mg)
1 milligram (mg)	=	1,000 micrograms (mcg)

Kilograms are used for the weight of patients. The prefix *kilo* means 1,000, so

$$1 \, \textbf{\textit{kilogram}} \, (\textbf{\textit{kg}}) = 1{,}000 \, \textit{grams} \, (\textit{g})$$

Milligrams are used for measuring the weight of drugs, and *micrograms* are used for very small weights of drugs.

The prefix *milli* means $\frac{1}{1{,}000}$, and *micro* means $\frac{1}{1{,}000{,}000}$, so

$$1 \, \textit{gram} \, (\textit{g}) = 1{,}000 \, \textbf{\textit{milligrams}} \, (\textbf{\textit{mg}})$$
$$1 \, \textit{milligram} \, (\textit{mg}) = 1{,}000 \, \textbf{\textit{micrograms}} \, (\textbf{\textit{mcg}})$$

The metric system for weight (*grams*) features the following format. Only the units in blue are needed for dosage calculations involving weight:

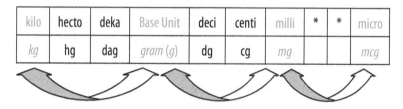

kilo	hecto	deka	Base Unit	deci	centi	milli	*	*	micro
kg	hg	dag	gram (g)	dg	cg	mg			mcg

For weight, the only units needed for medical dosage calculations are *kilogram (kg), gram (g), milligram (mg),* and *microgram (mcg)*. Because these units are all 3 places apart, the jumps between them will always be 3 places.

The following shortened version of the metric weight chart will be useful in the next few examples:

kilogram	gram	milligram	microgram
kg	g	mg	mcg

3 jumps   3 jumps   3 jumps

EXAMPLE 4.7

The order reads *125 mcg of Lanoxin (digoxin) PO* daily. How many *milligrams* of this cardiac medication would you administer to the patient?

$$125\ mcg = ?\ mg$$

> **NOTE**
>
> A dose is always expressed in the form of a number and a unit of measure. Both are important. For example:
>
> 150 *mcg*, 2.5 *mg*, 3 *tablets*, 1.5 *mL*, 0.5 *L*.
>
> When you write your answer, be sure to include the appropriate unit of measurement.

DIMENSIONAL ANALYSIS

Cancel the *micrograms* and obtain the equivalent amount in *milligrams*.

$$\frac{125\ mcg}{1} \times \frac{?\ mg}{?\ mcg} = ?\ mg$$

Because 1,000 *mcg* = 1 *mg*, you have

$$\frac{125\ \cancel{mcg}}{1} \times \frac{1\ \boxed{mg}}{1,000\ \cancel{mcg}} = 0.125\ mg$$

MOVING THE DECIMAL POINT

In this problem, you convert from *mcg* to *mg*. The movement from *mcg* to *mg* in the following chart is a movement of one column to the left.

Therefore, the conversion is accomplished by moving the decimal point three places to the left.

Kilo-	Fundamental Unit	Milli-	Micro-
kilogram (kg)	gram (g)	milligram (mg)	microgram (mcg)

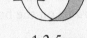

$$125\ mcg = 125.\ mcg = .125\ mg$$

$$= .125\ mg = 0.125\ mg$$

So, 125 *mcg* is the same amount as 0.125 *mg*, and you would administer 0.125 *mg* of digoxin.

EXAMPLE 4.8

The order reads *Glucotrol (glipizide) 15 mg PO daily ac breakfast.* How many *grams* of this hypoglycemic agent would you administer?

$$15\ mg = ?\ g$$

DIMENSIONAL ANALYSIS

Cancel the *milligrams* and obtain the equivalent amount in *grams*.

$$15\ mg \times \frac{?\ g}{?\ mg} = ?\ g$$

$$15\ \cancel{mg} \times \frac{1\ \text{(g)}}{1{,}000\ \cancel{mg}} = \frac{15}{1{,}000}\ g = 0.015\ g$$

MOVING THE DECIMAL POINT

In this problem, you convert from *mg* to *g*. The movement from *mg* to *g* in the following chart is a movement of one column to the left. Therefore, the conversion is accomplished by moving the decimal point three places to the left.

Kilo-	**Fundamental Unit**	**Milli-**	**Micro-**
kilogram (*kg*)	**gram** (*g*)	**milli**gram (*mg*)	**micro**gram (*mcg*)

$$15\ mg = 15.\ mg = .015\ g$$
$$= .015\ g = 0.015\ g$$

So, 15 *mg* is the same amount as 0.015 *g*, and you would administer 0.015 *g* of Glucotrol.

EXAMPLE 4.9

Convert 4.5 *kilograms* to an equivalent amount in *grams*.

BY DIMENSIONAL ANALYSIS

$$4.5\ kilograms = ?\ grams$$

You want to cancel the *kilograms* and get the answer in *grams*, so choose a fraction with *kilograms* on the bottom and *grams* on top.

You need a fraction in the form of $\frac{?\ g}{?\ kg}$

Because 1 *kg* = 1,000 *grams*, the fraction you need is $\frac{1{,}000\ g}{1\ kg}$

$$\frac{4.5\ \cancel{kg}}{1} \times \frac{1{,}000\ \text{(g)}}{1\ \cancel{kg}} = 4{,}500\ g$$

BY MOVING THE DECIMAL POINT

To convert *kg* to *g*, jump *3 places to the right.*

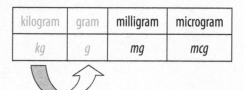

kilogram	gram	milligram	microgram
kg	*g*	*mg*	*mcg*

Move the decimal point *3 places to the right.*

$$4.5\ kg = 4.500\ kg = 4500.\ g = 4{,}500\ g$$

So, 4.5 *kilograms* is equivalent to 4,500 *grams*.

Length in the Metric System

The metric system for meters has the following format, but only the units in blue are used in measuring lengths.

Centimeters (cm) and *millimeters (mm)* are the only metric units of length used in this textbook. A patient's height might be measured in *centimeters*, and the diameter of a tumor might be measured in *centimeters* or *millimeters*.

kilo	hecto	deka	Base Unit	deci	centi	milli
km	hm	dam	meter (*m*)	dm	cm	mm

1 jump

Because *centimeters* and *millimeters* are adjacent units, conversion between them will require a movement of one decimal place.

Table 4.8 Metric Equivalents of Length

1 *centimeter* (*cm*) = 10 *millimeters* (*mm*)

EXAMPLE 4.10

A wound has a length of 0.7 *centimeters*. What is the length of this wound in *millimeters*?

$$0.7 \ cm = ? \ mm$$

BY DIMENSIONAL ANALYSIS

$$0.7 \ centimeters = ? \ millimeters$$

You want to cancel the *centimeters* and get the answer in *millimeters*, so choose a fraction with *centimeters* on the bottom and *millimeters* on top. You need a fraction in the form of $\dfrac{? \ mm}{? \ cm}$

Because 1 *centimeter* = 10 *millimeters*, the fraction you need is $\dfrac{10 \ mm}{1 \ cm}$

$$\frac{0.7 \ \cancel{cm}}{1} \times \frac{10 \ \cancel{mm}}{1 \ \cancel{cm}} = 7 \ mm$$

BY MOVING THE DECIMAL POINT

To convert *centimeters* to *millimeters*, jump *1 place to the right*.

meter	decimeter	centimeter	millimeter
m	dm	cm	mm

So, in 0.7 *cm* move the decimal point *1 place to the right*.

$$0.7 \ cm = 0 \underset{\curvearrowright}{7}. \ mm = 7. \ mm = 7 \ mm$$

So, the wound has a length of 7 *millimeters*.

Summary

In this chapter, the household and metric systems of measurement were introduced.

- The metric system is the dominant system used in healthcare.
- The apothecary system has been phased out.
- It is important to memorize the equivalences between the various units of measurement of the household and metric systems.
- It is important to memorize the abbreviations for the various units of measurement.
- To convert units of measure in the household system, use Dimensional Analysis.
- To convert units of measure in the metric system, use Dimensional Analysis or the shortcut method of moving the decimal point. Always jump 3 places except for *cm–mm* conversions, which use a 1-place jump.
- Remember, each jump is 3 places in this chart:

kilo	gram, liter	milli	micro
kg	g, L	mg, mL	mcg

- Abbreviations for units of measurement are not followed by periods.
  Example: *40 mg and 5 t* (not 40 *mg.* and 5 *t.*)

- Abbreviations for units of measurement are not made plural by adding the letter s.
  Example: *70 mcg and 3 oz*
  (not 70 *mcgs* and 3 *ozs*)
- Insert a leading zero for decimal numbers less than 1.
  Example: *0.05 g and 0.34 mL*
  (not *.05 g* and *.34 mL*)
- Omit trailing zeros for decimal numbers.
  Example: *7.3 mL and 0.07 g*
  (not *7.30 mL* and *0.070 g*)
- Numbers greater than 999 need commas.
  Example: *2,500 mL and 20,000 mcg*
  (not *2500 mL* and *20000 mcg*)
- Leave space between the number and the unit of measurement.
  Example: *60 mL and 100 g*
  (not *60mL* and *100g*)
- Avoid the use of fractions with metric units of measurement.
  Example: *0.5 mL and 1.5 g*
  (not $\frac{1}{2}$ *mL* and $1\frac{1}{2}$ *g*)

Practice Sets

Workspace

The answers to *Try These for Practice*, *Exercises*, and *Cumulative Review Exercises* are found in Appendix A. Ask your instructor for the answers to the *Additional Exercises*.

Try These for Practice

Test your comprehension after reading the chapter.

1. You need to memorize all the metric and household equivalents. To test yourself, fill in the missing numbers in the following chart.

Metric System

(a) 1 L   = _____ mL

(b) 1 mL   = _____ cc

(c) 1 L   = _____ cm³

(d) 1 kg   = _____ g

(e) 1 g   = _____ mg

(f) 1 mg   = _____ mcg

(g) 1 cm   = _____ mm

Household System

(h) 1 *qt*   = _____ *pt*

(i) 1 *pt*   = _____ *cups*

(j) 1 *measuring cup*   = _____ *oz*

(k) 1 *oz*   = _____ *T*

(l) 1 *T*   = _____ *t*

(m) 1 *ft*   = _____ *in*

(n) 1 *lb*   = _____ *oz*

2. How many *micrograms* of a drug are contained in one 15-*milligram* tablet of the drug?

3. Avonex (interferon beta-1a) is a drug used to treat multiple sclerosis (MS). A patient is to receive a 30 *mcg* injection of this drug once a week. How many *milligrams* of Avonex will the patient receive in one week?

4. A patient who has Crohn's disease is to receive *Tysabri (natalizumab) 300 mg IV once every four weeks.* How many *grams* of Tysabri will the patient receive in 12 weeks?

5. How many *tablespoons* are equivalent to 3 *ounces*?

Exercises

Reinforce your understanding in class or at home.

1. 56 *mg* = _____ *mcg*

2. 600 *mg* = _____ *g*

3. 16 *cups* = _____ *qt*

4. 5.6 *cm* = _____ *mm*

5. 4.5 *lb* = _____ *oz*

6. Use the label on the bottle in • **Figure 4.1** to determine the number of *micrograms* in one tablet of the drug.

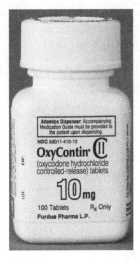

• **Figure 4.1**
Bottle of OxyContin.

Workspace

7. The prescriber ordered *ProBanthine (propantheline bromide) 30 mg PO ac and hs.* How many *grams* of ProBanthine will the patient receive in one week?

8. Order: *Benlysta (belimumab) 650 mg IV q 4 wk.* How many *grams* will the patient receive?

9. The urinary output of a patient with an indwelling Foley catheter is 1,400 *milliliters.* How many *liters* of urine are in the bag?

10. 42,000 *mcg* = ? *mg*

11. 2,650 *g* = ? *kg*

12. $4\frac{1}{2}$ *qt* = ? *pt*

13. Read the label in • **Figure 4.2** to determine the number of *micrograms* in 1 *milliliter* of Atgam.

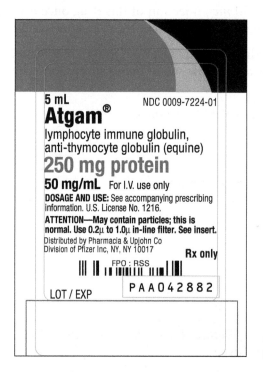

• **Figure 4.2**
Drug label for Atgam.

14. Order: *Nesina (alogliptin) 25 mg po daily.* This dipeptidyl peptidase-4 (DPP-4) inhibitor is used in the treatment of type II diabetes mellitus. How many *grams* of Nesina will the patient receive in 1 week?

15. According to the portion of the physician's order sheet in • **Figure 4.3,** how many *grams* of Avandia will the patient receive in 7 days?

Date	Time	Order
8/9/2016	1430 *h*	Avandia (rosiglitazone maleate) 2 *mg po b.i.d.*

• **Figure 4.3**
Portion of a physician's order sheet.

16. Order: *Amoxil (amoxicillin) oral susp 1 tsp po q8h.* How many *tablespoons* of Amoxil will the patient receive in 3 full days?

17. Read the label in • **Figure 4.4** to determine the number of *grams* of Norvir contained in 1 *mL* of the Norvir solution.

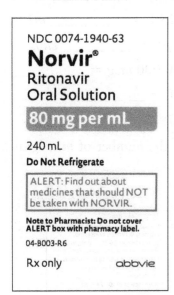

NDC 0074-1940-63

Norvir®
Ritonavir
Oral Solution

80 mg per mL

240 mL

Do Not Refrigerate

ALERT: Find out about
medicines that should NOT
be taken with NORVIR.

**Note to Pharmacist: Do not cover
ALERT box with pharmacy label.**

04-B003-R6

Rx only   abbvie

• **Figure 4.4**
Drug label for Norvir.

18. Read the label in • **Figure 4.5** and determine how many *grams* of Isentress are contained in one tablet.

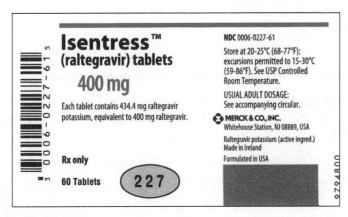

0006-0227-6115

Isentress™
(raltegravir) tablets

400 mg

Each tablet contains 434.4 mg raltegravir
potassium, equivalent to 400 mg raltegravir.

Rx only

60 Tablets   227

NDC 0006-0227-61

Store at 20-25°C (68-77°F);
excursions permitted to 15-30°C
(59-86°F). See USP Controlled
Room Temperature.

USUAL ADULT DOSAGE:
See accompanying circular.

⊕ **MERCK & CO., INC.**
Whitehouse Station, NJ 08889, USA

Raltegravir potassium (active ingred.)
Made in Ireland

Formulated in USA

9794800

• **Figure 4.5**
Drug label for Isentress.

19. An infant weighs 3.1 *kg.* How much does the infant weigh in *grams*?

20. Read the portion of the package insert in • **Figure 4.6** and determine whether or not this order is a safe starting dose: *Dilaudid (hydromorphone HCl) 1.7 mg IM q6h prn for pain.*

DOSAGE AND ADMINISTRATION

DILAUDID INJECTION
   The usual starting dose is 1–2 *mg* subcutaneously or intramuscularly every 4 to 6 *hours*
   as necessary for pain control.

• **Figure 4.6**
Portion of the package insert for Dilaudid.

Additional Exercises

Now, test yourself!

1. 9.6 *mg* = _____ *mcg*

2. 0.06 *g* = _____ *mg*

3. 40 *mg* = _____ *g*

4. 6.25 *L* = _____ *mL*

5. 21 *mm* = _____ *cm*

6. $2\frac{1}{2}$ *pt* = _____ *cups*

7. 24 *mL* = _____ *cc*

8. 250,000 *mcg* = _____ *mg*

9. 3.5 *qt* = _____ *pt*

10. 4 *T* = _____ *t*

11. 2 *cups* = _____ *oz*

12. 0.35 *kg* = _____ *g*

13. Use the label in • **Figure 4.7** to determine the number of *micrograms* in one Biaxin tablet.

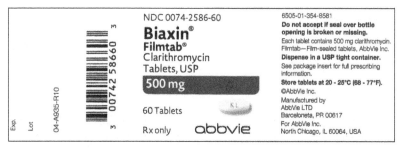

NDC 0074-2586-60

Biaxin®
Filmtab®
Clarithromycin
Tablets, USP

500 mg

60 Tablets

Rx only   abbvie

6505-01-354-8581
Do not accept if seal over bottle opening is broken or missing.
Each tablet contains 500 mg clarithromycin.
Filmtab—Film-sealed tablets, AbbVie Inc.
Dispense in a USP tight container.
See package insert for full prescribing information.
Store tablets at 20 - 25°C (68 - 77°F).
©AbbVie Inc.
Manufactured by
AbbVie LTD
Barceloneta, PR 00617
For AbbVie Inc.
North Chicago, IL 60064, USA

Exp.   Lot   04-A935-R10

• **Figure 4.7**
Drug label for Biaxin.

14. Order: *doxycycline 100 mg po b.i.d.* What is this dose in *grams*?

15. According to the package insert information in • **Figure 4.8**, would the following order be safe or not? *Uniphyl (theophylline, anhydrous) 400 mg po b.i.d.*

UNIPHYL®
Tablets
(theophylline, anhydrous)
400 mg and 600 mg

DOSAGE AND ADMINISTRATION
Uniphyl® 400 or 600 mg Tablets can be taken once a day in the morning or evening.

It is recommended that Uniphyl be taken with meals. Patients should be advised that if they choose to take Uniphyl with food it should be taken consistently with food and if they take it in a fasted condition it should routinely be taken fasted. It is important that the product whenever dosed be dosed consistently with or without food.

• **Figure 4.8**
Portion of the package insert for Uniphyl.

16. Read the label in • **Figure 4.9** to determine the number of *milligrams* in 2 tablets of Levothyroxine Sodium Tablets.

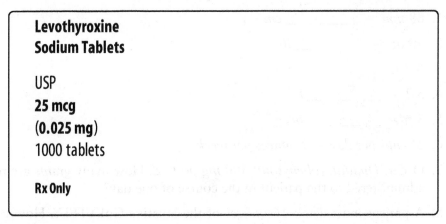

**Levothyroxine
Sodium Tablets**

USP
**25 mcg
(0.025 mg)**
1000 tablets

Rx Only

• **Figure 4.9**
Drug label for Levothyroxine Sodium Tablets.

17. According to the physician's order sheet in • **Figure 4.10**, what is the dose in *grams* of the chlorpromazine?

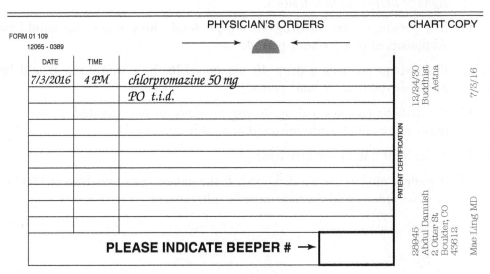

• **Figure 4.10**
Portion of a physician's order sheet.

18. A patient is drinking $\frac{1}{2}$ *pint* of orange juice every two hours. At this rate, how many *quarts* of orange juice will the patient drink in eight hours?

19. An infant weighs 3,400 *grams*. How much does the infant weigh in *kilograms*?

20. 5 *ft* = _____ *in*

Cumulative Review Exercises

Workspace

Reinforce your mastery of previous chapters.

1. 88 *mm* = _____ *cm*

2. 40 *oz* = _____ *lb*

3. 3.7 *L* = _____ *mL*

4. 5 *T* = _____ *t*

5. 5 *ft* = _____ *in*

6. $2\frac{1}{2}$ *cups per day* = ? *ounces per week*

7. Order: *Dilantin (phenytoin) 300 mg po t.i.d.* How many *grams* are to be administered to the patient in the course of one day?

8. A patient must drink 16 *ounces* of the laxative GoLYTELY. How many *cups* must the patient drink?

9. Order: *Ritalin (methylphenidate hydrochloride) 20 mg po daily in 2 divided doses.* How many *mg* of this psychostimulant drug will you administer to the patient with attention-deficit hyperactivity disorder (ADHD)?

10. What is missing from this order? *Sitavig (acyclovir) 50 mg apply within one hour after the onset of symptoms and before the appearance of any signs of herpes labialis lesions.*

11. If a patient receives a drug *40 mg po b.i.d.*, how many *mg* would be administered in a 24-hour period?

12. If a patient receives a drug *40 mg po q12h*, how many *mg* would be administered in a 24-hour period?

13. If a patient receives a drug *40 mg po daily in two divided doses*, how many *mg* would be administered in a 24-hour period?

14. Write 9:30 P.M. in military time.

15. A patient must receive a drug *q6h*. If the patient gets one dose at 1900 *h*, at what time would the next dose be administered?

Converting from One System of Measurement to Another

Learning Outcomes

1 *kilogram* (*kg*)
≈
2.2 *pounds* (lb)

After completing this chapter, you will be able to

1. State the equivalent units of weight between the metric and household systems.
2. State the equivalent units of volume between the metric and household systems.
3. State the equivalent units of length between the metric and household systems.
4. Convert a quantity measured in metric units to its equivalent measured in household units.
5. Convert a quantity measured in household units to its equivalent measured in metric units.

When calculating drug dosages, you will sometimes need to convert a quantity expressed in one system of measurement to an equivalent quantity expressed in a different system of measurement. For example, you might need to convert a quantity measured in ounces (household) to the same quantity measured in milliliters (metric). This chapter will show you how to accomplish such conversions.

Equivalents of Common Units of Measurement

To get started, you will need to learn some basic equivalent values of the various units in the different systems. Table 5.1 lists some common equivalent values for weight, volume, and length in the metric and household systems of measurement. Although these equivalents are considered standards, all of them are approximations.

A useful summary of the relationships you should know among all the equivalents of liquid volume is provided in Table 5.2.

NOtE

Some books use these approximations:

$250\,mL \approx 1\,cup$

$480\,mL \approx 1\,pt$

table 5.1 **Approximate Equivalents between Metric and Household Units of Volume, Weight, and Length**

	Metric		Household
Volume	5 milliliters (mL)	≈	1 teaspoon (t)
	15 milliliters (mL)	≈	1 tablespoon (T)
	30 milliliters (mL)	≈	1 ounce (oz)
	240 milliliters (mL)	≈	1 cup
	500 milliliters (mL)	≈	1 pint (pt)
	1,000 milliliters (mL)	≈	1 quart (qt)
Weight	1 kilogram (kg)	≈	2.2 pounds (lb)
Length	2.5 centimeters (cm)	≈	1 inch (in)

NOtE

Unlike all the approximations in Tables 5.1 and 5.2, an *inch* is defined to be exactly 2.54 *cm*.

table 5.2 **Summary table of Equivalents within and Approximate Equivalents between Metric and Household Units of Volume**

1 teaspoon	≈	5 mL
1 tablespoon = 3 teaspoons	≈	15 mL
1 ounce = 2 tablespoons = 6 teaspoons	≈	30 mL
1 cup = 8 ounces = 16 tablespoons	≈	240 mL
1 pint = 2 cups = 16 ounces	≈	500 mL
1 quart = 2 pints = 4 cups = 32 ounces	≈	1,000 mL = 1 L

You can use *Dimensional Analysis* to convert from one system to another in exactly the same way you converted from one unit to another within the same system. • **Figure 5.1** depicts medication cups with units of measurement from various systems.

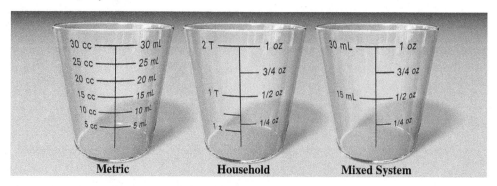

• **Figure 5.1**
Medication cups showing equivalent units.

The surface, called the meniscus, of a liquid in a medication cup is not flat (• **Figure 5.2**)—it is curved. Read the amount of liquid at the level of the bottom of the meniscus.

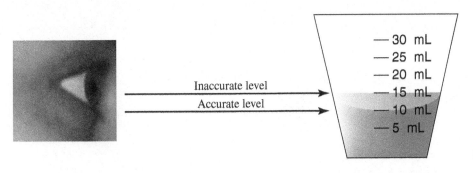

— 30 mL
— 25 mL
— 20 mL
— 15 mL
— 10 mL
— 5 mL

• **Figure 5.2**
Medication cup filled to 10 *mL*.

Metric-Household Conversions

Volume Conversions

ExAMpLE 5.1

A patient received 4 *teaspoons* of Robitussin in one day. How many *milliliters* of the drug did the patient receive?

$$4\ t = ?\ mL$$

You want to cancel the *teaspoons* and obtain the equivalent in *milliliters*.

$$\frac{4\ t}{1} \times \frac{?\ mL}{?\ t} = ?\ mL$$

Use the equivalence 5 *mL* = 1 *t*.

So, the unit fraction is $\dfrac{5\ mL}{1\ t}$

$$\frac{4\ \cancel{t}}{1} \times \frac{5\ mL}{1\ \cancel{t}} = 20\ mL$$

So, the patient received 20 *milliliters* of Robitussin.

NOtE

Although 1 *t* is approximately equal to 5 *mL*, in Example 5.1, for simplicity, the equal sign is used. This practice will be followed throughout the textbook.

ExAMpLE 5.2

Change $1\frac{1}{2}$ *pints* to an equivalent number of *milliliters*.

$$1\tfrac{1}{2}\ pt = ?\ mL$$

You want to cancel the *pints* and obtain the equivalent amount in *milliliters*.

$$\frac{3\ pt}{2} \times \frac{?\ mL}{?\ pt} = ?\ mL$$

Because $500 \; mL = 1 \; pt$, the fraction is $\dfrac{500 \; mL}{1 \; pt}$

$$\dfrac{3 \; \cancel{pt}}{\underset{1}{\cancel{2}}} \times \dfrac{\overset{250}{\cancel{500}} \; mL}{1 \; \cancel{pt}} = 750 \; mL$$

So, $1\frac{1}{2}$ *pints* is equivalent to 750 *milliliters*.

NOt E

Example 5.3 could be done mentally by understanding that, because 1 *ounce* = 30 *milliliters*, then twice as many *ounces* (2 oz) will equal twice as many *milliliters* (60 mL). That is, 2 oz = 60 mL.

ExAMpLE 5.3

A patient is to receive 60 *milliliters* of a medication. How many *ounces* will the patient receive?

$$60 \; milliliters = ? \; ounces$$

You want to cancel the *milliliters* and get the answer in *ounces*, so choose a fraction with *milliliters* on the bottom and *ounces* on top.

You need a fraction in the form of $\dfrac{? \; oz}{? \; mL}$

Because $1 \; oz = 30 \; mL$, the fraction you need is $\dfrac{1 \; oz}{30 \; mL}$

$$\dfrac{\overset{2}{\cancel{60}} \; \cancel{mL}}{1} \times \dfrac{1 \; oz}{\underset{1}{\cancel{30}} \; \cancel{mL}} = 2 \; oz$$

So, the patient will receive 2 *ounces* of the medication.

ExAMpLE 5.4

A medication cup contains 22.5 *milliliters* of a solution. How many *tablespoons* are in the medication cup?

$$22.5 \; milliliters = ? \; tablespoons$$

You want to cancel the *milliliters* and get the answer in *tablespoons*, so choose a fraction with *milliliters* on the bottom and *tablespoons* on top. You need a fraction in the form of $\dfrac{? \; T}{? \; mL}$

Because $15 \; milliliters = 1 \; tablespoon$, the fraction you need is $\dfrac{1 \; T}{15 \; mL}$

$$\dfrac{22.5 \; \cancel{mL}}{1} \times \dfrac{1 \; T}{15 \; \cancel{mL}} = 1.5 \; T$$

So, the medication cup contains $1\frac{1}{2}$ *tablespoons*.

Weight Conversions

ExAMpLE 5.5

A patient weighs 150 *pounds*. What is the patient's weight measured in *kilograms*?

$$150 \; pounds = ? \; kilograms$$

You want to cancel the *pounds* and get the answer in *kilograms*, so choose a fraction with *pounds* on the bottom and *kilograms* on top. You need a fraction in the form of $\dfrac{?\;kg}{?\;lb}$

Because 2.2 *pounds* = 1 *kilogram*, the fraction you need is $\dfrac{1\;kg}{2.2\;lb}$

$$\frac{150 \; \cancel{lb}}{1} \times \frac{1 \; kg}{2.2 \; \cancel{lb}} \approx 68.1818 \; kg$$

So, the patient weighs about 68 *kilograms*.

ExAMpLE 5.6

An obese patient weighs 355 *pounds*. Because the patient will receive medication based on his weight measured in *kilograms*, find the patient's weight in *kilograms*.

$$355 \; lb = ? \; kg$$

You want to cancel the *pounds* and obtain the equivalent in *kilograms*.

$$\frac{355 \; lb}{1} \times \frac{?\;kg}{?\;lb} = ? \; kg$$

Use the equivalence 1 *kg* = 2.2 *lb*

So, the unit fraction is $\dfrac{1\;kg}{2.2\;lb}$

$$\frac{355 \; \cancel{lb}}{1} \times \frac{1 \; kg}{2.2 \; \cancel{lb}} = 161 \; kg$$

So, the patient weighs 161 *kilograms*.

ExAMpLE 5.7

An infant weighs 4,200 *grams*. Convert this to *pounds* and *ounces*.

First change 4,200 *g* to *kilograms*, and then change the *kilograms* to *pounds*.

You could change 4,200 *grams* to *kilograms* by moving the decimal point 3 places to the right.

$$4,200 \; grams = 4.2 \; kilograms$$

Now the problem becomes

$$4.2 \ kg = ? \ lb$$

You want to cancel the *kilograms* and obtain the equivalent in *pounds*.

$$\frac{4.2 \ kg}{1} \times \frac{? \ lb}{? \ kg} = ? \ lb$$

Use the equivalence 1 *kg* = 2.2 *lb*

So, the unit fraction is $\dfrac{2.2 \ lb}{1 \ kg}$

$$\frac{4.2 \ kg}{1} \times \frac{2.2 \ lb}{1 \ kg} = 9.24 \ lb$$

Now, change the fraction of a *pound* (0.24 *lb*) to *ounces*.

$$0.24 \ lb = ? \ oz$$

You want to cancel the *pounds* and obtain the equivalent in *ounces*.

$$\frac{0.24 \ lb}{1} \times \frac{? \ oz}{? \ lb} = ? \ oz$$

Use the equivalence 1 *lb* = 16 *oz*

So, the unit fraction is $\dfrac{16 \ oz}{1 \ lb}$

$$\frac{0.24 \ lb}{1} \times \frac{16 \ oz}{1 \ lb} = 3.84 \ oz \approx 4 \ oz$$

So, the infant weighs 9 *pounds* 4 *ounces*.

Length Conversions

NOtE

In Example 5.8, the 6 *feet* could have been changed to 72 *inches* by understanding that because 1 *foot* = 12 *inches*, then 6 times as many *feet* (6 ft) will equal 6 times as many *inches* (72 in). That is, 6 ft = 72 in.

ExAMpLE 5.8

Adam is 6 *feet* 3 *inches* tall. What is his height in *centimeters*?

$$6 \ ft \ 3 \ in \quad \text{means} \quad 6 \ ft + 3 \ in$$

First, determine Adam's height in *inches*. To do this, convert 6 *feet* to *inches*.

$$6 \ ft = ? \ in$$

You want to cancel *feet* and obtain the equivalent height in *inches*.

$$6 \ ft \times \frac{? \ in}{? \ ft} = ? \ in$$

Because 1 *ft* = 12 *in*, the fraction is $\frac{12\ in}{1\ ft}$

$$6\ ft \times \frac{12\ in}{1\ ft} = 72\ in$$

Now, add the extra 3 *inches*.

$$72\ in + 3\ in = 75\ in$$

Now convert 75 *inches* to *centimeters*.

$$75\ in = ?\ cm$$

You want to cancel *inches* and obtain the equivalent length in *centimeters*.

$$75\ in \times \frac{?\ cm}{?\ in} = ?\ cm$$

Because 1 *in* = 2.5 *cm*, the unit fraction is $\frac{2.5\ cm}{1\ in}$

$$75\ in \times \frac{2.5\ cm}{1\ in} = 187.5\ cm$$

So, Adam is 187.5 *centimeters* tall.

ExAMpLE 5.9

A neonate's head circumference is 390 *mm*. The parents ask for the measurement in *inches*. What is the circumference in *inches*?

$$390\ mm = ?\ in$$

First change from *390 millimeters* to *centimeters* and then from *centimeters* to *inches*.

$$390\ mm \longrightarrow ?\ cm \longrightarrow ?\ in$$

You want to cancel the *millimeters* and obtain the equivalent in *centimeters*.

$$\frac{390\ mm}{1} \times \frac{?\ cm}{?\ mm} = ?\ in$$

Use the equivalence 1 *cm* = 10 *mm*

So, the unit fraction is $\frac{1\ cm}{10\ mm}$

$$\frac{390\ mm}{1} \times \frac{1\ cm}{10\ mm} = ?\ in$$

Now you want to cancel the *centimeters* and obtain the equivalent in *inches*.

$$\frac{390 \; \cancel{mm}}{1} \times \frac{1 \; cm}{10 \; \cancel{mm}} \times \frac{? \; in}{? \; cm} = ? \; in$$

Use the equivalence 1 *in* = 2.5 *cm*.

So, the unit fraction is $\dfrac{1 \; in}{2.5 \; cm}$

$$\frac{390 \; \cancel{mm}}{1} \times \frac{1 \; \cancel{cm}}{10 \; \cancel{mm}} \times \frac{1 \; in}{2.5 \; \cancel{cm}} = 15.6 \; in$$

So, the circumference is 15.6 *inches*.

Summary

In this chapter, quantities measured in one system of measurement were converted to equivalent quantities measured in a different system of measurement.

- It is important to memorize all the equivalences for volume, weight, and length between the metric and household systems of measurement.
- Dimensional Analysis can be used to perform conversions between the metric and household systems.

- The equivalences between systems are not exact—they are approximate.
- When performing conversions between two systems, your answers are not exact—they are approximate.
- When performing conversions between two systems, answers may differ somewhat, depending on which approximate equivalences are used.

practice Sets

Workspace

The answers to *Try These for Practice*, *Exercises*, and *Cumulative Review Exercises* are found in Appendix A. Ask your instructor for the answers to the *Additional Exercises*.

try these for practice

Test your comprehension after reading the chapter.

1. To do the exercises at the end of this chapter, you need to memorize all the equivalents presented so far. To test yourself, fill in the missing numbers in the following chart.

Metric System

(a) 1 *L* = _____ *mL*

(b) 1 *kg* = _____ *g*

(c) 1 *g* = _____ *mg*

(d) 1 *mg* = _____ *mcg*

(e) 1 *cm* = _____ *mm*

Household System

(f) 1 *qt* = _____ *pt*

(g) 1 *pt* = _____ *cups*

(h) 1 *cup* = _____ *oz*

(i) 1 *oz* = _____ *T*

(j) 1 *T* = _____ *t*

(k) 1 *lb* ≈ _____ *oz*

(l) 1 *ft* = _____ *in*

Mixed Systems

(m) 1 *in* ≈ _____ *cm*

(n) 1 *kg* ≈ _____ *lb*

(o) 1 *t* ≈ _____ *mL*

(p) 1 *T* ≈ _____ *mL*

(q) 1 *oz* ≈ _____ *mL*

(r) 1 *cup* ≈ _____ *mL*

(s) 1 *pt* ≈ _____ *mL*

(t) 1 *qt* ≈ _____ *mL*

(u) 1 *oz* = _____ *T* = _____ *t* ≈ _____ *mL*

(v) 1 *qt* = _____ *pt* = _____ *cups* = _____ *oz* ≈ _____ *mL*

2. Harold is 5 *feet* 3 *inches* tall. What is his height rounded off to the nearest whole *centimeter*?

3. Order: *Ravicti (glycerol phenylbutyrate) 15 mL po in three equally divided dosages, each rounded up to the nearest 0.5 mL.* How many *teaspoons* will you administer?

4. How many *milliliters* are contained in a 16-*ounce* bottle of water?

5. A patient must drink 1½ *ounces* of a prescribed solution. If only a *teaspoon* is available, how many *teaspoons* of the solution should the patient drink?

Exercises

Reinforce your understanding in class or at home.

1. 4 *t* ≈ _____ *mL*

2. 8 *oz* ≈ _____ *mL*

3. 45 *mL* ≈ _____ *T*

4. 120 *mL* ≈ _____ *cup*

5. 150 *lb* ≈ _____ *kg* (round off to tenth of a *kg*)

6. Use the label in • **Figure 5.3** to determine how many *teaspoons* of cephalexin will contain 125 *mg* of the drug.

Workspace

Workspace

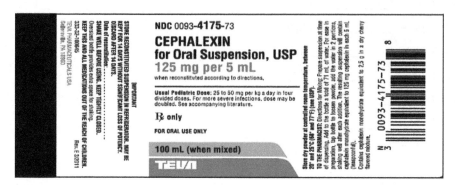

● **Figure 5.3**
Drug label for Cephalexin.

7. The diameter of a wound is *50 mm*. What is the diameter of the wound measured in *inches*?

8. 24 *t* = ? *T*

9. 120 *mL* ≈ ? *oz*

10. Read the label in ● **Figure 5.4** and determine how many *teaspoons* of dextromethorphan are in the container.

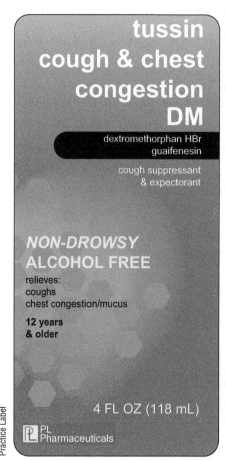

● **Figure 5.4**
Box for dextromethorphan.
(For educational purposes only)

11. General George Washington was 1.85 *meters* tall. What was his height in *feet* and *inches*?

12. Order: *Kynamro (mipomersen sodium) 200 milligrams subcut once weekly*. How many *grams* will the patient receive each week?

13. A neonate weighs 3,100 *grams*. Convert this weight to *pounds* and *ounces* (rounded off to the nearest *ounce*).

14. Use • **Figure 5.5** to determine the total number of *grams* of pseudoephedrine that are in the entire container.

Workspace

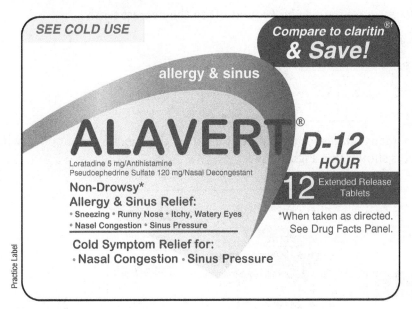

• **Figure 5.5**
Drug box for Alavert.

15. A nurse administers 30 *mL* of a drug by mouth t.i.d. to a patient. This patient is to be discharged and must continue to take the medication at home. How many *tablespoons* should the patient be advised to take daily?

16. The patient is required to take *Allegra (fexofenadine) 60 mg po b.i.d.* How many *grams* of this drug will the patient take in 3 days?

17. What is the patient's total fluid intake in *milliliters* for the day if he had the following fluid intake:
    Breakfast: 8 *oz* milk, 8 *oz* water
    Lunch: 6 *oz* juice, 3 *T* medication
    Dinner: 6 *oz* soup, 12 *oz* soda, 4 *oz* jello

18. The order for a patient is *Robitussin syrup (guaifenesin) 10 mL po q4h*. How many *ounces* of Robitussin would the patient have received by 10 P.M. if the first dose was administered at noon?

19. The patient must receive *Cipro (ciprofloxacin hydrochloride) 500 mg b.i.d. × 10 d* for acute sinusitis. How many *grams* of Cipro will the patient have received in total at the end of the 10 days?

20. A school nurse administers 2 *teaspoons* of Children's Tylenol to a child who has a fever. How many such doses are contained in an 8-*ounce* bottle of this medication?

Additional Exercises

Workspace

Now, test yourself!

1. 4.7 *mg* = _____ *mcg*

2. 400 *mL* = _____ *L*

3. 60 *mL* ≈ _____ *t*

4. 4 *T* ≈ _____ *mL*

5. 50 *lb* ≈ _____ *kg* (round off to the nearest tenth)

6. 50 *kg* ≈ _____ *lb*

7. 3.5 *pt* ≈ _____ *oz*

8. 4 *T* = _____ *oz*

9. 7.5 *cm* ≈ _____ *in*

10. How many *tablespoons* are contained in the Lexapro container whose label is shown in • **Figure 5.6**?

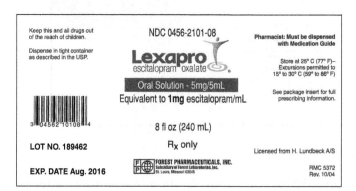

• **Figure 5.6**
Drug label for Lexapro.

11. A patient is 5 *feet* 9 *inches* tall. Find the height of the patient in *centimeters*.

12. Find the weight in *grams* of a 7-*pound* infant (round off to the nearest gram).

13. Harold weighs 250 *pounds* now. If Harold goes on a diet and loses 30 *pounds*, then how many *kilograms* will he weigh?

14. Use • **Figure 5.7** to determine how many *teaspoons* of Namenda will contain 2 *mg* of the drug.

15. A nurse administers KCl 30 *mL* by mouth daily to Mrs. M. This patient is to be discharged, and she must continue to take the medication at home. How many *tablespoons* should she be advised to take daily?

16. Read the information in • **Figure 5.8** and determine the number of *teaspoons* of the bronchodilator metaproterenol you will administer if the label reads "10 *mg*/5 *mL*."

17. A patient drank 12 *ounces* of orange juice. How many *milliliters* did the patient drink?

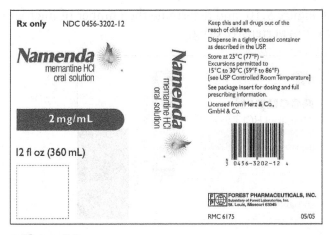

● **Figure 5.7**
Drug label for Namenda.

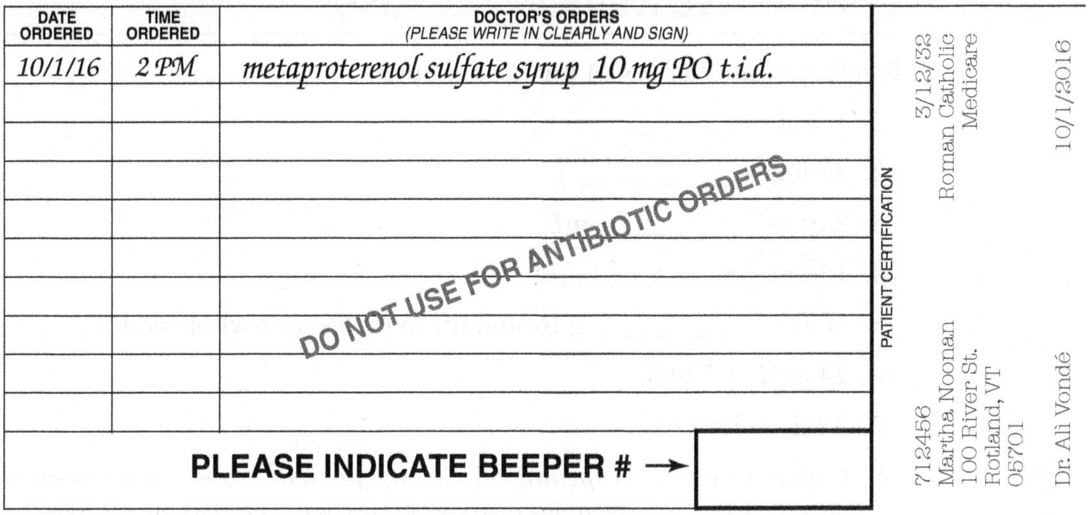

UNIVERSITY HOSPITAL
AUTHORIZATION IS HEREBY GIVEN TO DISPENSE THE GENERIC OR CHEMICAL EQUIVALENT UNLESS OTHERWISE INDICATED BY THE WORDS — **NO SUBSTITUTE**

DATE ORDERED	TIME ORDERED	DOCTOR'S ORDERS (PLEASE WRITE IN CLEARLY AND SIGN)	
10/1/16	2 PM	*metaproterenol sulfate syrup 10 mg PO t.i.d.*	
		PLEASE INDICATE BEEPER # →	

Patient certification (right margin):
3/12/32
Roman Catholic
Medicare

10/1/2016

712456
Martha Noonan
100 River St.
Rotland, VT
05701

Dr. Ali Vondé

● **Figure 5.8**
physician's order sheet.

18. The label indicates that in the container there are 120 metered sprays, each of which contains 32 *mcg* of Rhinocort. Use this information to determine the total number of *milligrams* of this corticosteroid inhalant that are in the container.

19. Using the label in ● **Figure 5.9**, determine the total number of *milliliters* of vaccine that are in the vial.

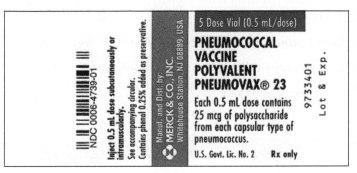

5 Dose Vial (0.5 mL/dose)

PNEUMOCOCCAL VACCINE POLYVALENT PNEUMOVAX® 23

Each 0.5 mL dose contains 25 mcg of polysaccharide from each capsular type of pneumococcus.

U.S. Govt. Lic. No. 2   **Rx only**

NDC 0006-4739-01

Inject 0.5 mL dose subcutaneously or intramuscularly.
See accompanying circular.
Contains phenol 0.25% added as preservative.

Manuf. and Dist. by
MERCK & CO., INC.
Whitehouse Station, NJ 08889, USA

9733401
Lot & Exp.

● **Figure 5.9**
Drug label for pneumococcal vaccine polyvalent pneumovax 23.

Workspace

Workspace

20. Read the label in • **Figure 5.10** and determine the number of micrograms in 1 tablet of this antihypertensive drug.

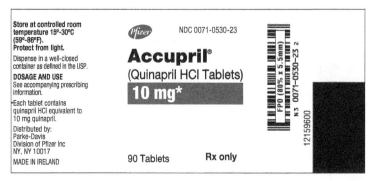

Store at controlled room
temperature 15°-30°C
(59°-86°F).
Protect from light.

Dispense in a well-closed
container as defined in the USP.

DOSAGE AND USE
See accompanying prescribing
information.

•Each tablet contains
quinapril HCl equivalent to
10 mg quinapril.

Distributed by:
Parke-Davis
Division of Pfizer Inc
NY, NY 10017

MADE IN IRELAND

Pfizer   NDC 0071-0530-23

Accupril®
(Quinapril HCl Tablets)
10 mg*

90 Tablets   Rx only

FPO (80% x 5.5mm)
N3 0071-0530-23 2
12159600

• **Figure 5.10**
Drug label for Accupril.

(Reg. Trademark of Pfizer Inc. Reproduced with permission.)

Cumulative Review Exercises

Reinforce your mastery of previous chapters.

1. $176\ lb\ \approx$ _____ kg

2. $80\ mg\ =$ _____ g

3. $2\ qt\ \approx$ _____ mL

4. $120\ mL\ =$ _____ L

5. $5\ lb\ \approx$ _____ g (round off to the nearest whole gram)

6. $24\ oz/d\ =\ ?\ pt/d$

7. $3\ t/d\ \approx\ ?\ mL/wk$

8. Order: *Osphena (ospemifene) 60 mg po with food daily*. How many *grams* of this estrogen agonist/antagonist will the patient receive in total in two weeks?

9. A patient enters the ICU at 5:30 A.M. and leaves 8 hours later. At what time did the patient leave the ICU (in military time)?

10. The maximum dose of VariZIG (varicella zoster immune globulin [human]) is 625 *IU* for all patients greater than 40 *kilograms* in weight. Harold weighs 70 *lb*. May Harold receive 625 *IU* of this drug?

11. A wound has a diameter of 1.7 *inches*. What is this diameter measured in *millimeters*?

12. How many *mL* are contained in 2 *t*?

13. Find the weight in *pounds* of a patient who weighs 90 *kg*.

14. Find the height of a 6-foot-tall patient in *centimeters*.

15. Convert $\frac{4\ mL}{min}$ to an equivalent rate in $\frac{cups}{hour}$

Unit

3

Oral and Parenteral Medications

Chapter

6 Oral Medications

Learning Outcomes

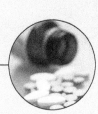

After completing this chapter, you will be able to

1. Calculate simple (one-step) problems for oral medications in solid and liquid form.
2. Calculate complex (multi-step) problems for oral medications in solid and liquid form.
3. Calculate doses for medications measured in milliequivalents.
4. Interpret drug labels to calculate doses for oral medication.
5. Calculate doses based on body weight.
6. Calculate body surface area (BSA).
7. Calculate doses based on body surface area (BSA).

In this chapter you will learn how to calculate doses of oral medications both in solid and liquid form. You will be introduced to *patient-specific* dosages that use the *size of the patient* (body weight or body surface area [BSA]) to determine the appropriate dose.

Simple (One-Step) problems

In the calculations you have done in previous chapters, all the equivalents have come from standard tables—for example, $1\ t = 5\ mL$. In this chapter, the equivalent used will depend on the *strength of the drug* that is available—for example, $1\ tab = 15\ mg$. In the following examples, the equivalent is found on the label of the drug container.

Medication in Solid Form

Oral medication is the most common type of prescription. As discussed in Chapter 2, oral medications come in many forms (tablets, capsules, caplets, and liquid), and drug manufacturers prepare oral medications in commonly prescribed dosages. Oral medications are often supplied in a variety of strengths.

Whenever possible, it is preferable to obtain the medication in the same strength as the dose ordered, or, if that is not available, choose a strength that equals a multiple of the prescribed dose. For example, if the order requires 100 *mg* to be administered, tablets with a strength of 100 *mg/tab* would make dosage computation unnecessary, and 1 *tablet* would be administered. However, tablets with a strength of 50 *mg/tab* would make dosage computation necessary, and 2 *tablets* would be administered.

It is best to *administer the fewest number of tablets or capsules possible.* For example, if a prescriber orders *ampicillin 750 mg po q12h* and you have both the 250-*mg* and 500-*mg* capsules available, then you would administer one 500-*mg* capsule and one 250-*mg* capsule rather than three 250-*mg* capsules.

In clinical settings, unit-dose medications are usually supplied by the pharmacist.

Suppose the order is *Tegretol 400 mg po b.i.d.* The Tegretol on hand is in the form of 200-*mg tablets*. How many tablets will you administer?

In this case you want to change the order of *400 mg* to the number of *tablets* to administer.

$$400\ mg = ?\ tab$$

The *strength of the drug* ($1\ tablet = 200\ mg$) will provide the unit fraction that is necessary. Because the *mg* must be cancelled, the denominator of the unit fraction must contain *mg*. Because you want the answer in *tablets*, the numerator of the unit fraction must contain *tab*.

$$400\ mg \times \frac{?\ tab}{?\ mg} = ?\ tab$$

The strength is $1\ tablet = 200\ mg$, so the unit fraction will be $\dfrac{1\ tab}{200\ mg}$

$$\frac{400\ mg}{1} \times \frac{1\ tab}{200\ mg} = ?\ tab$$

Now, cancel the *milligrams*, cancel the zeros, and finish the multiplication.

$$\frac{400\ \cancel{mg}}{1} \times \frac{1\ tab}{200\ \cancel{mg}} = 2\ tab$$

So, you would administer 2 *tablets* of Tegretol.

EXAMPLE 6.1

The order reads *Glucotrol XL (glipizide) 10 mg PO daily.* Read the drug label shown in • Figure 6.1. How many *tablets* of this blood glucose–lowering drug will you administer?

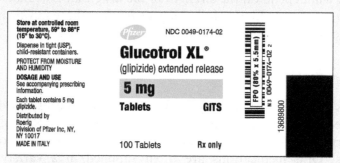

• **Figure 6.1**
Drug label for Glucotrol x L.

You want to convert the prescribed dose of 10 *mg* to the number of *tablets* to be administered.

$$10 \ mg = ? \ tab$$

Cancel the *milligrams* and calculate the equivalent amount in *tablets*.

$$\frac{10 \ mg}{1} \times \frac{? \ tab}{? \ mg} = ? \ tab$$

Because the strength on the label indicates that 1 *tablet* contains 5 *mg*, use the unit fraction $\frac{1 \ tab}{5 \ mg}$

$$\frac{10 \ mg}{1} \times \frac{1 \ tab}{5 \ mg} = ? \ tab$$

Now, cancel the *milligrams* and finish the multiplication.

$$\frac{10 \ \cancel{mg}}{1} \times \frac{1 \ tab}{5 \ \cancel{mg}} = 2 \ tab$$

So, you would administer 2 *tablets* of Glucotrol XL by mouth once a day to the patient.

EXAMPLE 6.2

The prescriber orders *Zoloft (sertraline HCl) 50 mg PO B.I.D.* Read the drug label in • Figure 6.2 and determine how many *tablets* of this antipsychotic drug you would give to the patient.

You must convert the order of 50 *milligrams* to *tablets*.

$$50 \ mg = ? \ tab$$

Cancel the *milligrams* and obtain the equivalent amount in *tablets*.

$$\frac{50 \ mg}{1} \times \frac{? \ tab}{? \ mg} = ? \ tab$$

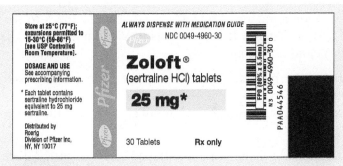

● **Figure 6.2**
Drug label for Zoloft.

Because the strength on the label is 1 *tab* = 25 *mg*, the unit fraction is $\dfrac{1\ tab}{25\ mg}$

$$\frac{50\ mg}{1} \times \frac{1\ tab}{25\ mg} = ?\ tab$$

Now, cancel the *milligrams* and finish the multiplication.

$$\frac{50\ \cancel{mg}}{1} \times \frac{1\ tab}{25\ \cancel{mg}} = 2\ tab$$

Because 2 *tablets* contain 50 *mg* of Zoloft, you would give 2 *tablets* by mouth to the patient twice a day.

EXAMPLE 6.3

Read the label in ● Figure 6.3. How many *tablets* of this narcotic analgesic will be needed for a dose containing 10 *mg* of hydrocodone bitartrate and 600 *mg* of acetaminophen?

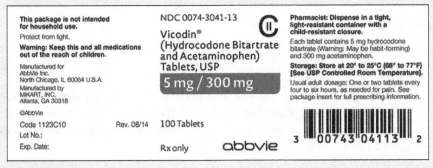

● **Figure 6.3**
Drug label for Vicodin.

Vicodin is a combination drug (see Figure 2.25 in Chapter 2) composed of hydrocodone bitartrate and acetaminophen. Therefore, for computational purposes, you need address only the first drug listed (hydrocodone bitartrate). Because the dose requires 10 *mg* of hydrocodone bitartrate, convert the 10 *mg* to the appropriate number of *tablets*.

However, before doing any calculations, you should check to see if the ratios of the amounts of the two drugs in Vicodin are equivalent in both the *dose* and on the *label*.

The hydrocodone bitartrate–acetaminophen ratio in the *dose* is 10:600, or 1:60.

The hydrocodone bitartrate–acetaminophen ratio on the *label* is 5:300, or 1:60.

Because the two ratios are the same (1:60), you can now proceed with the calculations.

You need consider only the amount of the first listed drug (10 *mg* of hydrocodone bitartrate) and convert that to *tablets*.

$$10 \; mg = ? \; tab$$

Cancel the *milligrams* and obtain the equivalent amount in *tablets*.

$$\frac{10 \; mg}{1} \times \frac{? \; tab}{? \; mg} = ? \; tab$$

The label indicates that one *tablet* contains 5 *mg* of hydrocodone bitartrate.

Because 1 *tab* = 5 *mg*, the unit fraction is $\frac{1 \; tab}{5 \; mg}$

$$\frac{10 \; mg}{1} \times \frac{1 \; tab}{5 \; mg} = ? \; tab$$

Now cancel the *milligrams* and finish the multiplication.

$$\frac{10 \; \cancel{mg}}{1} \times \frac{1 \; tab}{5 \; \cancel{mg}} = 2 \; tab$$

So, 2 *tablets* will contain 10 *mg* of hydrocodone bitartrate and 600 *mg* of acetaminophen, and 2 *tablets* will be needed for this dose.

NOTE

The chance of medication error increases as the number of *tablets* to be administered increases. Also, you need to consider the comfort of the patient who is required to swallow a large number of *tablets*. Many individuals do not like to take medication, and they may be reluctant to swallow large quantities of *tablets*.

EXAMPLE 6.4

The order is *tadalafil 20 mg PO prior to anticipated sexual activity*. The medication is available in three different strengths (• **Figure 6.4**). Determine how you would administer this dose using the fewest number of the available *tablets*.

The 20 *mg* dose could be administered in any of the following ways:

- One 20 *mg* tablet
- Two 10 *mg* tablets
- One 10 *mg* tablet and two 5 *mg* tablets
- Four 5 *mg* tablets

Because you want to administer the fewest number of *tablets*, you would choose to administer one 20 *mg* tablet.

tadalafil tablets

5 mg

30 Tablets

Rx Only

tadalafil tablets

10 mg

30 Tablets

Rx Only

tadalafil tablets

20 mg

30 Tablets

Rx Only

● **Figure 6.4**
t adalafil drug labels of differing strengths: 5, 10, and 20 *mg/tablet*.

Medication in Liquid Form

Because pediatric and geriatric patients, as well as patients with neurological conditions, may be unable to swallow medication in tablet form, sometimes oral medications are ordered in liquid form. The label states how much drug is contained in a given amount of liquid.

NOTE

Some liquid oral medications are supplied with special calibrated droppers or oral syringes that are used *only* for these medications (e.g., digoxin and Lasix). Some medication cups do not accurately measure amounts less than 5 *mL*.

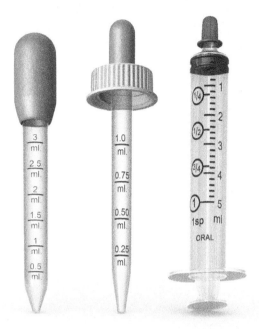

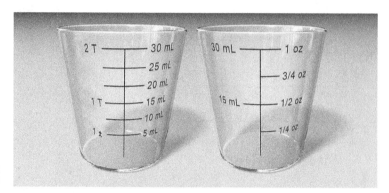

• **Figure 6.5**

Measuring drugs in liquid form (calibrated droppers, oral syringe, and measuring cups).

For medications supplied in liquid form, you must calculate the volume of the liquid that contains the prescribed drug dosage. Medication cups, oral syringes, or calibrated droppers are used to measure the dose. See • **Figure 6.5**.

NOTE

Recall the proper way to read the amount of liquid in a medication cup. See Figure 5.2.

EXAMPLE 6.5

The prescriber orders *alprazolam oral solution 0.25 mg PO b.i.d.* Read the label in • **Figure 6.6** and determine how many *milliliters* you will prepare.

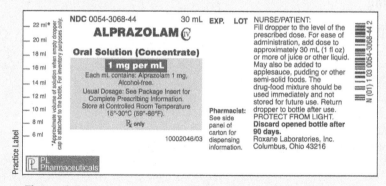

• **Figure 6.6**

Drug label for Alprazolam. (For educational purposes only)

You want to change the 0.25 *mg* dose prescribed to *milliliters*.

$$0.25 \ mg = ? \ mL$$

Cancel the *milligrams* and then calculate the equivalent amount in *mL*.

$$\frac{0.25 \ mg}{1} \times \frac{? \ mL}{? \ mg} = ? \ mL$$

NOTE

The critical thinker would recognize that because the strength in Example 6.5 is 1 *mg* = 1 *mL*, this example does not require computation—that is, 0.25 *mg* = 0.25 *mL*

Because the label indicates that every 1 *mL* of the solution contains 1 *mg* of alprazolam, use the unit fraction $\dfrac{1\ mL}{1\ mg}$

$$\frac{0.25\ mg}{1} \times \frac{1\ ml}{1\ mg} = 0.25\ mL$$

So, follow the directions on the label, and add 0.25 *mL* of a alprazolam to 30 *mL* of juice or other liquid.

EXAMPLE 6.6

The physician orders *furosemide 50 mg PO daily.* The strength of the solution is 10 mg/mL. Determine the number of *milliliters* of this diuretic you would administer to the patient.

Convert the order of 50 *milligrams* to *milliliters*.

$$50\ mg = ?\ mL$$

Cancel the *milligrams* and calculate the equivalent amount in *mL*.

$$\frac{50\ mg}{1} \times \frac{?\ mL}{?\ mg} = ?\ mL$$

Because the strength indicates that 1 *milliliter* of the solution contains 10 *mg* of furosemide, use the unit fraction $\dfrac{1\ mL}{10\ mg}$

$$\frac{50\ mg}{1} \times \frac{1\ mL}{10\ mg} = ?\ mL$$

Now, cancel the *milligrams* and finish the multiplication.

$$\frac{50\ mg}{1} \times \frac{1\ mL}{10\ mg} = 5\ mL$$

So, 5 *mL* will contain 50 *mg* of the drug, and you would give 5 *mL* of furosemide by mouth once a day to the patient. See • **Figure 6.7.**

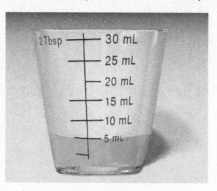

• **Figure 6.7**
**Medication cup with 50 *mg* (5 *mL*)
of furosemide.**

EXAMPLE 6.7

The physician orders *Biaxin (clarithromycin)   500 mg PO q12h.*
Read the label in • Figure 6.8. Determine the number of *mL* you
would administer to the patient.

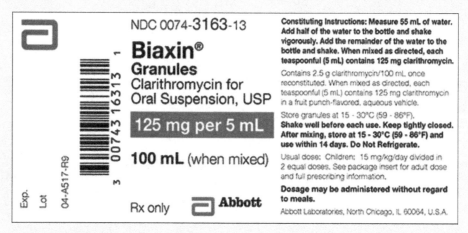

• **Figure 6.8**
Drug label for Biaxin

Convert 500 *mg* to *mL*.

$$500 \ mg = ? \ mL$$

Cancel the *milligrams* and calculate the equivalent amount in *milliliters*.

$$500 \ mg \times \frac{? \ mL}{? \ mg} = ? \ mL$$

Because the label indicates that every 5 *mL* of the solution contains

125 *mg* of Biaxin, use the unit fraction $\dfrac{5 \ mL}{125 \ mg}$

$$\overset{4}{500} \ mg \times \frac{5 \ mL}{\underset{1}{125} \ mg} = 20 \ mL$$

So, you would give 20 *mL* of this antibiotic by mouth every 12 *hours* to the patient. See • **Figure 6.9.**

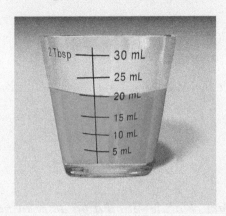

• **Figure 6.9**
**Medication cup with 500 *mg* (20 *mL*)
of Biaxin.**

Medications Measured in Milliequivalents

Some drugs are measured in **milliequivalents,** which are abbreviated *mEq.* A milliequivalent is an expression of the number of grams of a drug contained in one milliliter of solution. Pharmaceutical companies label electrolytes (sodium chloride, potassium chloride, and calcium chloride, for example) in milligrams as well as in milliequivalents.

EXAMPLE 6.8

Order: ***potassium chloride 30 mEq PO daily in three divided doses.*** Read the label in • **Figure 6.10** and determine how many *tablets* of this electrolyte supplement you should administer.

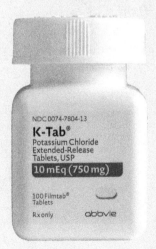

• **Figure 6.10**
Drug label for K-Tab.

NOTE

In Example 6.8, the order states "in three divided doses." This instructs the practitioner to separate the total daily dose into 3 equal parts over a 24-*hour* period. To ensure even distribution of the medication, the frequency of the doses should also be regular and consistent, so the drug is administered every 8 *hours.*

In this problem you want to change 30 *mEq* to *tablets.*

$$30 \text{ } mEq \longrightarrow \text{? } tab$$

You can do this on one line as follows:

$$30 \text{ } mEq \times \frac{\text{? } tab}{\text{? } mEq} = \text{? } tab$$

Because the label indicates that each *tablet* contains 10 *mEq*, the unit fraction is $\dfrac{1\ tab}{10\ mEq}$

$$\overset{3}{\cancel{30\ mEq}} \times \frac{\boxed{1\ tab}}{\cancel{10\ mEq}} = 3\ tab$$

Because the order indicates "three divided doses," you would administer 1 *tablet* of K-Tab every 8 *hours*.

EXAMPLE 6.9

The prescriber ordered *potassium chloride 40 mEq po daily in two divided doses*. The strength of the solution is 20 *mEq* per 15 *mL*. Determine the number of *milliliters* of this electrolyte supplement that you would administer.

You want to change the 40 *mEq* prescribed to *milliliters*.

$$40\ mEq = ?\ mL$$

Cancel the *mEq* and calculate the equivalent amount in *mL*.

$$\frac{40\ mEq}{1} \times \frac{?\ mL}{?\ mEq} = ?\ mL$$

Because the strength indicates that every 15 *mL* of the solution contains 20 *mEq* of potassium chloride, use the unit fraction $\dfrac{15\ mL}{20\ mEq}$

$$\frac{40\ \cancel{mEq}}{1} \times \frac{15\ mL}{20\ \cancel{mEq}} = 30\ mL$$

Because the 30 *mL* must be administered in "two divided doses," you would administer 15 *mL* to the patient every 12 *hours*.

Complex (Multi-Step) problems

Sometimes dosage calculations will require that multiplication by unit fractions be repeated one or more times. Recall that we examined complex (multi-step) problems in Chapter 3.

For example, if each *tablet* of a drug contains 1.25 *mg*, how many *tablets* would contain 0.0025 *gram*?

For complex problems, it helps to organize the information you will need for the computation as follows:

Given quantity: 0.0025 g [*single unit of measurement*]

Strength: 1 *tab* = 1.25 *mg* [*equivalence*]

Quantity you want to find: ? *tab* [*single unit of measurement*]

Because you want to find a *single unit of measurement* (? *tablets*), you must start with a *single unit of measurement* (0.0025 g). The *equivalence* (1 *tab* = 1.25 *mg*) will be used to form a unit fraction. So, the problem is

$$0.0025 \ g = ? \ tab$$

You do not know the direct equivalence between *grams* and *tablets*. This is a **complex** problem because you need to first convert 0.0025 *grams* to *milligrams* and then convert the *milligrams* to *tablets*.

$$0.0025 \ g \longrightarrow ? \ mg \longrightarrow ? \ tab$$

First, you want to cancel *grams (g)*. To do this you must use an equivalence containing *grams* to make a unit fraction with *grams* in the denominator.

Because the equivalence is 1 g = 1,000 *mg*, the unit fraction is $\dfrac{1,000 \ mg}{1 \ g}$

$$0.0025 \ g \times \frac{1,000 \ mg}{1 \ g} = ? \ tab$$

After the *grams* are cancelled, only *milligrams* remain on the left side. Now you need to change the *milligrams* to *tablets*. Because the strength is 1.25 *mg* = 1 *tab*, the unit fraction is $\dfrac{1 \ tab}{1.25 \ mg}$

$$0.0025 \ g \times \frac{1,000 \ mg}{1 \ g} \times \frac{1 \ tab}{1.25 \ mg} = ? \ tab$$

After cancelling the *milligrams*, only *tablets* remain on the left side. Now complete your calculation by multiplying the numbers.

$$0.0025 \ g \times \frac{1,000 \ mg}{1 \ g} \times \frac{1 \ tab}{1.25 \ mg} = \frac{2.5 \ tab}{1.25} = 2 \ tab$$

So, 2 *tablets* contain 0.0025 g.

EXAMPLE 6.10

How many 300-*mg* Ziagen (abacavir sulfate) *tablets* contain 0.9 g of Ziagen?

Given quantity: 0.9 g [*single unit of measurement*]

Strength: 1 *tab* = 300 *mg* [*equivalence*]

Quantity you want to find: ? *tab* [*single unit of measurement*]

Because you want to find a *single unit of measurement* (*tablets*), you must start with a *single unit of measurement* (0.9 g). The *equivalence* (1 *tab* = 300 *mg*) will be used to form a unit fraction. So, the problem is

$$0.9 \text{ g} = ? \text{ tab}$$

This is a **complex** problem because you need to convert 0.9 *g* to *milligrams* and then convert *milligrams* to *tablets*.

$$0.9 \text{ g} \longrightarrow ? \text{ mg} \longrightarrow ? \text{ tab}$$

First, you want to cancel *grams*. To do this you must use an equivalence containing *grams* to make a unit fraction with *grams* in the denominator.

Because the equivalence is 1 *g* = 1,000 *mg*, the unit fraction is $\dfrac{1,000 \text{ mg}}{1 \text{ g}}$

$$\frac{0.9 \ \cancel{g}}{1} \times \frac{1,000 \ \cancel{mg}}{1 \ \cancel{g}} = ? \text{ tab}$$

After the *grams* are cancelled, only *milligrams* remain on the left side. Now you need to change the *milligrams* to *tablets*. Because the strength is 300 *mg* = 1 *tab*, the unit fraction is $\dfrac{1 \text{ tab}}{300 \text{ mg}}$

$$\frac{0.9 \ \cancel{g}}{1} \times \frac{1,000 \ \cancel{mg}}{1 \ \cancel{g}} \times \frac{1 \text{ tab}}{300 \ \cancel{mg}} = \frac{9 \text{ tab}}{3} = 3 \text{ tab}$$

So, three 300 *mg* tablets contain 0.9 g of Ziagen.

EXAMPLE 6.11

Read the label in • Figure 6.11 to determine the number of Dilantin *capsules* that would contain a dose of 0.2 g.

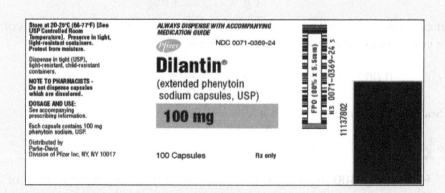

• **Figure 6.11**
Drug label for Dilantin.
(For educational purposes only)

Given quantity: 0.2 g
Strength: 1 *cap* = 100 *mg*
Quantity you want to find: ? *cap*

In this problem you want to convert 0.2 *gram* to *milligrams* and then convert *milligrams* to *capsules*.

$$0.2\ g \longrightarrow ?\ mg \longrightarrow ?\ cap$$

You can do this on one line as follows:

$$\frac{0.2\ g}{1} \times \frac{?\ mg}{?\ g} \times \frac{?\ cap}{?\ mg} = ?\ cap$$

Because 1,000 *mg* = 1 g, the first unit fraction is $\dfrac{1,000\ mg}{1\ g}$.

Because the strength is 100 *mg* = 1 *cap*, the second unit fraction is $\dfrac{1\ cap}{100\ mg}$

$$\frac{0.2\ g}{1} \times \frac{1,000\ mg}{1\ g} \times \frac{1\ cap}{100\ mg} = ?\ cap$$

Now cancel the grams, milligrams, and zeros.

$$\frac{0.2\ \cancel{g}}{1} \times \frac{1,000\ \cancel{mg}}{1\ \cancel{g}} \times \frac{1\ cap}{100\ \cancel{mg}} = 2\ cap$$

So, 2 *capsules* of this anticonvulsant drug would contain the dose.

EXAMPLE 6.12

The order is *Tikosyn (dofetilide) 0.5 mg PO b.i.d.* Read the label shown in • Figure 6.12. Calculate how many *capsules* of this antiarrythmic drug should be given to the patient. Although there are two strengths on the label (*mcg* and *mg*), calculate the problem using *microgram* strength.

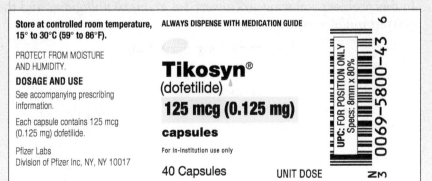

Store at controlled room temperature, 15° to 30°C (59° to 86°F).

PROTECT FROM MOISTURE AND HUMIDITY.

DOSAGE AND USE

See accompanying prescribing information.

Each capsule contains 125 mcg (0.125 mg) dofetilide.

Pfizer Labs
Division of Pfizer Inc, NY, NY 10017

ALWAYS DISPENSE WITH MEDICATION GUIDE

Tikosyn®
(dofetilide)

125 mcg (0.125 mg)

capsules

For in-institution use only

40 Capsules   UNIT DOSE

UPC: FOR POSITION ONLY
Specs: 8mm x 80%

0069-5800-43

• **Figure 6.12**
Drug label for Tikosyn.

(Reg. trademark of Pfizer Inc. Reproduced with permission.)

> **NOTE**
>
> Although Example 6.12 would be simpler using *milligrams*, we will do the calculation using *micrograms* to practice complex problems. For safety purposes, drug manufacturers often place both *microgram* and *milligram* concentrations on drug labels.

Dose: 0.5 *mg*
Strength: 1 *tab* = 125 *mcg*
Administer: ? *cap*

In this problem you want to convert 0.5 *milligrams* to *micrograms* and then convert *micrograms* to *capsules*.

$$0.5 \; mg \longrightarrow \; ? \; mcg \longrightarrow \; ? \; cap$$

You can do this on one line as follows:

$$0.5 \; mg \times \frac{? \; mcg}{? \; mg} \times \frac{1 \; cap}{? \; mcg} = \; ? \; cap$$

Because 1,000 *mcg* = 1 *mg*, the first unit fraction is $\dfrac{1{,}000 \; mcg}{1 \; mg}$

Because 1 *cap* = 125 *mcg*, the second unit fraction is $\dfrac{1 \; cap}{125 \; mcg}$

$$0.5 \; \cancel{mg} \times \frac{\overset{8}{\cancel{1{,}000}} \; \cancel{mcg}}{1 \; \cancel{mg}} \times \frac{1 \; \boxed{cap}}{\underset{1}{\cancel{125} \; \cancel{mcg}}} = 4 \; cap$$

So, you should give 4 *capsules* by mouth twice a day to the patient.

EXAMPLE 6.13

Order: *lithium carbonate 1.8 g PO daily in three divided doses.* The strength of the *lithium carbonate* is 600 *mg* per capsule. Calculate how many *capsules* of this antidepressant drug the patient will receive.

Order: 1.8 *g*
Strength: 1 *cap* = 600 *mg*
Administer: ? *cap*

In this problem you want to convert 1.8 *grams* to *milligrams* and then convert *milligrams* to *capsules*.

$$1.8 \; g \longrightarrow \; ? \; mg \longrightarrow \; ? \; cap$$

You can do this on one line as follows:

$$\frac{1.8\ g}{1} \times \frac{?\ mg}{?\ g} \times \frac{?\ cap}{?\ mg} = ?\ cap$$

Because 1,000 mg = 1 g, the first unit fraction is $\dfrac{1,000\ mg}{1\ g}$

Because the strength is 1 cap = 600 mg, the second unit fraction is $\dfrac{1\ cap}{600\ mg}$

$$\frac{1.8\ g}{1} \times \frac{1,000\ mg}{1\ g} \times \frac{1\ cap}{600\ mg} = ?\ cap$$

Now cancel and multiply.

$$\frac{1.8\ \cancel{g}}{1} \times \frac{1,000\ \cancel{mg}}{1\ \cancel{g}} \times \frac{1\ cap}{600\ \cancel{mg}} = 3\ cap$$

Because the order indicates "three divided doses," the patient would receive one 600-mg $capsule$ 3 times a day.

EXAMPLE 6.14

The physician orders *Norvir (ritonavir) 0.6 g PO b.i.d. with meals.* Read the label in • Figure 6.13 and determine the number of *mL* of this protease inhibitor your patient would receive.

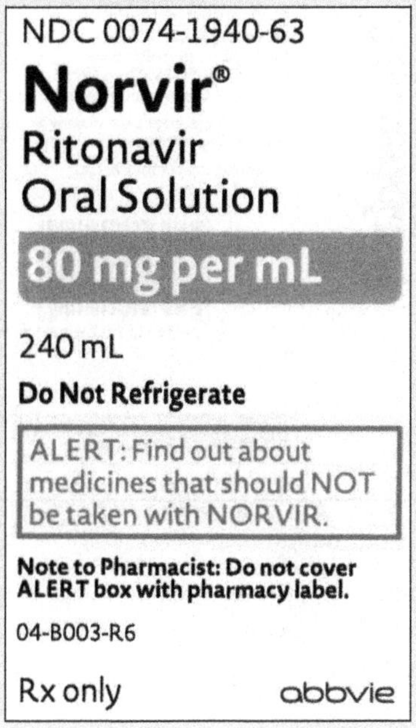

NDC 0074-1940-63

Norvir®
Ritonavir
Oral Solution

80 mg per mL

240 mL

Do Not Refrigerate

ALERT: Find out about medicines that should NOT be taken with NORVIR.

Note to Pharmacist: Do not cover ALERT box with pharmacy label.

04-B003-R6

Rx only   abbvie

• **Figure 6.13**
Drug label for Norvir.

Order: 0.6 g
Strength: 80 *mg/mL*
Administer: ? *mL*

In this problem you want to convert 0.6 *grams* to *milligrams* and then convert *milligrams* to *milliliters*.

$$0.6 \, g \longrightarrow ? \, mg \longrightarrow ? \, mL$$

You can do this on one line as follows:

$$0.6 \, g \times \frac{? \, mg}{? \, g} \times \frac{? \, mL}{? \, mg} = ? \, mL$$

Because 1,000 *mg* = 1 *g*, the first unit fraction is $\dfrac{1{,}000 \, mg}{1 \, g}$

Because 1 *mL* = 80 *mg*, the second unit fraction is $\dfrac{1 \, mL}{80 \, mg}$

$$0.6 \, \cancel{g} \times \frac{1{,}000 \, \cancel{mg}}{1 \, \cancel{g}} \times \frac{1 \, mL}{80 \, \cancel{mg}} = \frac{60}{8} \, mL = 7.5 \, mL$$

So, you would give 7.5 *mL* by mouth to the patient twice a day with meals.

NOTE

In Example 6.15, the order states "in 2 divided doses." This instructs the practitioner to separate the total daily dose into 2 equal parts over a 24-hour period. To ensure even distribution of the medication, the frequency of the doses should also be regular and consistent, so the drug is administered every 12 hours.

EXAMPLE 6.15

The order is for *Namenda (memantine HCL) oral solution 20 mg PO in 2 divided doses.* Read the label in • Figure 6.14 and determine the number of *teaspoons* of this dementia drug you should administer.

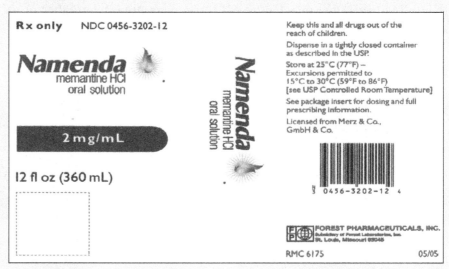

• Figure 6.14
Drug label for Namenda.

Order:	20 *mg*
Strength:	2 *mg* per 1 *mL*
Administer:	? *t*

In this problem you want to convert 20 *milligrams* to *milliliters* and then convert *mL* to *teaspoons*.

$$20 \, mg \longrightarrow ? \, mL \longrightarrow ? \, t$$

You can do this on one line as follows:

$$\frac{20\ mg}{1} \times \frac{?\ mL}{?\ mg} \times \frac{?\ t}{?\ mL} = ?\ t$$

Because the strength is $2\ mg = 1\ mL$, the first unit fraction is $\dfrac{1\ mL}{2\ mg}$

Because $5\ mL = 1\ t$, the second unit fraction is $\dfrac{1\ t}{5\ mL}$

$$\frac{20\ mg}{1} \times \frac{1\ mL}{2\ mg} \times \frac{1\ t}{5\ mL} = ?\ t$$

Now cancel and multiply.

$$\frac{20\ \cancel{mg}}{1} \times \frac{1\ \cancel{mL}}{2\ \cancel{mg}} \times \frac{1\ t}{5\ \cancel{mL}} = 2\ t$$

Because the order specifies "2 divided doses," the 2 *t* must be divided into 2 equal amounts over 24 *hours*. Therefore, you would give 1 *teaspoon* of Namenda to the patient every 12 *h* by mouth.

Dosages Based on the Size of the patient

Sometimes the amount of medication prescribed is based on the patient's size. A patient who is larger will receive a larger dose of the drug, and a patient who is smaller will receive a smaller dose of the drug. The size of a patient is measured by either *body weight* or *body surface area* (*BSA*). In general, when the order is based on the size of the patient, if you multiply the *size of the patient* by the *order*, you will obtain the *dose*. This can be expressed by the shortcut formula

$$Size\ of\ patient \times Order = Dose$$

Dosages Based on Body Weight

When an order is based on the body weight of the patient, the patient's weight is expressed in *kilograms*. For example, an order might indicate that the patient should receive "*5 g/kg*", this is read "*5 grams per kilogram*", and it means that the patient should receive *5 grams* of the drug for each kilogram of the patient's body weight. Based on such an order, a neonate weighing *1 kg* should receive *5 g* of the drug, one weighing *2 kg* should receive *10 g* of the drug, a baby weighing *3 kg* should receive *15 g* of the drug, and so on.

Because the amount of drug to be administered is proportional to the patient's weight, Dimensional Analysis methods can be used to determine the appropriate drug dosage. It is easier, however, to use the shortcut formula. Both methods are shown in Example 6.16, but throughout the remainder of this book, the shortcut formula will be preferred.

EXAMPLE 6.16

Order: *Dilantin (phenytoin) 15 mg/kg loading dose PO, then 300 mg/d.* For the loading dose, how many *mg* of this anticonvulsant would you administer to a patient who weighs 80 *kg*?

Body weight: 80 *kg*

Order: 15 *mg/kg*

Dose: ? *mg*

You want to "change" the body weight of the patient (80 *kg*) to *milligrams* of drug. The order is 15 *mg/kg*, so use the formula

$$Size\ of\ patient \times Order = Dose$$

$$80\ kg \times \frac{15\ mg}{1\ kg} = 1,200\ mg$$

Therefore, the patient should receive 1,200 *mg* of Dilantin for the loading dose.

EXAMPLE 6.17

Order: *Vibramycin (doxycycline calcium) 2 mg/lb daily PO for 10 days.* Read the label in • Figure 6.15 and determine how many *milliliters* of this antibiotic you would administer to a patient who weighs 90 *lb*.

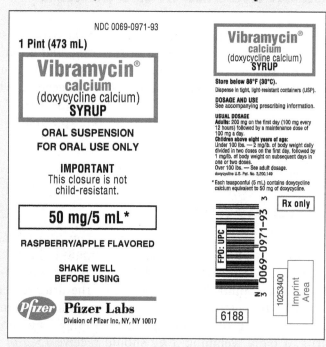

• Figure 6.15
Drug label for Vibramycin.

Patient weight: 90 *lb*

Order: 2 *mg/lb*

Strength: 50 *mg/5 mL*

Administer: ? *mL*

When an order is based on the size of the patient, you can use this formula:

Size of the Patient × *Order* = *Dose*

$$\frac{90 \; \cancel{lb}}{1} \times \frac{2 \; mg}{\cancel{lb}} = 180 \; mg$$

Now convert the dose of 180 *mg* to *mL*.

$$180 \; mg = ? \; mL$$

Because each 5 *mL* of the solution contains 50 *mg* of the drug, the unit fraction is $\dfrac{5 \; mL}{50 \; mg}$

$$\frac{180 \; \cancel{mg}}{1} \times \frac{5 \; mL}{50 \; \cancel{mg}} = 18 \; mL$$

So, the patient should receive 18 *mL* of Vibramycin daily for 10 days.

EXAMPLE 6.18

The physician orders *Biaxin (clarithromycin) 7.5 milligrams per kilogram PO q12h.* If the drug strength is 250 *milligrams* per 5 *mL*, how many *mL* of this antibiotic drug should be administered to a patient who weighs 154 *pounds*?

Patient weight: 154 *lb*

Order: 7.5 *mg/kg*

Strength: 250 *mg/5 mL*

Administer: ? *ml*

The first step is to change the body weight of the patient from 154 *pounds* to an equivalent weight in *kilograms*.

$$154 \; lb = ? \; kg$$

Because 1 *kg* = 2.2 *lb*, the unit fraction will be $\dfrac{1 \; kg}{2.2 \; lb}$.

$$\frac{154 \; \cancel{lb}}{1} \times \frac{1 \; kg}{2.2 \; \cancel{lb}} = 70 \; kg$$

When the order is based on the size of the patient, use the formula:

Size of the Patient × *Order* = *Dose*

$$\frac{70 \; \cancel{kg}}{1} \times \frac{7.5 \; mg}{\cancel{kg}} = 525 \; mg$$

Now convert 525 *mg* to *mL*.
   Because the strength is 250 *mg* per 5 *mL*, the unit fraction will be $\dfrac{5 \; mL}{250 \; mg}$

$$\frac{525 \; \cancel{mg}}{1} \times \frac{5 \; mL}{250 \; \cancel{mg}} = 10.5 \; mL$$

The problem could have been done in one line as follows:

$$\frac{154 \, lb}{1} \times \frac{1 \, kg}{2.2 \, lb} \times \frac{7.5 \, mg}{kg} \times \frac{5 \, mL}{250 \, mg} = 10.5 \, mL$$

So, the patient should receive 10.5 *mL* of Biaxin by mouth every 12 hours.

Dosages Based on Body Surface area (BSA)

NOTE

Use a search engine, such as Google, to search the Web for "body surface area calculators" to obtain links to online BSA calculators.

In some cases, *body surface area (BSA)* may be used rather than *weight* in determining appropriate drug dosages. This is particularly true when calculating dosages for children, those receiving cancer therapy, burn patients, and patients requiring critical care. A patient's BSA can be estimated by using formulas.

BSA Formulas

Body surface area can be approximated by formula using either a handheld calculator or an online Web site. BSA, which is measured in square *meters* (m^2), can be determined by using either of the following two mathematical formulas:

Formula for metric units:

$$BSA = \sqrt{\frac{\text{weight in kilograms} \times \text{height in centimeters}}{3,600}}$$

Formula for household units:

$$BSA = \sqrt{\frac{\text{weight in pounds} \times \text{height in inches}}{3,131}}$$

NOTE

In Example 6.19, the metric formula for BSA was used, and in Example 6.20, the household formula for BSA was used. However, each formula provided the BSA measured in square meters (m^2). In this book, we will round off BSA to two decimal places.

EXAMPLE 6.19

Find the BSA of an adult who is 183 *cm* tall and weighs 92 *kg*.

Because this example has metric units (kilograms and centimeters), we use the following formula:

$$BSA = \sqrt{\frac{\text{weight in kilograms} \times \text{height in centimeters}}{3,600}}$$

$$= \sqrt{\frac{92 \times 183}{3,600}}$$

At this point we need a calculator with a square-root key.

$$= \sqrt{4.6767}$$
$$= 2.16256$$

Therefore, the BSA of this adult is 2.16 m^2.

EXAMPLE 6.20

What is the BSA of a man who is 5 *feet* 6 *inches* tall and weighs 168 *pounds*?

First you convert 5 *feet* 6 *inches* to 66 *inches*.

Because the example has household units (*pounds* and *inches*), we use the following formula:

$$BSA = \sqrt{\frac{\text{weight in pounds} \times \text{height in inches}}{3,131}}$$

$$= \sqrt{\frac{168 \times 66}{3,131}}$$

$$= \sqrt{3.5414}$$

$$= 1.8819$$

Therefore, the BSA of this adult is 1.88 m^2.

EXAMPLE 6.21

The physician orders 40 *mg/m*^{2} of a drug PO once daily. How many *milligrams* of the drug would you administer to an adult patient weighing 88 *kg* with a height of 150 *cm*?

The first step is to determine the BSA of the patient.

Using the formula, you get

$$BSA = \sqrt{\frac{88 \times 150}{3,600}}$$

$$= \sqrt{3.6667}$$

$$= 1.91 \ m^2$$

BSA: 1.91 m^2

Order: 40 *mg/m*^{2}

Find: ? *mg*

The patient's BSA is 1.91 m^2, and the order is for 40 *mg/m*^{2}. Multiply the *size of the patient* by the *order* to determine how many *milligrams* of the drug to give the patient.

$$1.91 \ m^2 \times \frac{40 \ mg}{m^2} = 76.4 \ mg$$

You would administer 76.4 *mg* of the drug to the patient.

ALERT

Before a medication is administered, it is the responsibility of the healthcare practitioner administering the medication to check the *safe dosage and administration range* for the drug in the *Physicians' Desk Reference* (PDR), in a designated drug book, on the manufacturer's Web site, or with the pharmacist.

EXAMPLE 6.22

The prescriber ordered 30 mg/m^2 of a drug PO stat for a patient who has a BSA of 1.65 m^2. The "safe dose range" for this drug is 20 to 40 mg per day. Calculate the prescribed dose in *milligrams* and determine if it is within the safe range.

BSA: 1.65 m^2
Order: 30 mg/m^2
Find: ? mg

The patient's BSA is 1.65 m^2, and the order is for 30 mg/m^2. Multiply the *size of the patient* by the *order* to determine how many *milligrams* of the drug to give the patient.

$$1.65 \; m^2 \times \frac{30 \; mg}{m^2} = 49.5 \; mg$$

The safe dose range is 20–40 mg per day.

So, the dose prescribed, 49.5 mg, is higher than the upper limit (40 mg) of the daily safe dose range. It is an overdose. Therefore, the prescribed dose is not safe, and you may not administer this drug. You must consult with the prescriber.

EXAMPLE 6.23

Order: *leucovorin calcium 10 mg/m^2 PO q6h until serum methotrexate level is less than* . The strength of the *leucovorin calcium* is 15 mg per tablet. Calculate how many *tablets* you will administer to a patient who has a BSA of 1.49 m^2. The package information states that these are scored *tablets*.

BSA: 1.49 m^2 [single unit of measurement]

Order: 10 mg/m^2 [equivalence]

Strength: 1 tab = 15 mg [equivalence]

Administer: ? tab [single unit of measurement]

The patient's BSA is 1.49 m^2, and the order is 10 mg/m^2. First, multiply the *size of the patient* by the *order* to determine how many *milligrams* of the drug to give the patient, and then use the strength to change the resulting *milligrams* to tablets. This can be done in one line as follows:

$$1.49 \; \cancel{m^2} \times \frac{10 \; mg}{\cancel{m^2}} \times \frac{1 \; tab}{15 \; \cancel{mg}} = 0.993 \; tab$$

So, you will administer 1 *tablet* to the patient by mouth every 6 hours.

Summary

In this chapter, you learned the computations necessary to calculate dosages of oral medications in liquid and solid form. You also learned about the equipment used to accurately measure liquid medication.

- It is crucial to ensure that every medication administered is within the recommended safe dosage range.

Calculating doses for oral medications in solid and liquid form

- The label states the strength of the drug (e.g., 10 mg/tab, 15 mg/mL).
- Sometimes oral medications are ordered in liquid form for special populations such as pediatrics, geriatrics, and patients with neurological conditions.
- Some medication cups cannot accurately measure volumes less than 5 mL.
- Special calibrated droppers or oral syringes that are supplied with some liquid oral medications may be used to administer *only those medications*.
- Some drugs, such as electrolytes, are measured in *milliequivalents* (*mEq*).

Calculating doses based on body weight

- Dosages based on body weight are generally measured in *milligrams* per *kilogram* (*mg/kg*).
- Start calculations with the weight of the patient.
- To change pounds to *kilograms* quickly, merely divide by 2.2.
- Multiply the size of the patient (*kg*) by the order to obtain the dose.
- Size of the Patient × Order = Dose
- Medications may be prescribed by body weight in special populations such as pediatrics and geriatrics.

Calculating doses based on body surface area

- Body surface area (BSA) is measured in square *meters* (*m^2*).
- Start calculations with the BSA of the patient.
- Multiply the size of the patient (*m^2*) by the order to obtain the dose.
- Size of the Patient × Order = Dose
- BSA is estimated by using a formula.
- BSA may be used to determine dosages for special patient populations such as those receiving cancer therapy or burn therapy and for patients requiring critical care.

Case Study 6.1

Read the case study and answer the questions. Answers can be found in Appendix A.

A 58-year-old male who has a history of angina, type II diabetes mellitus, hypertension, and hyperlipidemia has had a cardiac catheterization. He is 6 *feet* tall and weighs 325 *pounds* and has a very stressful job in financial services. His vital signs are stable, there is no bleeding from the catheterization site, and he is awaiting his discharge. Review his discharge orders, and use the labels to answer the questions if required.

Discharge Orders

- 2,200 calorie ADA diet
- Follow-up with PMD in one week
- Janumet (sitagliptin/metformin HCl) 50/1,000 *mg* PO B.I.D.
- lansoprazole 30 *mg* PO daily before breakfast
- Xanax (alprazolam) 2 *mg* PO prn anxiety
- Lipitor (atorvastatin calcium) 40 *mg* PO daily
- Lovaza (omega-3-acid ethyl esters) 2 *g* PO B.I.D.
- lisinopril/hydrochlorothiazide 20/12.5 *mg* PO daily
- Tricor (fenofibrate) 48 *mg* PO daily
- Amaryl (glimepiride) 2 *mg* PO daily with breakfast
- Plavix (clopidogrel bisulfate) 75 *mg* PO daily

- Coreg (carvedilol) 12.5 *mg* PO B.I.D.
- Sumaycin (tetracycline HCl) 500 *mg* PO B.I.D.

1. Select the appropriate label and calculate how many *tablets* of sitagliptin/metformin the patient must take for each dose.
2. How many *capsules* of omega-3-acid ethyl esters contain the dose?
3. How many *tablets* of atorvastatin will the patient take each day?
4. Calculate the number of *tablets* of carvedilol the patient will take per day.
5. How many *tablets* of alprazolam may the patient take per dose?
6. What is the dose of clopidogrel in *grams*?
7. How many *tablets* of fenofibrate will the patient take in four weeks?
8. The strength of the glimepiride is 1 *mg/tab*. How many *tablets* contain the dose?
9. How many *capsules* of lansoprazole contain the dose?
10. The strength of the tetracycline is 250 *mg/cap*. How many *capsules* will the patient take per day?
11. Calculate the patient's BSA.

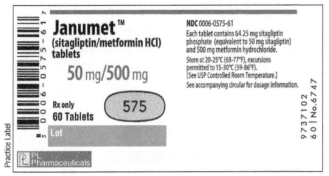

(a) **(For educational purposes only)**

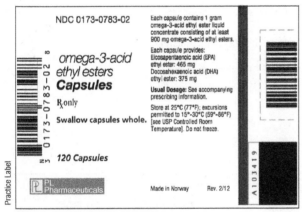

(b) **(For educational purposes only)**

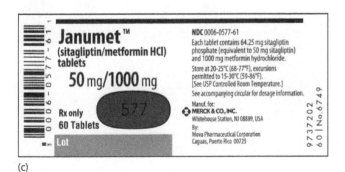

(c)

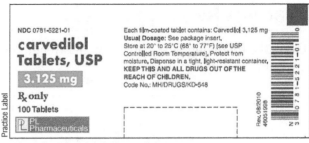

(e) **(For educational purposes only)**

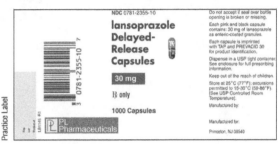

(f) **(For educational purposes only)**

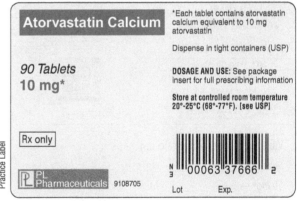

(g) **(For educational purposes only)**

(d)

(h)

Drug labels for Case Study 6.1

Practice Reading Labels

Using the following labels, identify the strength of the medication and calculate the doses indicated. The answers are found in Appendix A .

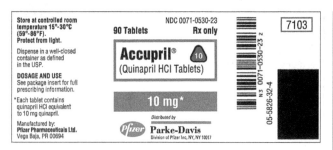

1. Accupril (quinapril HCl)

   Strength: _____

   10 mg = _____ tab

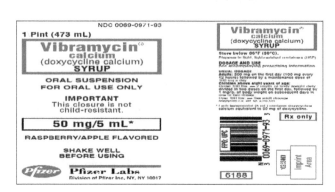

2. Vibramycin (doxycycline calcium)

   Strength: _____

   50 mg = _____ mL

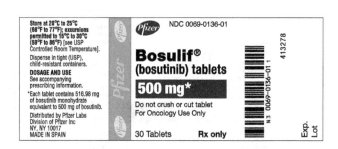

3. Bosulif (bosutinib)

   Strength: _____

   1 g = _____ tab

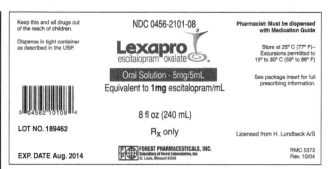

4. Lexapro (escitalopram oxalate)

   Strength: _____

   15 mg = _____ mL

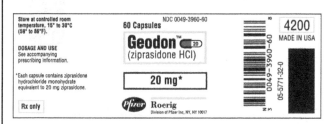

5. Geodon (ziprasidone HCl)

   Strength: _____

   40 mg = _____ cap

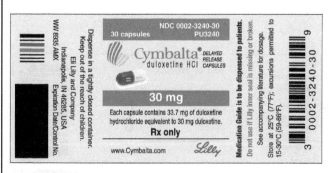

6. Cymbalta (duloxetine HCl)

   Strength: _____

   60 mg = _____ cap

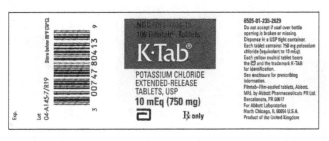

7. K-Tab (potassium chloride)

Strength: _____

20 *mEq* _____ *tab*

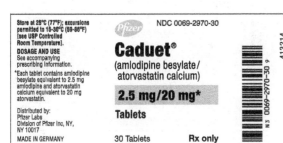

8. Caduet (amlodipine besylate/atorvastatin calcium)

Strength: _____

5 *mg*/40 *mg* = _____ *tab*

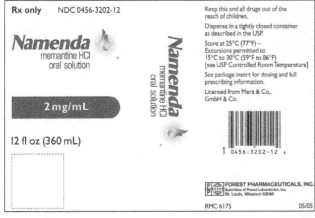

9. Namenda (memantine HCl)

Strength: _____

4 *mg* = _____ *mL*

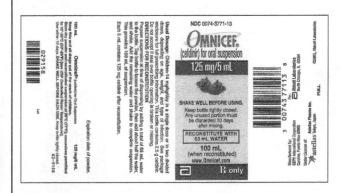

10. Vicodin ES (hydrocodone bitartrate and acetaminophen)

Strength: _____

15 *mg*/600 *mg* = _____ *tab*

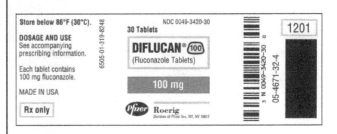

11. Omnicef (cefdinir) oral suspension

Strength: _____

500 *mg* = _____ *mL*

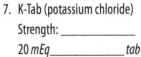

12. Diflucan (fluconazole)

Strength: _____

300 *mg* = _____ *tab*

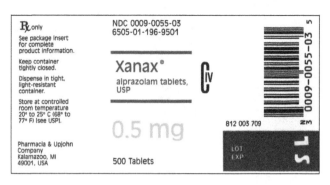

13. Xanax (alprazolam)

Strength: _____

1 *mg* = _____ *tab*

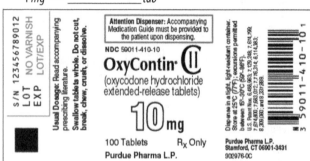

14. Oxycontin (oxycodone hydrochloride extended release)

Strength: _____

20 *mg* = _____ *tab*

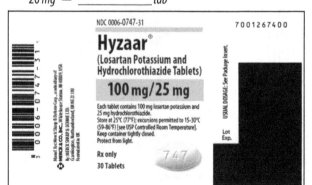

15. Hyzaar (lorsartan potassium and hydrochlorothiazide)

Strength: _____

300 *mg*/75 *mg* = _____ *tab*

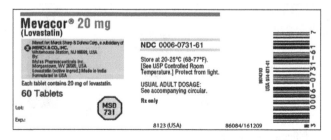

16. Mevacor (lovastatin)

Strength: _____

40 *mg* = _____ *tab*

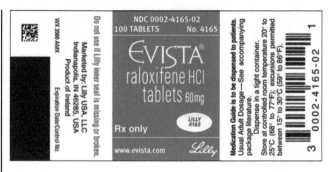

17. Evista (raloxifene HCl)

Strength: _____

60 *mg* = _____ *tab*

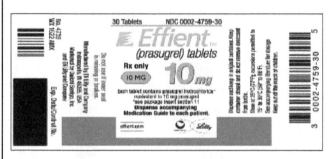

18. Effient (prasugrel)

Strength: _____

60 *mg* = _____ *tab*

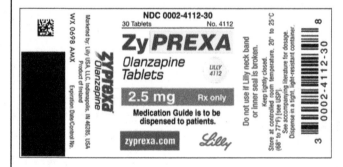

19. ZyPREXA (olanzapine)

Strength: _____

5 *mg* = _____ *tab*

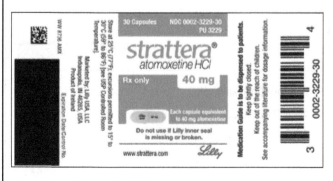

20. Strattera (atomoxetine HCl)

Strength: _____

80 *mg* = _____ *cap*

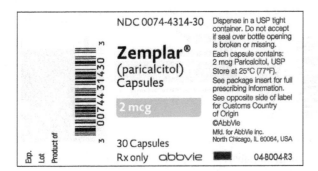

21. Zemplar (paricalcitol)

Strength: _____

6 *mcg* = _____ *cap*

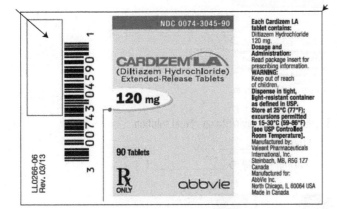

22. Cardizem LA (diltiazem HCl)

Strength: _____

480 *mg* = _____ *tab*

Singulair® 10 mg
(Montelukast Sodium) TABLETS
For Adults 15 Years of Age and Older

23. Singulair (montelukast sodium)

Strength: _____

20 *mg* = _____ *tab*

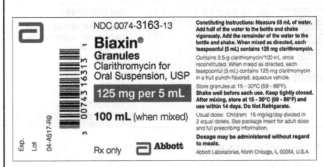

24. Depakene (valproic acid)

Strength: _____

750 *mg* = _____ *mL*

25. Biaxin (clarithromycin)

Strength: _____

500 *mg* = _____ *mL*

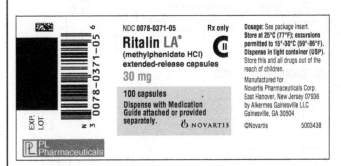

26. Ritalin (methylphenidate HCl)

Strength: _____

60 *mg* = _____ *cap*

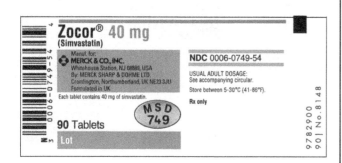

27. Zocor (simvastatin)

    Strength: _____

    80 *mg* = _____ *tab*

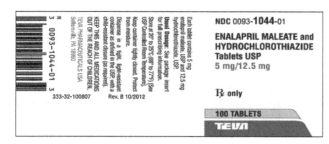

28. enalapril maleate and hydrochlorothazide

    Strength: _____

    10 *mg*/25 *mg* = _____ *tab*

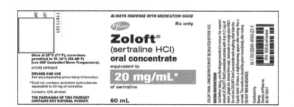

29. Zoloft (sertraline HCl)

    Strength: _____

    120 *mg* = _____ *mL*

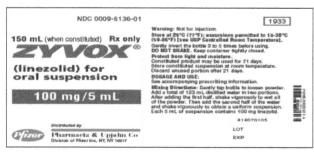

30. Zyvox (linezolid)

    Strength: _____

    400 *mg* = _____ *t*

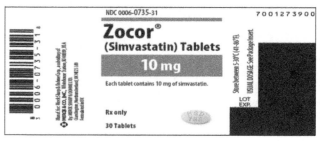

31. Zocor (simvastatin)

    Strength: _____

    20 *mg* = _____ *tab*

NDC 0074-3956-46

Kaletra®

Lopinavir/Ritonavir
Oral Solution

80 mg/20 mg per mL

160 mL

ALERT: Find out about medicines
that should NOT be taken with
KALETRA

Attention Pharmacist: Do not cover
ALERT box with pharmacy label.
Dispense the enclosed Medication
Guide to each patient.
04-B092-R5
Rx only   abbvie

32. Kaletra (lopinavir/ritonavir) oral solution

    Strength: _____

    400 *mg*/100 *mg* = _____ *t*

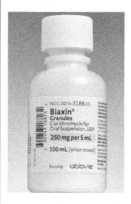

33. Biaxin (clarithromycin oral suspension)

    Strength: _____

    500 *mg* = _____ *t*

34. Dilantin (extended phenytoin sodium)

    Strength: _____

    300 *mg* = _____ *cap*

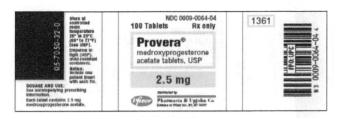

35. Provera (medroxyprogesterone acetate)

    Strength: _____

    5 mg = _____ tab

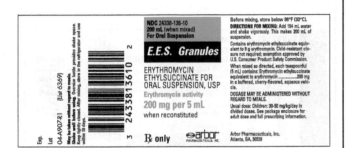

36. E.E.S. Granules (erythromycin ethylsuccinate)

    Strength: _____

    400 mg = _____ mL

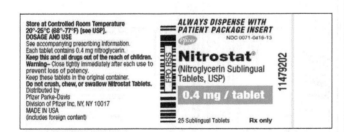

37. Nitrostat (nitroglycerin)

    Strength: _____

    0.4 mg = _____ tab

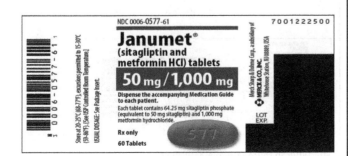

38. Janumet (sitagliptin and metformin)

    Strength: _____

    100 mg/2,000 mg = _____ tab

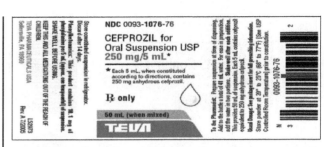

39. cefprozil

    Strength: _____

    500 mg = _____ mL

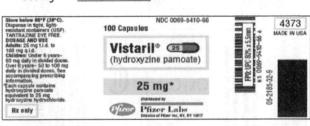

40. Vistaril (hydroxyzine pamoate)

    Strength: _____

    75 mg = _____ cap

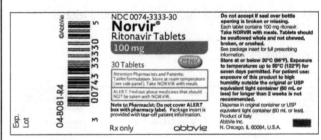

41. Norvir (ritonavir)

    Strength: _____

    600 mg = _____ tab

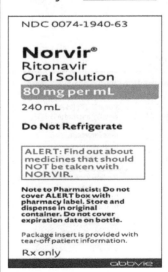

42. Norvir (ritonavir)

    Strength: _____

    600 mg = _____ mL

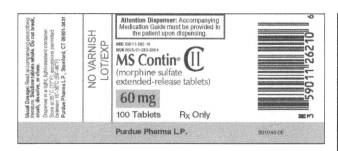

43. MS Contin (morphine sulfate controlled-release)

Strength: _____

60 *mg* = _____ tab

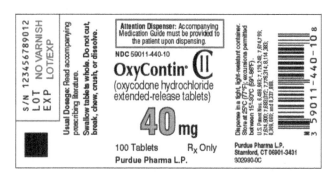

44. OxyContin (oxycodone hydrochloride controlled-release)

Strength: _____

80 *mg* = _____ tab

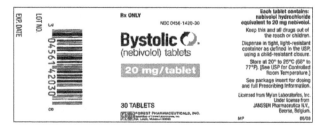

45. Bystolic (nebivolol)

Strength: _____

40 *mg* = _____ tab

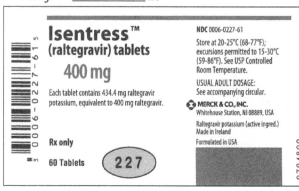

46. Isentress (raltegravir)

Strength: _____

400 *mg* = _____ tab

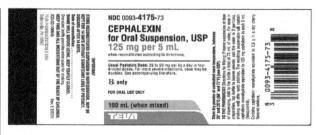

47. cephalexin for oral suspension

Strength: _____

500 *mg* = _____ mL

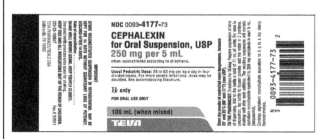

48. cephalexin for oral suspension

Strength: _____

500 *mg* = _____ mL

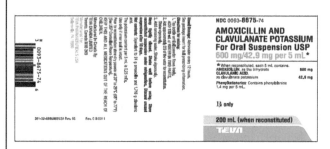

49. amoxicillin and clavulanate potassium oral suspension

Strength: _____

1,200 *mg*/85.8 *mg* = _____ mL

50. Diflucan (fluconazole) oral suspension

Strength: _____

100 *mg* = _____ mL

Practice Sets

The answers to *Try These for Practice*, *Exercises*, and *Cumulative Review Exercises* are found in Appendix A. Ask your instructor for the answers to the *Additional Exercises*.

Note: Remember that throughout this text when you are asked to calculate the amount of drug to administer, it is assumed to be the amount "per administration"—unless specified otherwise.

Try These for Practice

Test your comprehension after reading the chapter.

1. Use the formula to estimate the BSA of a person who is 153 *centimeters* tall and who weighs 72 *kilograms*.

2. Order: *Dilantin (phenytoin suspension) 250 mg po t.i.d.* The strength of the drug is 125 *mg/5 mL.* How many *teaspoons* will you administer?

3. Order: *calcitriol oral solution 0.5 mcg PO every other day.* The strength of the *calcitriol* is 1 *mcg/mL.* Determine how many *milliliters* contain the dose.

4. The prescriber ordered 150 *mg/m²* of a drug PO q6h for *5 days* for a patient who has a BSA of 1.4 *m².* How many *grams* will the patient receive in total for the 5 days?

5. Order: *paregoric 10 mL PO prn after loose bowel movement, maximum 4 times daily.* The strength of this antidiarrheal drug is 2 *mg/5 mL.* How many *milligrams* will the patient receive?

Exercises

Reinforce your understanding in class or at home.

1. Order: *Coumadin (warfarin sodium) 7.5 mg po daily.* The strength of the scored *tablets* is 2.5 *mg/tablet.* How many *tablets* of this vitamin K antagonist would be given to the patient who has venous thrombosis?

2. Order: *Dynapen (dicloxacillin sodium) 250 mg po q6h for 7 days.* The strength of the oral suspension is 62.5 *mg/5 mL.* How many *teaspoons* will you administer to the patient who has an upper respiratory tract infection?

3. The dosage range for the antineoplastic agent Mithracin (plicamycin) is 25–30 *mcg/kg* daily. What is the safe dosage range in *mg* per day for a patient who weighs 190 *pounds* and has a malignant tumor?

4. The daily safe dose range for a certain drug is 1–5*mg/m²*. A 6-foot-tall patient who weighs 200 *pounds* is scheduled to receive 40 *mg* of the drug each day. Is the scheduled dose safe for this patient?

5. Order: *Tegretol (carbamazepine) 200 mg po b.i.d.* The strength of the oral suspension is 100 *mg/5 mL*. How many *teaspoons* will you give the patient who has bipolar disorder?

6. Use the formula to estimate the BSA of a person who is 160 *cm* tall and weighs 83 *kg*.

7. Order: *Anadrol-50 (oxymetholone) 200 mg po daily.* The recommended dose for this anabolic steroid is 1–5 *mg/kg/d*. Is the prescribed order in the recommended range for a patient who has aplastic anemia and weighs 75 *kg*?

8. The prescribed order is *120 mg/m²/d × 14 days PO.* How many *grams* will the patient who has a BSA of 1.4 *m²* receive in total after this two-week regimen?

9. See • Figure 6.16 to determine the number of capsules of Cymbalta (duloxetine hydrochloride) that you would administer each day after the first week to a patient who has fibromyalgia.

ROUTE & DOSAGE

Depression
Adult: PO 40–60 mg/d in one or two divided doses

Generalized Anxiety/Diabetic Neuropathy
Adult: PO 60 mg once daily

Fibromyalagia
Adult: PO 30 mg/d in × 1 wk then 60 mg/d

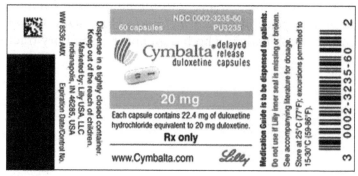

• **Figure 6.16**
Exerpt from a drug guide and the drug label for Cymbalta.

10. A drug is ordered 100 *mg/m²* PO B.I.D. How many *milliliters* will a patient receive if her BSA is 1.80 *m²* and the concentration of the solution is 100 *mg/5 mL*?

11. Order: *Aldactazide (spironolactone and hydrochlorothiazide) 100 mg/100 mg PO B.I.D.* Read the label in • **Figure 6.17** and determine how many *tablets* of this diuretic you will administer.

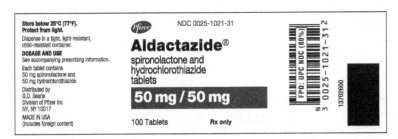

• **Figure 6.17**
Drug label for Aldactazide.

12. Order: *alprazolam 0.25 mg PO T.I.D.* The strength of the *alprazolam* is 1 *mg/mL.* Determine how many *milliliters* of this antianxiety drug you will administer.

13. The prescriber ordered *Bosulif (bosutinib) 500 mg PO daily to be given with food for a patient who has chronic myelogenous leukemia (CML).* Read the label in • **Figure 6.18** and determine how many *tablets* to administer.

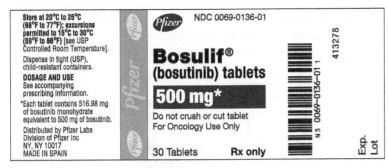

• **Figure 6.18**
Drug label for Bosulif.

Workspace

14. The prescriber ordered *lithium citrate 0.6 g po T.I.D.* for a patient with acute mania. The recommended dosage range is 600 *mg* to 1200 *mg* daily in three or four divided doses. Read the label in • **Figure 6.19** and

    (a) Determine if the prescribed dose is safe.
    (b) If the dose is safe, determine how many *milliliters* you will administer.

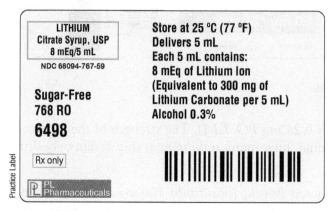

• **Figure 6.19**
Drug label for lithium. (For educational purposes only)

15. Read the label in • **Figure 6.20** and determine the number of *grams* of OxyContin (oxycodone HCl) that are contained in the entire bottle.

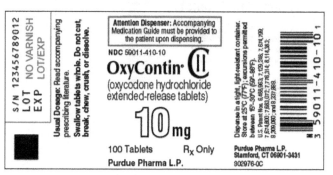

• **Figure 6.20**
Drug label for OxyContin.

16. Estimate the body surface area of a patient who is *5 feet* tall and weighs *60 kg*.

17. A drug is ordered *50 mg/m² po b.i.d.* How many *mL* will a patient receive if her BSA is 1.44 m^2 and the concentration of the solution is *2 mg/mL*?

18. Order: *Lexapro (escitalopram oxalate) 10 mg po daily.* Read the label in • **Figure 6.21** and determine the number of *milliliters* of this antidepressant that a geriatric patient who has generalized anxiety will receive in a week.

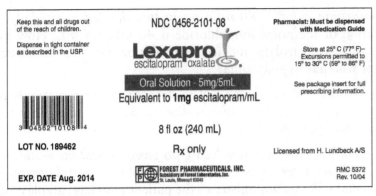

● **Figure 6.21**
Drug label for Lexapro.

19. Order: *digoxin 0.75 mg po stat*. How many *0.25 mg tablets* of this antiarrhythmic drug will you administer to the patient?

20. Order: *Percocet (oxycodone/acetaminophen) 10/650 mg po prn pain q6h*. How many *5/325 mg tablets* of this opioid analgesic will you administer to the patient?

Additional Exercises

Now, test yourself!

1. Order: *Depakene (valproic acid) 750 mg/day po in three divided doses*. Read the label in ● **Figure 6.22**. How many *capsules* of this anticonvulsant will you administer to the patient who has mania?

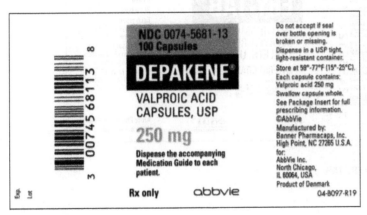

● **Figure 6.22**
Drug label for Depakene.

2. Order: *Xanax (alprazolam) 1.5 mg po t.i.d.* How many *0.5 mg tablets* of this antianxiety drug will you administer to the patient who suffers from panic attacks?

3. Order: *amoxicillin oral suspension 500 mg po q8h*. The concentration of the amoxicillin solution is *125 mg/5 mL*. How many *milliliters* of this antibiotic will you administer to the patient who has a mild infection?

4. Order: *potassium chloride 80 mEq po in two divided doses daily*. The concentration of the potassium chloride is *40 mEq/15 mL*. How many *milliliters* of this electrolytic replacement solution will you administer to the patient who has hypokalemia?

5. Order: *furosemide 50 mg po b.i.d.* The strength of the *furosemide* is 10 *mg/mL*. How many teaspoons of this diuretic will you administer to the patient who has high blood pressure?

6. Order: *Xyrem (sodium oxybate) 2.25 g po given at bedtime while in bed and repeat 4 hours later*. How many *milliliters* of this central nervous system depressant will you administer to the patient who has cataplexy if the strength of the Xyrem solution is 500 *mg/mL*?

7. Basketball player Shaquille O'Neal stands 7 *feet* 1 *inch* in height and weighs 325 *pounds*. Estimate his BSA.

8. Entertainer Madonna weighs 52 *kg* and is 160 *cm* in height. Estimate her BSA.

9. A drug is ordered 6 *mg/kg po b.i.d.* How many *tablets* will a patient receive if he weighs 148 *pounds* and the strength of the *tablet* is 200 *mg/tab*?

10. A drug is ordered 200 *mg/m²* po b.i.d. How many *mL* will a patient receive if her BSA is 1.34 *m²*, and the concentration of the solution is 5 *mg/mL*?

11. Order: *ERY-TAB (erythromycin) 333 mg po q8h*. Read the label in • **Figure 6.23**. How many *tablets* of this macrolide antibiotic will you administer to the patient who has a severe infection?

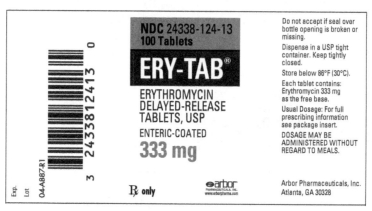

• **Figure 6.23**
Drug label for ERY-TAB.

12. Order: *Kaletra (lopinavir/ritonavir) 800/200 mg po daily*. Read the label in • **Figure 6.24**. How many *mL* of this antiretroviral agent will you administer to the patient who has HIV infection?

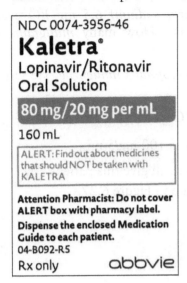

• **Figure 6.24**
Drug label for Kaletra.

13. Order: *metformin hydrochloride 750 mg po b.i.d. with meals*. Read the label in • **Figure 6.25**. How many *tablets* of this antidiabetic drug will you administer to the patient?

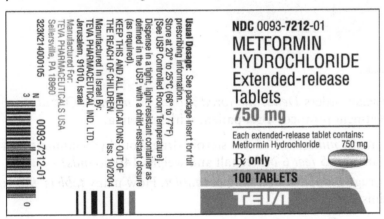

• **Figure 6.25**
Drug label for metformin HCl.

14. Order: *phenobarbitol sodium 400 mg po in two divided doses daily*. The recommended dosage of this anticonvulsant is *1–3 mg/kg/d*. Is the prescribed dose safe for the patient who weighs 203 *pounds*?

15. The physician orders *Detrol LA (tolterodine tartrate) 4 mg PO daily* for a patient with an overactive bladder. Read the label in • **Figure 6.26** and determine how many *capsules* you will give this patient.

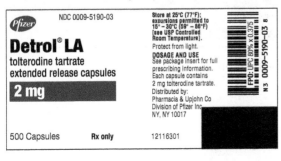

• **Figure 6.26**
Drug label for Detrol LA.

Workspace

16. A patient who has difficulty sleeping is medicated for insomnia with 0.25 *g* of a drug PO at bedtime. The drug is available as *500 mg* per scored *tablet*. How many *tablets* will you administer to your patient?

17. The physician orders *Coumadin (warfarin sodium) 6.5 mg* PO every other day from Monday through Sunday. How many *milligrams* of Coumadin will your patient receive in the week?

18. A physician is treating a patient for *Haemophilus influenzae*. He writes the following prescription:

    cefpodoxime proxetil 200 mg PO q12h for 14 days

    The strength of the cefpodoxime proxetil is 100 mg/5 mL.

    (a) Calculate the number of *milliliters* you will give this patient.
    (b) Indicate the dose on the medication cup in Figure 6.27.

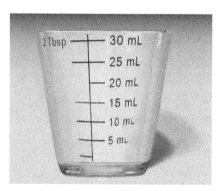

• **Figure 6.27**
Medication cup.

19. The physician orders *Deltasone (prednisone) 60 mg/m²* PO *daily* as part of the treatment protocol for a patient with leukemia.

    (a) How many *milligrams* of this steroid drug would you administer if the patient is *5 feet 6 inches* tall and weighs 140 *pounds*?
    (b) The drug is supplied in *50 mg* per *tablet*. How many *tablets* will you administer?

20. The antibiotic Zithromax (azithromycin) is ordered to treat a patient who has a diagnosis of chronic obstructive pulmonary disease (COPD). The order is:

    Zithromax (azithromycin) 500 mg PO as a single dose on day one, followed by 250 mg once daily on days 2 through 5

    How many *milligrams* will the patient receive by the completion of the prescription?

Cumulative Review Exercises

Review your mastery of previous chapters.

1. $4\ T = ?\ mL$

2. $44\ lb = ?\ kg$

3. $480\ oz = ?\ pt$

4. 47 *mm* = ? *cm*

5. Order: *Ceclor (cefaclor) 100 mg po q.i.d.* The label states *125 mg* per *5 mL*. How many *milliliters* of this antibiotic will you administer?

6. Order: *Zyprexa (olanzapine) 5 mg po daily*. Read the label in • **Figure 6.28** and determine how many tablets of this anti-psychotic drug will administer.

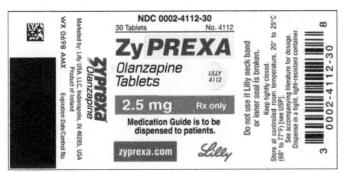

• **Figure 6.28**
Drug label for Zyprexa.

7. Order: *Augmentin* (amoxicillin and clavulanate potassium) *500 mg PO q12h*. The strength on the label is *125 mg* per *5 mL*. How many *milliliters* of this antibiotic will you administer? Draw a line at the correct measurement on the medication cup in • **Figure 6.29**.

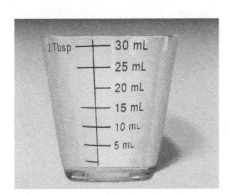

• **Figure 6.29**
Medication cup for question 7.

8. The prescriber ordered *donepezil HCl 10 mg PO daily at bedtime* for a patient who has Alzheimer's disease. Read the label in • **Figure 6.30** and determine how many *tablets* you will administer.

donepezil HCl tablets

5 mg
30 Tablets

• **Figure 6.30**
Drug label for donepezil HCL.

Workspace

9. Estimate the BSA for a person who is 6 *ft* 3 *in* tall and weighs 200 *lb*.

10. James is 150 *cm* and 85 *kg*; Tristan is 165 *cm* and 93 *kg*. Who has the larger BSA?

11. Order: *Flagyl (metronidazole) 7.5 mg/kg po q6h*. How many *mg* of this amebicide would you administer to a patient who weighs 150 *lb*?

12. Order: *codeine sulfate 10 mg po q4h prn pain*. The strength of the codeine sulfate is 15 *mg/5 mL*. How many *mL* of this narcotic drug will you administer to the patient?

13. Convert *0.5 mL/min* to an equivalent rate in *mL/h*.

14. Order: *Micro-K (potassium chloride) 16 mEq po stat*. How many 8 *mEq* tablets would you administer?

15. Write 10:30 P.M. in military time.

Syringes

Chapter 7

Learning Outcomes

After completing this chapter, you will be able to

1. Identify the parts of a syringe and needle.
2. Identify various types of syringes.
3. Interpret the calibrations on syringes of various sizes.
4. Select the most appropriate syringe to administer a prescribed dose.
5. Measure single insulin dosages.
6. Combine two different types of insulin in one syringe.

In this chapter you will learn how to use various types of syringes to measure medication dosages. You will also discuss the difference between the types of insulin and how to measure single insulin dosages and combined insulin dosages.

A **syringe** is a device used to draw in or eject either air or liquid. When fitted with a needle, it is called a hypodermic syringe and may be used to inject medication into the body. Oral syringes (without the needles) are used to administer medication orally. Syringes are made of plastic or glass, designed for one-time use, and packaged either separately or together with needles of appropriate sizes. After use, syringes must be discarded in special puncture-resistant containers. See • **Figure 7.1**.

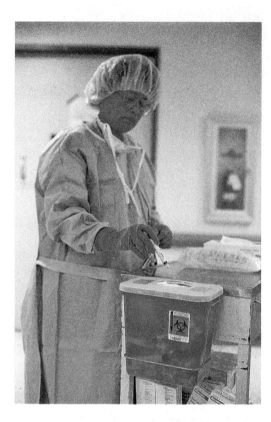

● **Figure 7.1**
Puncture-resistant container for needles, syringes, and other "sharps."

Parts of a Syringe

A syringe consists of a barrel, a plunger, and a tip.

- **Barrel:** a hollow cylinder that holds the medication. It has calibrations (graduated markings) on the outer surface.
- **Plunger:** fits in the barrel and is moved back and forth. A rubber stopper attached to the plunger has two rings that fit snugly into the barrel. Pulling back on the plunger draws liquid or air into the syringe. Pushing in the plunger forces air or liquid out of the syringe.
- **Tip:** the end of the syringe that holds the needle. The needle slips onto the tip or can be twisted and locked in place (Luer-Lok™).

The inside of the barrel, plunger, and tip must always be sterile.

Needles

Needles are thin stainless steel tubes that come in various lengths and diameters. They are packaged with a protective cover that keeps them from being contaminated. The parts of a needle are the **hub**, which attaches to the syringe; the **shaft**, the long tube that is embedded in the hub; and the **bevel**, the slanted portion that makes the sharp point on the end of the needle. The **length** of the needle is the distance from the point to the hub. Needles most commonly used in medication administration range from $\frac{3}{8}$ *inch* to 2 *inches*. The **gauge** of the needle refers to the thickness of the needle and varies from 18 to 28 (the larger the gauge, the thinner the needle). The parts of a syringe and needle are shown in ● **Figure 7.2.**

ALERT

The amount of fluid to be put in the syringe, the patient's size, the type of tissue being injected, and the viscosity of the medication are factors that determine the size of the needle to be used. The inside of the barrel, the plunger, the tip of the syringe, and the needle should never come in contact with anything unsterile.

Parts of a 10 *mL* Luer-Lok™ Hypodermic Syringe and Needle

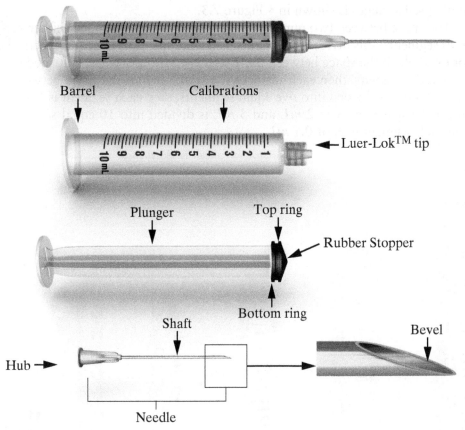

Barrel   Calibrations

Luer-Lok™ tip

Plunger   Top ring

Rubber Stopper

Bottom ring

Shaft   Bevel

Hub

Needle

• **Figure 7.2**
Parts of a syringe and needle.

Commonly Used Sizes of Hypodermic Syringes

The two major types of syringes are hypodermic and oral. In 1853, doctors Charles Pravaz and Alexander Wood were the first to develop a syringe with a needle that was fine enough to pierce the skin. This is known as a **hypodermic syringe.** Use of oral syringes (without needles) will be discussed in Chapter 12.

Hypodermic syringes are calibrated (marked) in cubic centimeters (cc), milliliters (*mL*), or units. Practitioners often refer to syringes by the volume they contain—for example, a 3-cc syringe. Although some syringes are still labeled in cubic centimeters, manufacturers are now phasing in syringes labeled in milliliters. In this text, we will generally show *mL* instead of cc on the syringes.

The smaller-capacity syringes (0.5, 1, and 3 *mL*) are used most often for intradermal, subcutaneous, or intramuscular injections of medication. The larger sizes (5, 12, and 35 *mL*) are commonly used to draw blood or prepare medications for intravenous administration. A representative sample of commonly used syringes is shown in • **Figure 7.3**.

The space between two numbers on a syringe is broken up into either 2, 5, or 10 segments; this divides the space into halves, fifths, or tenths, respectively. For example, if the space between 2 *mL* and 3 *mL* on a syringe is divided into two equal segments, then each segment is $\frac{1}{2}$ or 0.5 *mL*. If the space between 2 *mL* and 3 *mL* is divided into five equal segments, then each segment is $\frac{1}{5}$ or 0.2 *mL*. If the space between 2 *mL* and 3 *mL* is divided into 10 equal segments, then each segment is $\frac{1}{10}$ or 0.1 *mL*.

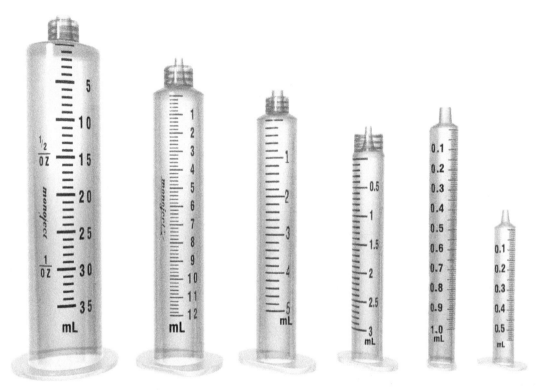

• **Figure 7.3**

A sample of commonly used hypodermic syringes (35 *mL*, 12 *mL*, 5 *mL*, 3 *mL*, 1 *mL*, and 0.5 *mL*).

A 35 *mL* syringe is shown in • **Figure 7.4**. Each line on the barrel represents 1 *mL*, and the longer lines represent 5 *mL*.

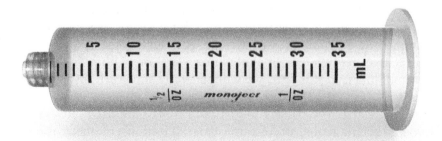

• **Figure 7.4**

A 35 *mL* syringe.

A 12 *mL* syringe is shown in • **Figure 7.5.** Each line on the barrel represents 0.2 *mL*, and the longer lines represent 1 *mL*.

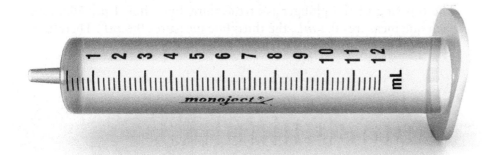

• **Figure 7.5**
A 12 *mL* syringe.

EXAMPLE 7.1

How much liquid is in the partially filled 12 *mL* syringe shown in • Figure 7.6?

The top ring of the plunger is at the second line after the 5 *mL* line. Because each line measures 0.2 *mL*, the second line measures 0.4 *mL*. Therefore, the amount in the syringe is 5.4 *mL*.

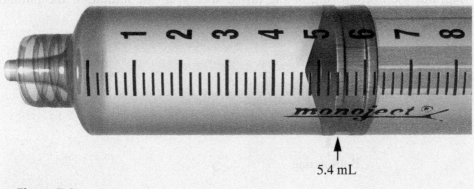

5.4 mL

• **Figure 7.6**
A partially filled 12 *mL* syringe.

A 5 *mL* syringe is shown in • **Figure 7.7.** Each line on the barrel represents 0.2 *mL*, and the longer lines represent 1 *mL*.

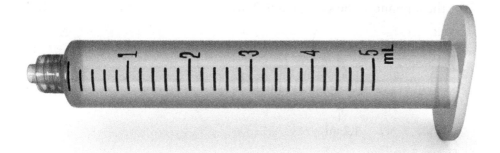

• **Figure 7.7**
A 5 *mL* syringe.

EXAMPLE 7.2

How much liquid is in the 5 *mL* syringe shown in • Figure 7.8?

The top ring of the plunger is at the third line after 4 *mL*. Because each line measures 0.2 *mL*, the third line measures 0.6 *mL*. Therefore, the amount of liquid in the syringe is 4.6 *mL*.

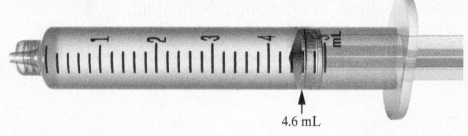

4.6 mL

• **Figure 7.8**
A partially filled 5 *mL* syringe.

In • **Figure 7.9**, a 3 *mL* syringe is shown. There are 10 spaces between the largest markings. This indicates that the syringe is measured in tenths of a milliliter. So, each of the lines is 0.1 *mL*. The longer lines indicate half and full milliliter measures. The liquid volume in a syringe is read from the *top ring*, **not** the bottom ring or the raised section in the middle of the plunger. Therefore, this syringe contains 0.9 *mL*.

Top ring

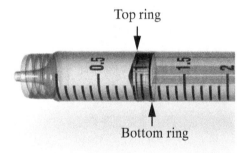

Bottom ring

• **Figure 7.9**
A partially filled 3 *mL* syringe.

EXAMPLE 7.3

How much liquid is in the 3 *mL* syringe shown in • Figure 7.10?

The top ring of the plunger is at the second line after 1 *mL*. Because each line measures 0.1 *mL*, the two lines measure 0.2 mL. Therefore, the amount in the syringe is 1.2 *mL*.

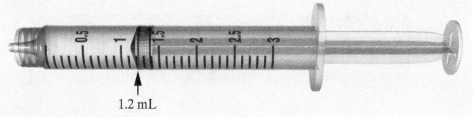

1.2 mL

• **Figure 7.10**
A partially filled 3 *mL* syringe.

When small volumes of 1 *milliliter* or less are required, a low-volume syringe provides the greatest accuracy. The 1 *mL* syringe, also called a tuberculin syringe, shown in • **Figure 7.11** is calibrated in hundredths of a milliliter. Because there are 100 lines on the syringe, each line represents 0.01 *mL*. The 0.5 *mL* syringe shown in • **Figure 7.12** has 50 lines, and each line also represents 0.01 *mL*. For doses of 0.5 *mL* or less, this syringe should be used. These syringes are used for intradermal injection of very small amounts of substances in tests for tuberculosis and allergies, as well as for intramuscular injections of small quantities of medication.

0.52 mL

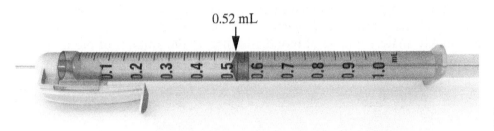

• **Figure 7.11**
A partially filled 1 *mL* safety tuberculin syringe.

The top ring of the plunger in Figure 7.11 is at the second line after 0.5 *mL*. Therefore, the amount in the syringe is 0.52 *mL*.

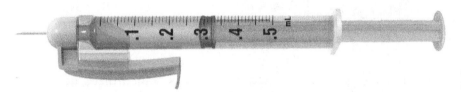

• **Figure 7.12**
A partially filled 0.5 *mL* safety syringe.

The top ring of the plunger in Figure 7.12 is at the first line before 0.3 *mL* (0.30 *mL*). Therefore, the syringe contains 0.29 *mL*.

EXAMPLE 7.4

How much liquid is shown in the portion of the 1 *mL* tuberculin syringe shown in • **Figure 7.13**?

0.36 mL

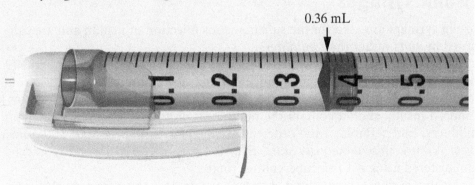

• **Figure 7.13**
A portion of a partially filled 1 *mL* safety syringe.

The top ring of the plunger is 6 lines after the 0.3 *mL* calibration. Because each line represents 0.01 *mL*, the amount of liquid in the syringe is 0.36 *mL*.

ALERT

The calibrations on the 1 *mL* syringe are very small and close together. Use caution when drawing up medication in this syringe.

NOTE

Because 0.5 *mL* and 1 *mL* tuberculin syringes can accurately measure amounts to hundredths of a milliliter, the volume of fluid to be measured in these syringes is rounded to the nearest hundredth; for example, 0.358 *mL* is rounded off to 0.36 *mL*. The 3 *mL* syringe can accurately measure amounts to tenths of a milliliter. The volume of fluid to be measured in this syringe is rounded to the nearest tenth of a milliliter; for example, 2.358 *mL* is rounded off to 2.4 *mL*.

Insulin

Insulin is a hormone used to treat patients who have insulin-dependent diabetes mellitus (IDDM). Diabetes is fast becoming the epidemic of the 21st century.

Insulin is a high-risk medication. Therefore, a thorough understanding of the various types of insulins and insulin syringes is essential in preventing medication errors. Depending on its form, insulin can be administered via subcutaneous injection, via intravenous route, or continuously via an insulin pump.

Insulin dosage is determined by the patient's daily blood-glucose readings, frequently referred to as a "fingerstick." A blood-glucose monitor is small and can quickly analyze a drop of blood and display the amount of blood glucose measured in milligrams per deciliter (*mg/dL*). See • **Figure 7.14**.

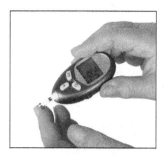

• **Figure 7.14**
A blood-glucose monitor.

Insulin is supplied as a liquid measured in standardized units of potency rather than by weight or volume. These standardized units are called **USP** *units*, often shortened to *units*. The most commonly prepared concentration of insulin is 100 *units* per milliliter, which is referred to as *units 100 insulin* and is abbreviated as U-100. Although a 500 *units/mL* concentration of insulin (U-500) is also available, it is used only for the rare patient who is markedly insulin resistant. U-40 insulin is used in some countries; however, in the United States, insulin is standardized at U-100.

Insulin Syringes

Insulin syringes are used for the subcutaneous injection of insulin and are calibrated in *units* rather than *milliliters*.

Insulin syringes are calibrated for the administration of standard U-100 insulin only. Therefore, insulin syringes should not be used for administering nonstandard strengths of insulin. To ensure patient safety, an order for nonstandard insulin should contain the number of units as well as the volume in milliliters. For example, if the order were "*Regular Insulin U-500, 100 units, inject 0.2 mL subcutaneously stat*," then 0.2 *mL* of U-500 insulin would be administered using a 1 *mL* tuberculin syringe.

Insulin syringes have three different capacities: the standard 100-*unit* capacity, and the **Lo-Dose** 50-*unit* or 30-*unit* capacities.

• **Figure 7.15** shows a *single-scale standard* 100-*unit* insulin syringe calibrated in 2-*unit* increments. Any odd number of units (e.g., 23, 35) is measured halfway between the even calibrations. These calibrations and spaces are very small, so this is not the syringe of choice for a person with impaired vision.

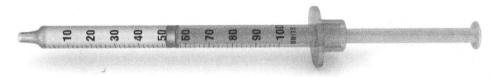

● **Figure 7.15**
A single-scale standard 100-*unit* insulin syringe with 52 *units* of insulin.

The dual-scale version of the 100-*unit* insulin syringe is easier to use. • **Figure 7.16** shows both sides of a *dual-scale* 100-*unit* insulin syringe, also calibrated in 2-*unit* increments. However, it has a scale with *even* numbers on one side and a scale with *odd* numbers on the opposite side. Both the even and odd sides are shown. Even-numbered doses are measured using the "even" side of the syringe, whereas odd numbered doses are measured using the "odd" side.

Each line on the barrel represents 2 *units*.

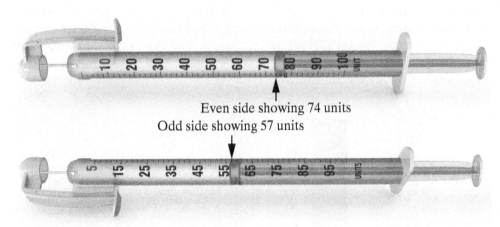

Even side showing 74 units
Odd side showing 57 units

● **Figure 7.16**
Two views of the same dual-scale standard 100-*unit* insulin safety syringe.

For small doses of insulin (50 *units* or fewer), Lo-Dose insulin syringes more accurately measure the doses and should be used. A 50-*unit* Lo-Dose insulin syringe, shown in • **Figure 7.17**, is a single-scale syringe with 50 *units*. It is calibrated in 1-*unit* increments.

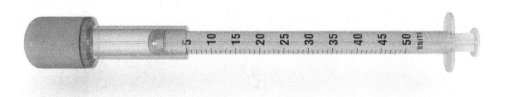

● **Figure 7.17**
A 50-*unit* Lo-Dose insulin syringe with protective cap.

A 30-*unit* Lo-Dose insulin syringe, shown in • **Figure 7.18**, is a syringe with a capacity of 30 *units*. It is calibrated in 1-*unit* increments and is used when the dose is less than 30 *units*.

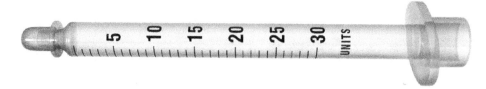

• **Figure 7.18**
A 30-*unit* Lo-Dose insulin syringe.

Types of Insulin

Insulin is available in 100-*unit/mL* multidose vials. The major route of administration of insulin is by subcutaneous injection. *Insulin is never given intramuscularly.* It can also be administered with an insulin pen that contains a cartridge filled with insulin or with a Continuous Subcutaneous Insulin Infusion (CSII) pump. The CSII pump is used to administer a programmed dose of a rapid-acting 100-*unit* insulin at a set rate of *units* per hour.

The *source* (animal or human) and *type* (rapid-, short-, intermediate-, or long-acting) are indicated on the insulin label. Today, the most commonly used *source* is human insulin. Insulin from a human source is designated on the label as recombinant DNA (rDNA origin). The *type* of insulin relates to both the *onset and duration of action*. See • **Figure 7.19** for examples of drug labels for various types of insulin.

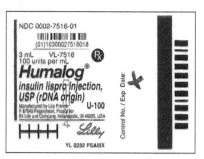

(a) rapid-acting

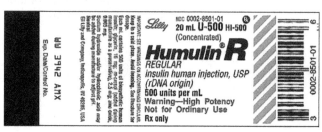

(b) short-acting

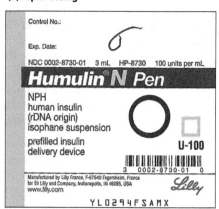

(c) intermediate-acting

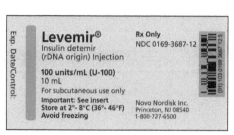

(d) long-acting

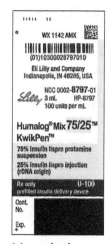

(e) premixed combination

• **Figure 7.19**
Drug labels for various types of insulin.

Healthcare providers must be familiar with the various **types of insulin,** as summarized in Table 7.1. Insulins are classified according to how fast they begin to work, when they reach maximum effect, and how long their effects last:

- **onset of action:** the length of time before insulin reaches the bloodstream and begins to lower blood glucose
- **peak of action:** the time period in which the insulin is the most effective in lowering blood glucose
- **duration of action:** the period of time during which the insulin continues to lower blood glucose

Because each person responds differently to insulin, the prescriber will determine which insulin schedule is best for the particular patient.

Table 7.1 Types of Insulin

Type	Examples	Approximate Time	
Rapid-acting	Apidra (insulin glulisine) Humalog (insulin lispro) Novolog (insulin aspart)	Onset: Peak: Duration:	15 *min* 30–90 *min* 3–5 *h*
Short-acting	Novolin R (insulin regular) Humulin R (insulin regular)	Onset: Peak: Duration:	0.5–1 *h* 2–4 *h* 5–8 *h*
Intermediate-acting	Novolin N (insulin isophane NPH) Humulin N (insulin isophane NPH)	Onset: Peak: Duration:	1–3 *h* 8 *h* 12–16 *h*
Long-acting	Lantus (insulin glargine) Levemir (insulin detemir)	Onset: Peak: Duration:	1 *h* none 20–26 *h*
Pre-mixed NPH (intermediate-acting) and regular (short-acting)	Humulin 70/30 (70% NPH & 30% regular) Novolin70/30 (70% NPH & 30% regular)	Onset: Peak: Duration:	30–60 *min* varies 10–16 *h*
	Humulin 50/50 (50% NPH & 50% regular)	Onset: Peak: Duration:	30–60 *min* varies 10–16 *h*
Pre-mixed insulin lispro protamine suspension (intermediate-acting) and insulin lispro (rapid-acting)	Humalog Mix 75/25 (75% insulin lispro protamine & 25% insulin lispro)	Onset: Peak: Duration:	10–15 *min* varies 10–16 *h*
	Humalog Mix 50/50 (50% insulin lispro protamine & 50% insulin lispro)	Onset: Peak: Duration:	10–15 *min* varies 10–16 *h*
Pre-mixed insulin aspart protamine suspension (intermediate-acting) and insulin aspart (rapid-acting)	NovoLog Mix 70/30 (70% insulin aspart protamine & 30% insulin aspart)	Onset: Peak: Duration:	5–15 *min* varies 10–16 *h*

This table was adapted from the National Diabetes Information Clearinghouse (NDIC), Feb. 16, 2012.

Insulin Pens

An insulin pen is an insulin delivery system that looks like a pen, uses an insulin cartridge, and has disposable needles. Compared to the traditional syringe and vial, a pen device is easier to use, provides greater dose accuracy, and is more acceptable to patients.

Some pens are disposed of after one use, whereas others have replaceable insulin cartridges. All pens use needles that minimize the discomfort of injection because they are extremely short and very thin.

The parts of an insulin pen are shown in • **Figure 7.20.** The dose selector knob is used to "dial" the desired dose of insulin. Once the pen has been "primed" (cleared of any air in the cartridge) and the dose set, the insulin is injected by pressing on the injection button. Because preparing a dose with a pen involves dialing a mechanical device and not looking at the side of a syringe, insulin users with reduced visual acuity can be more assured of accurate dosing. Some pens have a "memory" that records the date, time, and amount of doses administered.

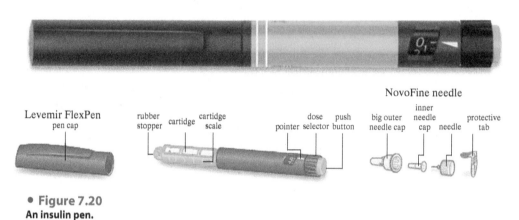

NovoFine needle

Levemir FlexPen pen cap | rubber stopper | cartidge | cartridge scale | dose pointer | push selector | button | big outer needle cap | inner needle cap | needle | protective tab

• **Figure 7.20**
An insulin pen.

See video demo of the FlexPen at http://www.levemir-us.com/about-levemir-FlexPen-demo.asp?WLac=LevemirFlexPen

Insulin Pumps

An insulin pump, shown in • **Figure 7.21,** is a beeperlike, external, battery-powered device that delivers rapid-acting insulin continuously for 24 *hours* a day through a **cannula** (a small, hollow tube) inserted under the skin. The pump contains an insulin cartridge that is attached to tubing with a cannula or

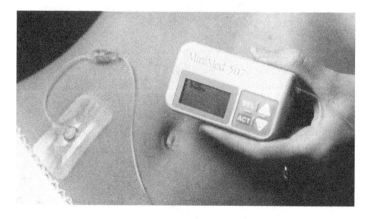

• **Figure 7.21**
An insulin pump.

needle on the end. The needle is inserted under the skin of the abdomen, and it can remain in place for two to three days. The insulin is delivered through this "infusion set." This eliminates the need for multiple daily injections of insulin.

The pump can be programmed to deliver a basal rate and/or a bolus dose. **Basal** insulin is delivered continuously over 24 *hours* to keep blood-glucose levels in range between meals and overnight. The basal rate can be programmed to deliver different rates at different times. **Bolus** doses can be delivered at mealtimes to provide control for additional food intake. The insulin pump currently on the market is the closest approximation to an artificial pancreas.

EXAMPLE 7.5

What is the dose of insulin in the single-scale 100-*unit* insulin syringe shown in • Figure 7.22?

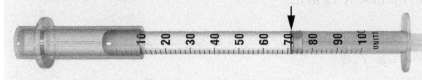

• **Figure 7.22**
A single-scale 100-*unit* insulin syringe.

The top ring of the plunger is one line after 70. Because each line represents 2 *units*, the dose is 72 *units* of insulin.

EXAMPLE 7.6

What is the dose of insulin in the dual-scale 100-*unit* insulin syringe shown in • Figure 7.23?

100-unit dual-scale syringe

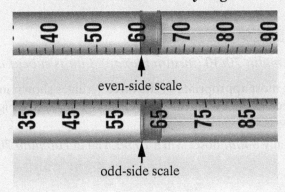

• **Figure 7.23**
Two views of a dual-scale insulin syringe.

The top ring of the plunger is between calibrations and is slightly more than 2 lines after 55 on the odd-side scale. Notice how difficult it would be to determine where 60 *units* would measure using the odd-side scale of the syringe. However, on the even-side scale, the plunger falls exactly on the 60. So, the dose is 60 *units*.

EXAMPLE 7.7

What is the dose of insulin in the 50-*unit* insulin syringe shown in
• Figure 7.24?

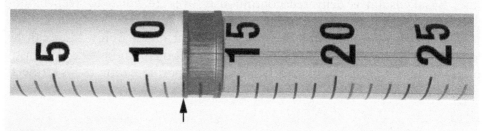

• **Figure 7.24**
A 50-*unit* insulin syringe.

The top ring of the plunger is at 12. Because each line represents
1 *unit*, the dose is 12 *units*.

EXAMPLE 7.8

What is the dose of insulin in the 30-*unit* insulin syringe shown in
• Figure 7.25?

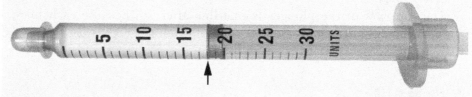

• **Figure 7.25**
A 30-*unit* Lo-Dose insulin syringe.

The top ring of the plunger is three lines after 15. Because each line
represents one unit, the dose is 18 *units* of insulin.

EXAMPLE 7.9

Order: *Humulin 70/30 (insulin human) 8 units subcut daily.*

(a) Choose most appropriate of the three syringes shown in Figure 7.26,
and place an arrow at the correct dosage level. See Figure 7.27 for
the answer.

(b) How many 8-*unit* doses will a *10 mL* vial of *Humulin 70/30* contain?

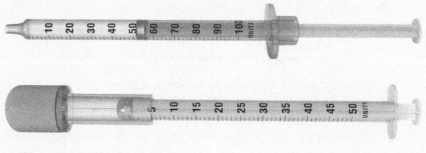

• **Figure 7.26**
Syringe choices for Example 7.9.

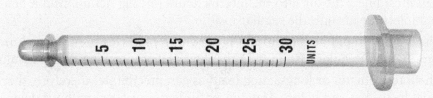

● **Figure 7.26**
(*Continued*)

(a) The best choice would be the smallest syringe that contains the dose, that is, the 30 *mL* Lo-Dose insulin syringe.

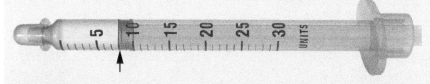

● **Figure 7.27**
Insulin syringe showing 8 *units* for Example 7.9.

(b) You want to know how many doses would be contained in the vial. That is,

$$1 \; Vial = ? \; doses$$

You know the following:

- 1 *vial* contains a volume of 10 *mL*
- the standard strength of U-100 insulin is 100 *units/mL*
- 1 *dose* = 8 *units*

The above three items will provide the three unit fractions needed to do the problem as follows:

$$\frac{1 \; vial}{1} \times \frac{10 \; mL}{1 \; vial} \times \frac{100 \; units}{1 \; mL} \times \frac{1 \; dose}{8 \; units} = 125 \; doses$$

So, the vial contains 125 *doses*.

Measuring Two Types of Insulin in One Syringe

Individuals who have insulin-dependent diabetes mellitus (IDDM) often must have two different types of insulin administered at the same time. This combination is usually composed of a *rapid-acting* insulin with either an *intermediate-* or *long-acting* insulin; this can be accomplished by using an appropriate premixed combination drug. However, often the different insulin types are mixed in a single syringe just before administration, and the important points to remember in this process are:

- The *total volume* in the syringe is the *sum of the two insulin* amounts.
- The smallest-capacity syringe containing the dose should be used to measure the insulins because the enlarged scale is easier to read and therefore more accurate.
- The *amount of air equal to the amount of insulin to be withdrawn* from each vial must be injected into each vial.

- You must inject the air into the intermediate- or long-acting insulin before you inject the air into the regular insulin.

- The *regular* (rapid-acting) insulin is drawn up *first*; this prevents contamination of the regular insulin with the intermediate- or long-acting insulin.

- The intermediate- or long-acting insulins can precipitate; therefore, they must be well mixed before drawing up and administered without delay.

- Only insulins from the same source should be mixed together; for example, Humulin R and Humulin N are both human insulin and can be mixed.

- If you draw up too much of the intermediate- or long-acting insulin, you must discard the entire medication and start over.

The steps for preparing two types of insulin in one syringe are shown in Example 7.10.

EXAMPLE 7.10

The prescriber ordered 10 *units* Humulin R insulin and 30 *units* Humulin N insulin subcutaneously, 30 *minutes* before breakfast. Explain how you would prepare to administer this in one injection. • Figures 7.28 and • 7.29.

The total amount of insulin is 40 *units* (10 + 30). To administer this dose, use a 50-*unit* Lo-Dose syringe. Inject 30 *units* of air into the Humulin N vial and 10 *units* of air into the Humulin R vial. Withdraw 10 *units* of the Humulin R (rapid-acting) first and then withdraw 30 *units* of the Humulin N (intermediate-acting).

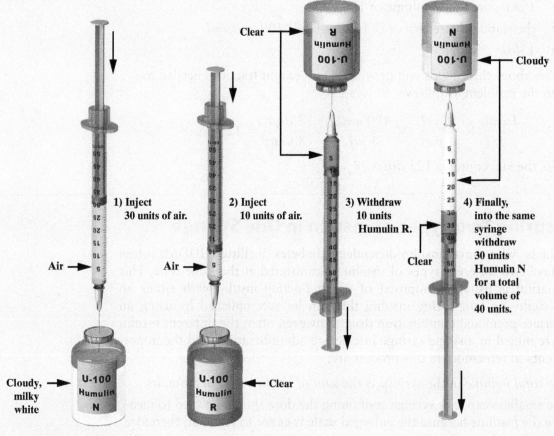

1) Inject 30 units of air.

2) Inject 10 units of air.

3) Withdraw 10 units Humulin R.

4) Finally, into the same syringe withdraw 30 units Humulin N for a total volume of 40 units.

• **Figure 7.28**
Mixing two types of insulin in one syringe.

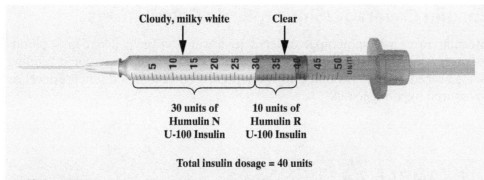

Total insulin dosage = 40 units

● **Figure 7.29**
Combination of 30 *units* Humulin N and 10 *units* of Humulin R.

Premixed Insulin

Using premixed insulin (see Table 7.1) eliminates errors that may occur when mixing two types of insulin in one syringe (Figure 7.28).

EXAMPLE 7.11

Order: Give 35 *units* of Humalog Mix 50/50 insulin subcutaneously 30 *minutes* before breakfast. Use the label shown in ● Figure 7.30, and place an arrow at the appropriate calibration on the syringe.

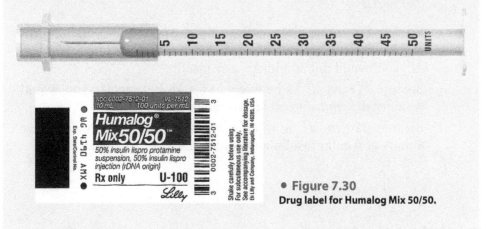

● **Figure 7.30**
Drug label for Humalog Mix 50/50.

In the syringe in ● **Figure 7.31**, the top ring of the plunger is at the 35-*unit* line.

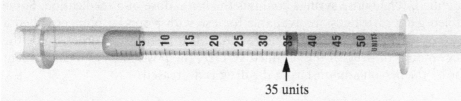

35 units

● **Figure 7.31**
A 50-*unit* Lo-Dose insulin syringe with protective cap measuring 35 *units*.

Insulin Coverage/Sliding-Scale Calculations

Regular insulin is sometimes ordered to lower ("cover") a patient's blood-sugar level. The prescriber may order regular insulin to be given on a "sliding scale" schedule that is related to the patient's current blood-glucose level as measured by a fingerstick.

EXAMPLE 7.12

Order: *fingersticks Q.I.D., at breakfast, lunch, and dinner, and at bedtime. Give regular insulin as follows:*

glucose less than 150 mg/dL	*—no insulin*
glucose of 150–200 mg/dL	*—2 units*
glucose of 201–250 mg/dL	*—3 units*
glucose of 251–300 mg/dL	*—5 units*
glucose of more than 300 mg/dL	*—give 6 units and contact the prescriber stat*

Use the sliding scale to determine how much insulin you will give the patient if the glucose level before lunchtime is:

(a) *125 mg/dL*

(b) *278 mg/dL*

(c) *350 mg/dL*

(a) You need to compare the patient's level with the information provided in the sliding scale. Because 125 *mg/dL* is less than 150 *mg/dL*, you would not administer any insulin.

(b) Because 278 *mg/dL* is between 251 and 300 *mg/dL*, you would administer 5 *units* of regular insulin immediately.

(c) Because 350 *mg/dL* is more than 300 *mg/dL*, you would give 6 units of regular insulin and contact the prescriber stat.

Prefilled Syringes

A prefilled, single-dose syringe contains the usual dose of a medication. Some prefilled glass cartridges are available for use with a special plunger called a Tubex or Carpuject syringe (• **Figure 7.32**). If a medication order is for the exact amount of drug in the prefilled syringe, the possibility of measurement error by the person administering the drug is decreased.

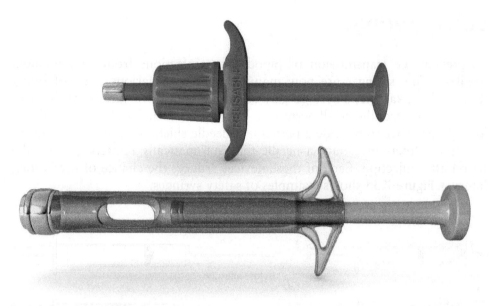

● **Figure 7.32**
Carpuject and Tubex prefilled cartridge holders.

EXAMPLE 7.13

The prefilled syringe cartridge shown in ● Figure 7.33 is calibrated so that each line measures $0.1\ mL$, and it has a capacity of $2.5\ mL$. How many milliliters are indicated by the arrow shown in Figure 7.33?

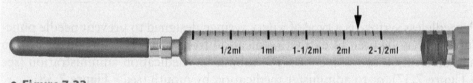

● **Figure 7.33**
Prefilled cartridges.

The cartridge has a total capacity of $2.5\ mL$, and the arrow is at $2.2\ mL$.

EXAMPLE 7.14

How much medication is in the prepackaged cartridge shown in ● Figure 7.34?

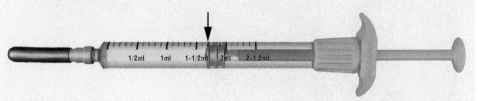

● **Figure 7.34**
Prefilled cartridge in holder.

The top of the plunger is at two lines after the $1.5\ mL$ line. Because each line measures $0.1\ mL$, the two lines measure $0.2\ mL$. Therefore, there are $1.7\ mL$ of medication in this prefilled cartridge.

NOTE

To view an animation of the operation of a safety syringe, go to http://www.bd.com/hypodermic/products/integra/

Safety Syringes

To prevent the transmission of blood-borne infections from contaminated needles, many syringes are now manufactured with various types of safety devices. For example, a syringe may contain a protective sheath (a) that can be used to protect the needle's sterility. This sheath is then pulled forward and locked into place to provide a permanent needle shield for disposal following injection. Others may have a needle that automatically retracts (b) into the barrel after injection. Each of these devices reduces the chance of needlestick injury. • **Figure 7.35** shows examples of safety syringes.

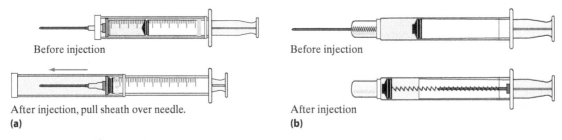

Before injection

Before injection

After injection, pull sheath over needle.

After injection

(a)

(b)

• **Figure 7.35**
Safety syringes with (a) an active safety device and (b) a passive safety device.

Needleless Syringes

A needleless syringe is a type of safety syringe designed to prevent needle punctures. It may be used to extract medication from a vial (see • **Figure 7.36**), to add medication to intravenous (IV) tubing for medication administration (see • **Figure 7.37**), or to administer medication by mouth (see • **Figure 7.38**).

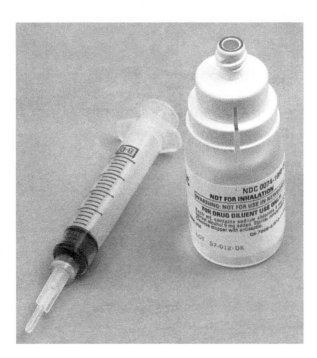

• **Figure 7.36**
A needleless syringe and vial.

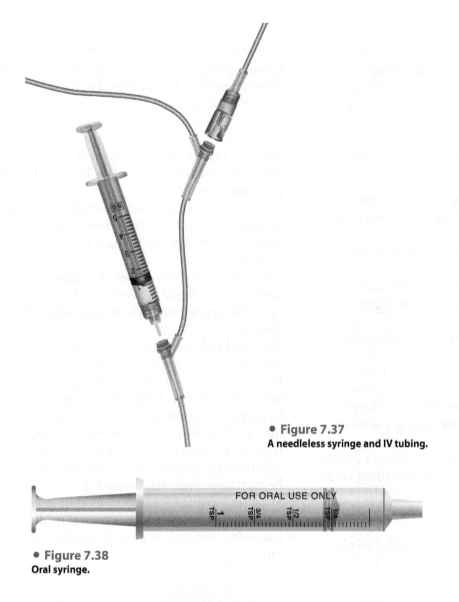

• **Figure 7.37**
A needleless syringe and IV tubing.

FOR ORAL USE ONLY

1 TSP 3/4 TSP 1/2 TSP 1/4 TSP

• **Figure 7.38**
Oral syringe.

Dosing Errors with Syringes

Care must be taken when filling a syringe. Being off by even a small amount on the syringe scale can be critical. This is especially true when a syringe contains a relatively small portion of its capacity. For example, say a 3 *mL* syringe should correctly be filled to the prescribed 2.8 *mL* and by mistake it is filled to 2.9 *mL* (one extra tick on the scale). This results in about a 4% overdose [Change/Original = 0.1/2.8]. On the other hand, if a 3 *mL* syringe should correctly be filled to 1 *mL* and by mistake it is filled to 1.1 *mL* (one extra tick), this results in a more serious, 10% overdose [Change/Original = 0.1/1].

Rounding your final calculations also may lead to concerns. For example, say your computation yields a correct dose of 0.985 *mL*. If you correctly round off this result and administer 0.99 *mL*, you have increased the dose by about 0.5% [Change/Original = 0.005/0.985]. On the other hand, if your computation yields 0.025 *mL* and you correctly round off this result and administer 0.03 *mL*, then you have increased the dose by 20% [Change/Original = 0.005/0.025]. With pediatric and high-alert drugs, sometimes *rounding down* is used to avoid the possibility of overdose; consult the rounding protocols at your facility.

Summary

In this chapter, the various types of syringes were discussed. You learned how to measure the amount of liquid in various syringes. The types of insulin, how to measure a single dose, and how to mix two insulins in one syringe were explained. Prefilled, single-dose, and safety syringes were also presented.

- Milliliters (*mL*), rather than cubic centimeters (cc), are the preferred unit of measure for volume.
- All syringe calibrations must be read at the top ring of the plunger.
- Large-capacity hypodermic syringes (5, 12, 35 *mL*) are calibrated in increments from 0.2 *mL* to 1 *mL*.
- Small-capacity 3 *mL* hypodermic syringes are calibrated in tenths of a milliter (0.1 *mL*).
- The very small-capacity 0.5 *mL* and 1 *mL* hypodermic (tuberculin) syringes are calibrated in hundredths of a milliliter. They are the preferred syringes for use in measuring a dose of less than 1 *millimeter*.
- The calibrations on hypodermic syringes differ; therefore, be very careful when measuring medications in syringes.
- Amounts less than 1 *mL* are rounded to two decimal places.
- Amounts more than 1 *mL* are rounded to one decimal place.

- Insulin syringes are designed for measuring and administering U-100 insulin. They are calibrated for 100 *units* per *mL*.
- Standard insulin syringes have a capacity of 100 *units*.
- Lo-Dose insulin syringes are used for measuring small amounts of insulin. They have a capacity of 50 *units* or 30 *units*.
- For greater accuracy, use the smallest-capacity syringe possible to measure and administer doses. However, avoid filling a syringe to its capacity.
- When measuring two types of insulin in the same syringe, Regular insulin is always drawn up in the syringe first. Think: *first clear, then cloudy.*
- The total volume when mixing insulins is the sum of the two insulin amounts.
- Insulin syringes are for measuring and administering insulin only. Tuberculin syringes are used to measure and administer other medications that are less than 1 *mL*. Confusion of the two types of syringes can cause a medication error.
- The prefilled single-dose syringe cartridge is to be used once and then discarded.
- Syringes intended for injections should not be used to measure or administer oral medications.
- Use safety syringes to prevent needlestick injuries.

Case Study 7.1

Read the Case Study and answer the questions. Answers can be found in Appendix A.

A 55-year-old male with a medical history of obesity, hypertension, hyperlipidemia, and diabetes mellitus comes to the emergency department complaining of constant abdominal pain, nausea, vomiting, and constipation. He states that his pain is a 10 (on a 0–10 pain scale). His abdomen is distended, bowel sounds are hypoactive, and stool is positive for blood. Vital signs are: B/P 154/94; T 101.4° F; P 110; and R 26. The diagnostic workup confirms a bowel obstruction, and he is admitted for a bowel resection.

Pre-op orders:
- NPO
- NG (nasogastric) tube to low suction
- V/S q 2h
- Morphine sulfate 2 *mg* subcut stat
- IV R/L @ 125 *mL/h*
- **Pre-op meds:** Demerol (meperidine hydrochloride) 75 *mg* and Phenergan (promethazine 25 *mg* IM 30 *minutes* before surgery
- Cefoxitin 2 g IV 30 *minutes* before surgery

Post-op orders:

- NPO
- NG tube to low suction
- PCA as per pain management service
- V/S q2h

- IV D5RL@ 125 *mL/h*
- cefoxitin 1 *g* IVPB q8h for 3 *doses*, infuse in 100 *mL* D5W over 30 *min*
- octreotide 50 *mcg* subcut q8h
- haloperidol 1 *mg* subcut q6h

1. Read the morphine label and:
   - (a) Draw a line indicating the dose on each of the following syringes.
   - (b) Which syringe will most accurately measure the dose?

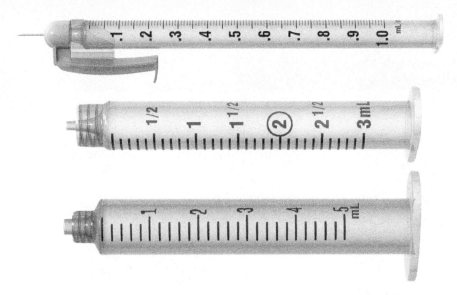

2. Calculate the pre-op dose of the Phenergan and Demerol to be administered 30 minutes before surgery. Phenergan is available in 25 *mg/mL* vials. Demerol is available in 2.5 *mL*–capacity prefilled syringes, each containing 1 *mL* of Demerol. The Demerol prefilled syringes have strengths of 10 *mg/mL*, 25 *mg/mL*, and 75 *mg/mL*.
   - (a) How many milliliters of Phenergan will you prepare?
   - (b) Which prepackaged syringe of Demerol will you use?
   - (c) Indicate, on the appropriate syringe given, the dose of each of these drugs that you will administer.

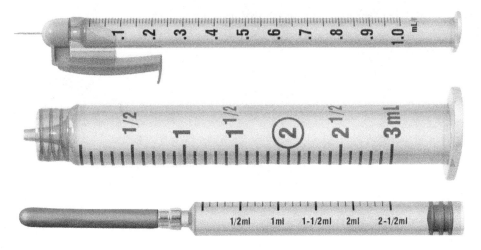

3. The label on the cefoxitin states: "add 10 *mL* of diluent to the 2 *g* vial." Draw a line on the appropriate syringe given, indicating the amount of diluent you will add to the vial.

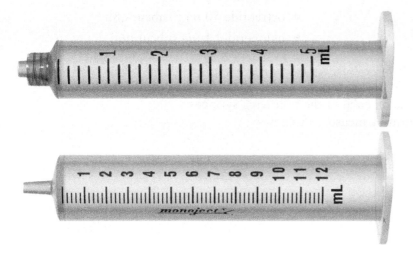

4. Read the octreotide label. Draw a line on the appropriate syringe, indicating the dose of octreotide.

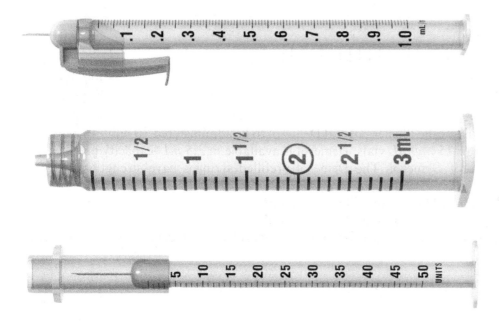

5. Read the haloperidol label and draw a line on the appropriate syringe, indicating the dose.

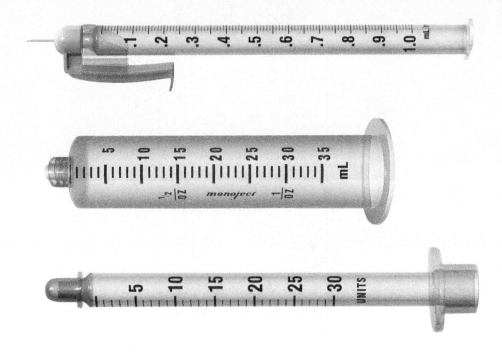

6. The patient has progressed to a regular diet and is ordered Humulin N 13 *units* and Humulin R 6 *units* subcutaneous 30 *minutes* ac breakfast, and Humulin N 5 *units* and Humulin R 5 *units* subcutaneous 30 *minutes* ac dinner.
   (a) How many units will the patient receive before breakfast?
   (b) Indicate on the appropriate syringe given the number of units of each insulin required before breakfast.

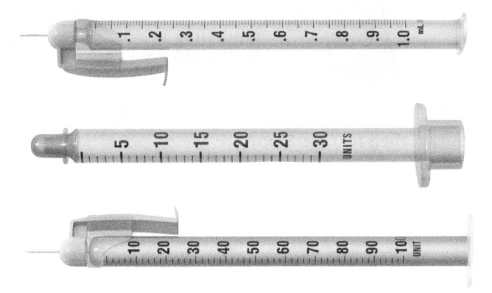

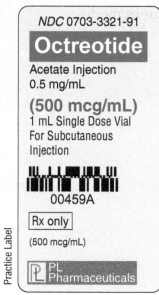

NDC 0703-3321-91

Octreotide

Acetate Injection
0.5 mg/mL

(500 mcg/mL)
1 mL Single Dose Vial
For Subcutaneous
Injection

00459A

Rx only

(500 mcg/mL)

PL
Pharmaceuticals

Practice Label

(a) **(For educational purposes only)**

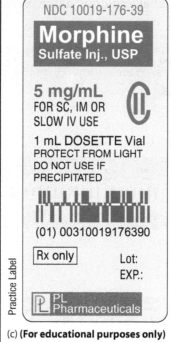

NDC 10019-176-39

Morphine
Sulfate Inj., USP

5 mg/mL
FOR SC, IM OR
SLOW IV USE

1 mL DOSETTE Vial
PROTECT FROM LIGHT
DO NOT USE IF
PRECIPITATED

(01) 00310019176390

Rx only   Lot:

                 EXP.:

PL
Pharmaceuticals

Practice Label

(c) **(For educational purposes only)**

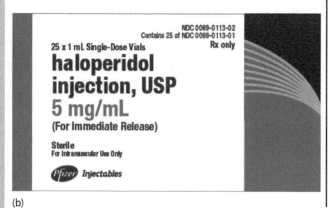

NDC 0069-0113-02
Contains 25 of NDC 0069-0113-01
Rx only

25 x 1 mL Single-Dose Vials

haloperidol injection, USP
5 mg/mL

(For Immediate Release)

Sterile
For Intramuscular Use Only

Pfizer Injectables

(b)

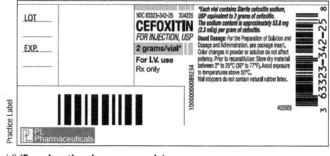

LOT _____

EXP. _____

NDC 63323-342-25   304225

CEFOXITIN
FOR INJECTION, USP

2 grams/vial*

For I.V. use
Rx only

*Each vial contains Sterile cefoxitin sodium,
USP equivalent to 2 grams of cefoxitin.
The sodium content is approximately 53.8 mg
(2.3 mEq) per gram of cefoxitin.
Usual Dosage: For the Preparation of Solution and
Dosage and Administration, see package insert.
Color changes in powder or solution do not affect
potency. Prior to reconstitution: Store dry material
between 2° to 25°C (36° to 77°F). Avoid exposure
to temperatures above 50°C.
Vial stoppers do not contain natural rubber latex.

402609

3 63323-342-25 8

PL
Pharmaceuticals

Practice Label

(d) **(For educational purposes only)**

Labels for Case Study 7.1

Practice Sets

The answers to *Try These for Practice, Exercises,* and *Cumulative Review Exercises* are found in Appendix A. Ask your instructor for the answers to the *Additional Exercises.*

Try These for Practice

Test your comprehension after reading the chapter.

In problems 1 through 4, identify the type of syringe shown in the figure. Place an arrow at the appropriate level of measurement on the syringe for the volume given.

1. _____ syringe; 0.68 *mL*

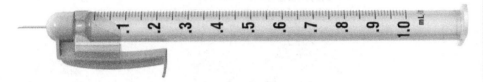

2. _____ syringe; 5.6 *mL*

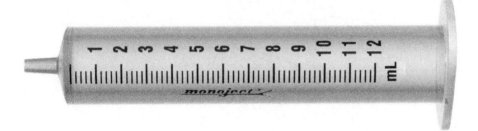

3. _____ syringe; 1.8 *mL*

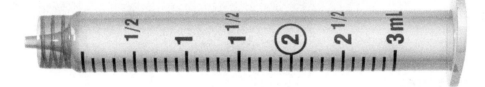

4. _____ syringe; 4.4 *mL*

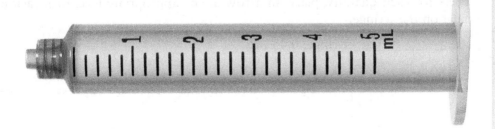

Workspace

Workspace

5. Order: *meperidine 150 mg IM q4h prn severe pain.*
   Read the label and calculate the number of milliliters to administer.
   Draw an arrow to show the dose on the most appropriate of the safety syringes.

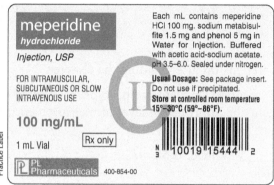

meperidine
hydrochloride

Injection, USP

FOR INTRAMUSCULAR,
SUBCUTANEOUS OR SLOW
INTRAVENOUS USE

100 mg/mL

1 mL Vial   Rx only

Each mL contains meperidine HCl 100 mg. sodium metabisulfite 1.5 mg and phenol 5 mg in Water for Injection. Buffered with acetic acid-sodium acetate. pH 3.5–6.0. Sealed under nitrogen.

Usual Dosage: See package insert. Do not use if precipitated. **Store at controlled room temperature 15°–30°C (59°–86°F).**

N 3 10019 15444 2

PL Pharmaceuticals   400-854-00

For educational purposes only

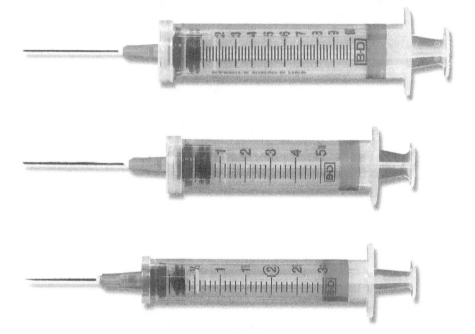

Exercises

Reinforce your understanding in class or at home.

In problems 1 through 14, identify the type of syringe shown in the figure. Then, for each quantity, place an arrow at the appropriate level of measurement on the syringe.

1. _____ syringe; 0.45 *mL*

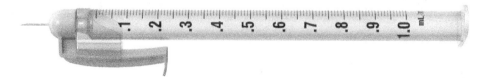

2. _____ syringe; 17 *units*

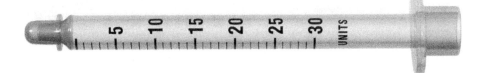

3. _____ syringe; 1.8 *mL*

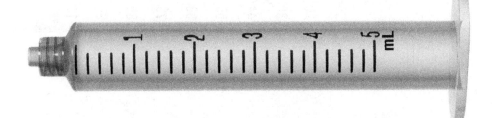

4. _____ syringe; 1.8 *mL*

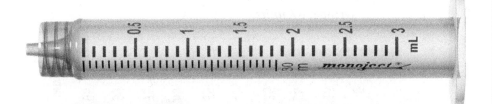

5. _____ syringe; 18 *mL*

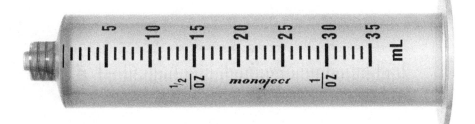

6. _____ syringe; 9.2 *mL*

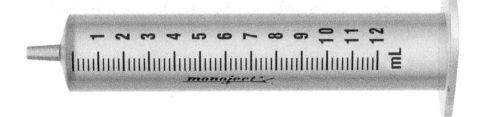

Workspace

Workspace

7. _____ syringe; 33 *units*

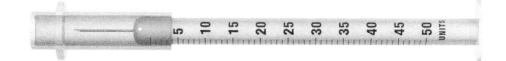

8. _____ syringe; 66 *units*

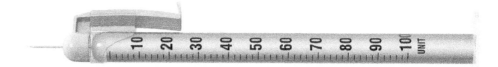

9. _____ syringe; 0.09 *mL*

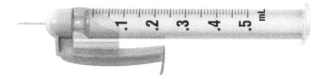

10. _____ syringe; 67 *units*

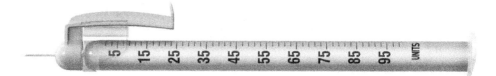

11. _____ syringe; 10.4 *mL*

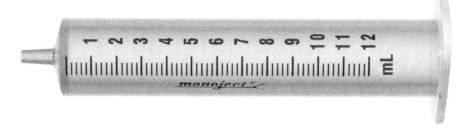

12. _____ syringe; 0.75 *mL*

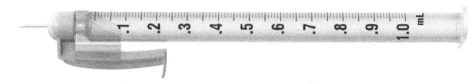

13. _____ syringe; 11.2 *mL*

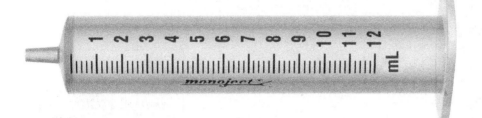

14. _____ syringe; 24 *mL*

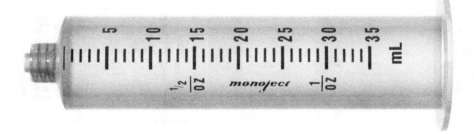

In problems 15 through 20, read the order, use the appropriate label in
• **Figure 7.39**, calculate the dosage if necessary, and place an arrow at the
appropriate level of measurement on the syringe.

2.5 mL

**Streptomycin Sulfate
Injection, USP**

1 g/2.5 mL
(400 mg/mL)
(of streptomycin)
*For **IM** use only*
**Store under refrigeration at
36° to 46°F (2° to 8°C)**
CAUTION: Federal law
prohibits dispensing
without prescription.

LOT   8E31A
EXP

Pfizer **Roerig**
Division of Pfizer Inc, NY, NY 10017

(a)

NAFCILLIN SODIUM

(naf-sill'in)

Classifications: BETA-LACTAM ANTI-
BIOTIC; PENICILLIN
Therapeutic: ANTISTAPHYLOCOCCAL
PENICILLIN

Staphylococcal Infections
Adult: **IV** 500 mg–1 g q4h (max:
12 g/day) **IM** 500 mg q4–6h
Child: **IV** 50–200 mg/kg/day
divided q4–6h (max: 12 g/day)
IM *Weight greater than 40 kg,
500 mg q4–6h; weight less than
40 kg, 25 mg/kg b.i.d.*
Neonate: **IV** 50–100 mg/kg/day
divided q6–12h **IM** 25–50 mg/
kg b.i.d.

(b)

NALBUPHINE HYDROCHLORIDE

(nal'byoo-feen)
Nubain
Classifications: ANALGESIC; NAR-
COTIC (OPIATE) AGONIST-ANTAGONIST
Therapeutic: NARCOTIC ANALGESIC

Moderate to Severe Pain
Adult: **IV/IM/Subcutaneous** 10
mg/70 kg q3–6h prn (max: 160
mg/day)

Surgery Anesthesia Supplement
Adult: **IV** 0.3–3 mg/kg, then
0.25–0.5 mg/kg as required

(c)

• **Figure 7.39**
Drug labels and drug guide information for Exercises 15–20.

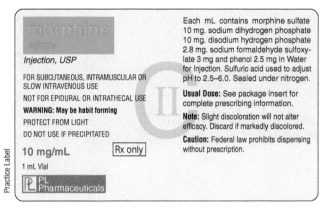

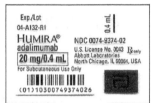

(d) **(For educational purposes only)**

(e)

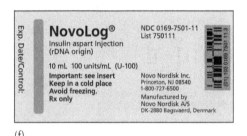

(f)

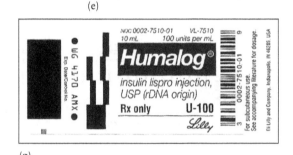

(g)

● **Figure 7.39**
(*Continued*)

Workspace

15. Order: *morphine sulfate 15 mg subcut q4h prn pain.*

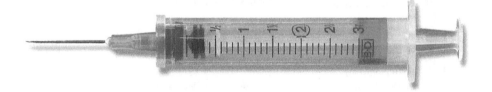

16. The patient weighs 220 *pounds*. The order is *insulin aspart 0.5 units/kg subcut daily 10 min ac.*

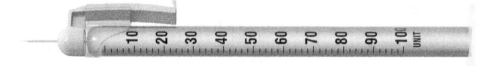

17. Order: *Streptomycin 800 mg IM daily*

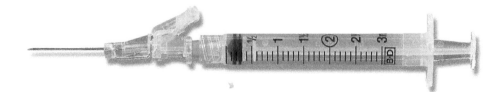

18. Order: *Humira 20 mg subcut stat*

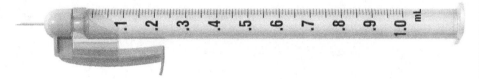

19. Nafcillin sodium is ordered IM for an adult patient. The strength of the nafcillin sodium on hand is 250 *mg/mL*. Is the amount shown by the arrow on the syringe the correct dose to administer?

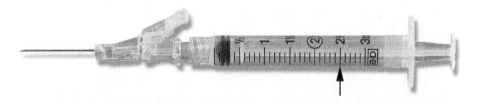

20. Indicate, by placing an arrow on the syringe, the dose of nalbuphine HCl to be administered IM for severe pain. The strength available is 10 *mg/mL*, and the adult patient weighs 105 *kg*.

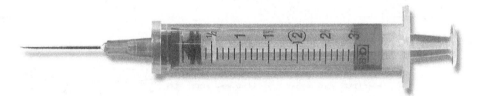

Additional Exercises

Now, test yourself!

In problems 1 through 15, identify the type of syringe shown in the figure. Then, for each quantity, place an arrow at the appropriate level of measurement on the syringe.

1. _____ syringe; 66 *units*

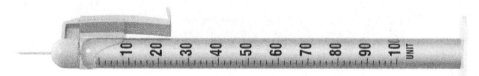

2. _____ syringe; 21 *units*

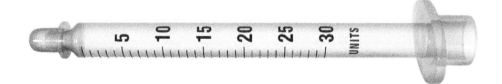

Workspace

3. _____ syringe; 1.4 *mL*

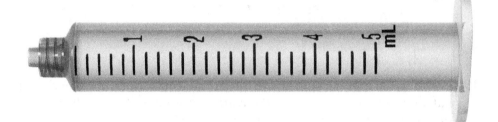

4. _____ syringe; 1.4 *mL*

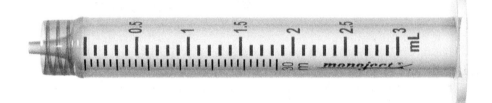

5. _____ syringe; 8.3 *mL*

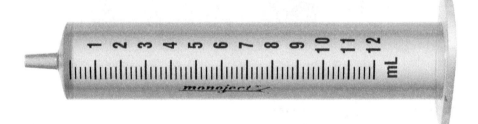

6. _____ syringe; 14 *mL*

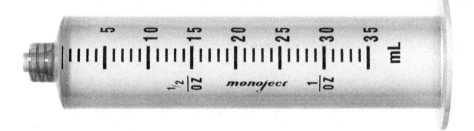

7. _____ syringe; 29 *units*

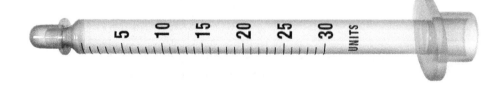

8. _____ syringe; 78 *units*

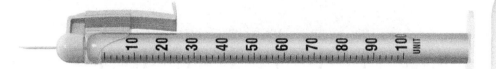

9. _____ syringe; 0.43 *mL*

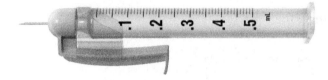

10. _____ syringe; 81 *units*

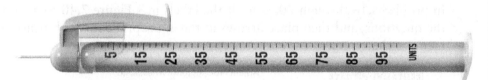

11. _____ syringe; 8.6 *mL*

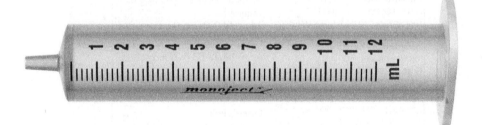

12. _____ syringe; 0.56 *mL*

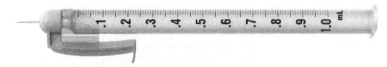

13. _____ syringe; 9.2 *mL*

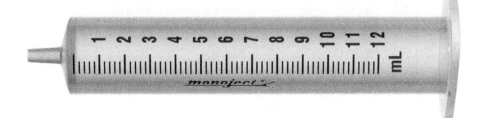

Workspace

Workspace

14. _____ syringe; 33 *mL*

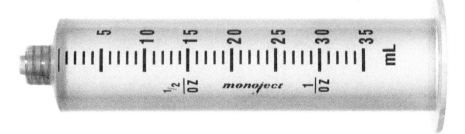

15. _____ syringe; 0.29 *mL*

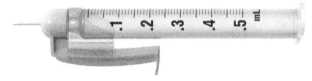

In problems 16 through 20, consult the labels in • **Figure 7.40** to answer the questions, and then place arrows at the appropriate level of measurement on the syringes.

FENTANYL CITRATE

(fen′ta-nil)

Actiq Oralet, Duragesic, Fentora, Ionsys, Onsolis, Sublimaze

Classifications: ANALGESIC; NARCOTIC (OPIATE AGONIST)

Therapeutic: NARCOTIC ANALGESIC

Prototype: Morphine

Pregnancy Category: C (B for fentanyl injection)

Controlled Substance: Schedule II

AVAILABILITY 0.05 mg/mL injection; 100 mcg, 200 mcg, 300 mcg, 400 mcg lozenges; 200 mcg, 400 mcg, 600 mcg, 800 mcg, 1200 mcg, 1600 mcg lozenges on a stick; 12 mcg/h, 25 mcg/h, 50 mcg/h, 75 mcg/h, 100 mcg/h transdermal patch; 100 mcg, 200 mcg, 300 mcg, 400 mcg, 600 mcg, 800 mcg buccal tablet; 0.2 mg, 0.4 mg. 0.6 mg, 0.8 mg, 1.2 mg buccal film

Adjunct for Regional Anesthesia

Adult: **IM/IV** 50–100 mcg

General Anesthesia

Adult: **IV** 2–20 mcg/kg, additional doses of 25–100 mcg as required

Child: **IV** 2–3 mcg/kg as needed

Postoperative Pain

Adult: **IM/IV** 50–100 mcg q1–2h prn

Child: **IM** 1.7–3.3 mcg/kg q1–2h prn

Chronic Pain

Adult: **Transdermal** Individualize and regularly reassess doses of transdermal fentanyl; for patient not already receiving an opioid, the initial dose is 25 mcg/h patch q3days; for patients already on opioids, see package insert for conversions **Stick lozenge (Actiq)** Place in mouth between cheek and lower gum and suck on lozenge; should be consumed over 15-min period

(a)

(b)

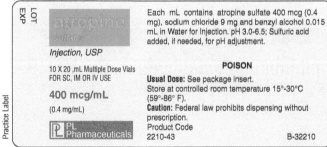

Each mL contains atropine sulfate 400 mcg (0.4 mg), sodium chloride 9 mg and benzyl alcohol 0.015 mL in Water for Injection. pH 3.0-6.5; Sulfuric acid added, if needed, for pH adjustment.

LOT
EXP

atropine
sulfate

Injection, USP

10 X 20 ,mL Multiple Dose Vials
FOR SC, IM OR IV USE

400 mcg/mL

(0.4 mg/mL)

PL Pharmaceuticals

Practice Label

POISON

Usual Dose: See package insert.
Store at controlled room temperature 15°-30°C (59°-86° F).
Caution: Federal law prohibits dispensing without prescription.
Product Code
2210-43   B-32210

For educational purposes only

• **Figure 7.40**

Drug labels for Additional Exercises 16–20.

Workspace

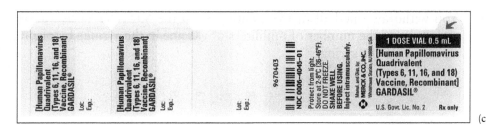

(c)

HYDROMORPHONE HYDROCHLORIDE

(hye-droe-mor′fone)

Dilaudid, Dilaudid-HP

Classifications: NARCOTIC (OPIATE) AGONIST; ANALGESIC

Therapeutic: NARCOTIC ANALGESIC; ANTITUSSIVE

Prototype: Morphine

Pregnancy Category: C; D in prolonged use or high doses at term

Controlled Substance: Schedule II

AVAILABILITY 2 mg, 4 mg, 8 mg tablets; 5 mg/5 mL oral liquid; 1 mg/mL, 10 mg/mL injection

ACTION & *THERAPEUTIC EFFECT*
Has more rapid onset and shorter duration of action than morphine, and is reported to have less hypnotic effect. *An effective narcotic analgesic that controls mild to moderate pain. Also has antitussive properties.*

ROUTE & DOSAGE

Moderate to Severe Pain

Adult: **PO** 2–4 mg q4–6h prn in naïve patients **Subcutaneous/IM/IV** 0.75–2 mg q4–6h depending on patient response

Child: **PO** 0.03–0.08 mg/kg q4–6h (max: 5 mg/dose) **IV** 0.015 mg/kg q4–6h prn

(d)

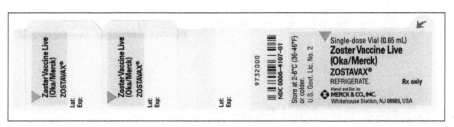

(e)

(f)

● **Figure 7.40**
(*Continued*)

16. Order: *atropine sulfate 0.5 mg IM 30–60 min before surgery.*

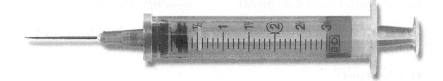

17. Order: *Zostavax 0.65 mL subcut stat.*

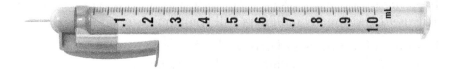

18. You withdraw one-half of the solution from the Varicella Virus Vaccine vial. Indicate the number of milliliters of vaccine in the syringe by placing an arrow on the syringe.

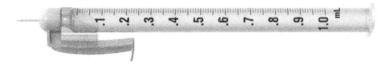

19. Fentanyl citrate has been ordered for an adult with postoperative pain. The strength of the drug is 0.05 *mg/mL*. Is the dose indicated by the arrow on the syringe in the safe dose range?

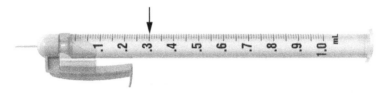

20. An adult has an order for Dilaudid for moderate pain, to be administered subcutaneously. The strength of the Dilaudid is 10 *mg/mL*. Indicate with two arrows the safe dose range in milliliters on the syringe.

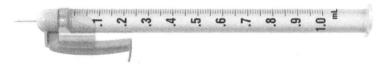

Cumulative Review Exercises

Review your mastery of previous chapters.

1. Prescriber's order: *Administer Humulin R (regular insulin [rDNA origin]) subcutaneously as per the following blood-glucose results*:

For glucose less than 160 mg/dL	*—no insulin*
glucose 160 mg/dL–220 mg/dL	*—give 2 units*
glucose 221 mg/dL–280 mg/dL	*—give 4 units*
glucose 281 mg/dL–340 mg/dL	*—give 6 units*
glucose 341 mg/dL–400 mg/dL	*—give 8 units*
glucose greater than 400 mg/dL	*—notify MD stat*

How many units will you administer if the patient's glucose level at lunchtime is

(a) *140 mg/dL?*

(b) *200 mg/dL?*

(c) *450 mg/dL?*

2. If *40 mg* of a drug is ordered *po daily* and the strength of the drug is 10 *mg/mL*, how many milliliters will you administer?

3. If *40 mg* of a drug is ordered *po b.i.d.* and the strength of the drug is 10 *mg/mL*, how many milliliters will you administer?

Workspace

4. If *40 mg* of a drug is ordered *po daily in two divided doses* and the strength of the drug is *10 mg/mL,* how many milliliters will you administer?

5. If *40 mg* of a drug is ordered *po q12h* and the strength of the drug is *10 mg/mL,* how many milliliters will you administer?

6. Order: *Dilantin (phenytoin) 250 mg po stat.* The concentration of the Dilantin is 125 *mg/5 mL.* How many teaspoons will you administer?

7. Order: *Camptosar (irinotecan) 350 mg/m² IV over 90 minutes on day 1 every 3 weeks.* How many g will be administered to a patient who has a BSA of 1.95 *m²*?

8. Find the weight, to the nearest tenth of a kilogram, of a patient who weighs 200 *pounds.*

9. Order: *Glucotrol (glipizide) 15 mg po daily.* Available tablets are *5 mg* per tablet. How many tablets will you administer?

10. A drug is ordered *50 mg b.i.d.* How many grams will be administered in 10 days?

11. Order: *Cytovene (ganciclovir) 5 mg/kg IV q12h for 14 d.* The patient weighs 110 *pounds.* How many *grams* of this antiviral drug will the patient receive over the 14-*day* period?

12. Using the formula, find the BSA of a patient who is *5 feet* tall and weighs 140 *pounds.*

13. Order: *Natulan (procarbazine HCl) 50 mg/m² /d po.* How many *mg* of this antineoplastic drug would be administered daily to a patient whose BSA is 1.5 *m²*?

14. What is the most appropriate syringe that would be used to administer 67 *units* of insulin subcut?

15. Your initial calculations indicate that you need to administer 0.66666 *mL* of a drug IM to a geriatric patient. To what volume would you round off, and what size syringe would you use?

Chapter

8 Solutions

Learning Outcomes

After completing this chapter, you will be able to

1. Find the strength of a solution as a ratio, as a fraction, and as a percent.
2. Determine the amount of solute in a given amount of solution.
3. Determine the amount of solution that would contain a given amount of solute.
4. Do the calculations necessary to prepare solutions from pure drugs.
5. Do the calculations necessary to prepare solutions for irrigations, soaks, and nutritional feedings.

**lidocaine
hydrochloride**
Topical Solution USP

4%

In this chapter you will learn about solutions. Although medicinal solutions are generally prepared by the pharmacist, others may be required to prepare solutions for irrigations, soaks, and nutritional feedings.

Drugs are manufactured in both pure and diluted forms. A pure drug contains only the drug and nothing else. A pure drug can be diluted by dissolving a quantity of the pure drug in a liquid to form a **solution.** The pure drug (either dry or liquid) is called the **solute.** The liquid added to the pure drug to form the solution is called the **solvent** or **diluent.**

Introduction

To make a cup of coffee, you might dissolve 2 *teaspoons* of instant coffee granules in a cup of hot water. The instant coffee granules (*solute*) are added to the hot water (*solvent*) to form the cup of coffee (*solution*). If instead of 2 teaspoons of instant coffee granules, you add either 1 or 3 teaspoons of instant coffee granules to the cup of hot water, the coffee solution will taste quite different. The **strength** or **concentration** of the coffee could be described in terms of *teaspoons per cup* (*t/cup*). Thus, a coffee solution with a strength of *1 t/cup* is a *"weaker"* solution than a coffee solution with a strength of *2 t/cup*, and a strength of *3 t/cup* is *"stronger" than a strength of 2 t/cup*.

Important terms for the elements of a solution:

- The **solute** is the solid or liquid to be dissolved or diluted. Some solutes are powdered drugs, chemical salts, and liquid nutritional supplements.
- The **solvent** (**diluent**) is the liquid that dissolves the solid solute or dilutes the liquid solute. Two commonly used solvents are sterile water and normal saline.
- The **solution** is the liquid resulting from the combination of the solute and the solvent.

Strengths of Solutions Using Explicit Units of Measurement

The strength of a drug is stated on the label. Liquid drugs are solutions. The strength of these solutions compares the *amount of drug (solute)* in the solution to the *volume of solution*. Some examples of drug strengths or concentrations are: *Lanoxin 500 mcg/2 mL, KCl 2 mEq/mL, Garamycin 80 mg/2 mL,* and *heparin 10,000 units/mL.*

Suppose a vial is labeled *furosemide 5 mg/mL.* This means that there are 5 milligrams of furosemide in each milliliter of the solution. If a second vial is labeled *furosemide 10 mg/mL,* then this second solution is "stronger" than the first because there are 10 *mg* of furosemide in each milliliter of the solution. If an order is *furosemide 10 mg po stat,* then to receive 10 *mg* of the drug, the patient would receive either 2 *mL* of the "weaker" first solution or 1 *mL* of the "stronger" second solution.

Strengths of Solutions as Ratios, Fractions, and Percents

Sometimes the strength of a solution is specified *without using explicit units of measurement such as milligrams* or *milliliters* but by comparing the number of parts of *solute* to the number of parts of *solution*. This method of stating strength is generally expressed by using either *ratios, fractions,* or *percents.* Some examples of these strengths are *epinephrine 1:1,000 (ratio), Enfamil $\frac{1}{2}$ strength (fraction),* and *0.9% NaCl (percent).* In fractional form, the strength of a solution equals the amount of solute (drug) over the amount of solution.

$$\text{STRENGTH} = \frac{\text{SOLUTE}}{\text{SOLUTION}}$$

NOTE

This textbook does not make a distinction between the words *strength* and *concentration.* Some references call *5 g/100 mL* a "concentration" because it contains units of measurement, and *5%* a "strength" because it contains no units of measurement.

If a solution contains *1 part solute* in *2 parts of solution*, the strength could be expressed in the form of the *ratio 1:2* (read "1 to 2"), the *fraction* $\frac{1}{2}$ *strength* or, (because $\frac{1}{2} = 50\%$) the *percentage 50%*. See • **Figure 8.1**.

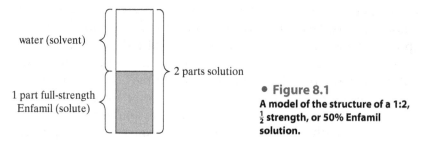

water (solvent)

2 parts solution

1 part full-strength
Enfamil (solute)

• **Figure 8.1**
A model of the structure of a 1:2, $\frac{1}{2}$ strength, or 50% Enfamil solution.

The ratio *1:5* means that there is 1 part *solute* in 5 parts *solution*. This solution is also referred to as a $\frac{1}{5}$ strength solution or as a *20% solution*. See • **Figure 8.2**.

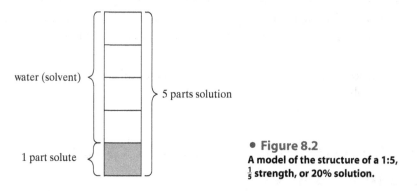

water (solvent)

5 parts solution

1 part solute

• **Figure 8.2**
A model of the structure of a 1:5, $\frac{1}{5}$ strength, or 20% solution.

A $\frac{1}{3}$ strength solution can be expressed as a *1:3* solution. This has 1 part *solute* for 3 parts *solution*. Because $\frac{1}{3} = 33\frac{1}{3}\%$, this is a $33\frac{1}{3}\%$ solution. See • **Figure 8.3**.

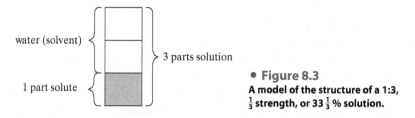

water (solvent)

3 parts solution

1 part solute

• **Figure 8.3**
A model of the structure of a 1:3, $\frac{1}{3}$ strength, or $33\frac{1}{3}$% solution.

A *60% solution* can be referred to (in fractional form) as a 60/100 solution, and after reducing, this fraction becomes $\frac{3}{5}$. In ratio form this strength would be *3:5*. This solution has 3 parts *solute* for 5 parts *solution*. See • **Figure 8.4**.

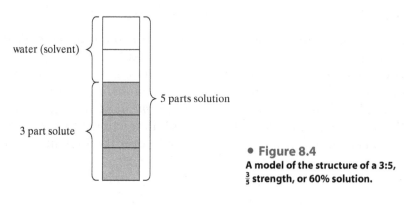

water (solvent)

5 parts solution

3 part solute

• **Figure 8.4**
A model of the structure of a 3:5, $\frac{3}{5}$ strength, or 60% solution.

EXAMPLE 8.1

Fill in the missing items in each line by following the pattern of the first line.

The solution contains:	The strength of the solution is		
	ratio	fraction	percent
1 part solute in 2 parts solution	1:2	$\frac{1}{2}$	50%
	1:4		
		$\frac{1}{5}$	
			3%
			5%
		$\frac{2}{5}$	
1 part solute in 1,000 parts solution			

Here are the answers.

The solution contains:	The strength of the solution is		
	ratio	fraction	percent
1 part solute in 2 parts solution	1:2	$\frac{1}{2}$	50%
1 part solute in 4 parts solution	1:4	$\frac{1}{4}$	25%
1 part solute in 5 parts solution	1:5	$\frac{1}{5}$	20%
3 parts solute in 100 parts solution	3:100	$\frac{3}{100}$	3%
1 part solute in 20 parts solution	1:20	$\frac{1}{20}$	5%
2 parts solute in 5 parts solution	2:5	$\frac{2}{5}$	40%
1 part solute in 1,000 parts solution	1:1,000	$\frac{1}{1,000}$	0.1%

Liquid Solutes

For a solute that is in liquid form, the ratio *1:40* means there is 1 part of solute in every 40 parts of solution. This could be 1 ounce of solute in every 40 ounces of solution, 1 *cup* of solute in every 40 *cups* of solution, or 1 *milliliter* of solute in every 40 *milliliters* of solution. For most solutions, milliliters will be used. So 40 *milliliters* of a *1:40* acetic acid solution means that 1 *milliliter* of pure acetic acid is diluted with water to make a total of 40 *milliliters* of solution. You would prepare this solution by placing 1 *milliliter* of pure acetic acid in a graduated cylinder and adding water until the level in the graduated cylinder reaches 40 *milliliters*. See • **Figure 8.5**.

A 1% solution means that there is 1 part of the solute in 100 parts of solution. So you would prepare 100 *mL* of a 1% creosol solution by placing

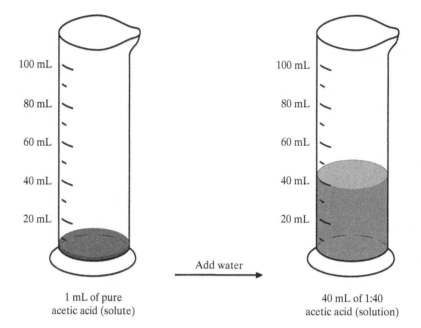

● **Figure 8.5**
**Preparing a 1:40 solution
from a liquid solute.**

1 mL of pure
acetic acid (solute)

Add water

40 mL of 1:40
acetic acid (solution)

1 *milliliter* of pure creosol in a graduated cylinder and adding water until the
level in the graduated cylinder reaches 100 *mL*. See ● **Figure 8.6.**

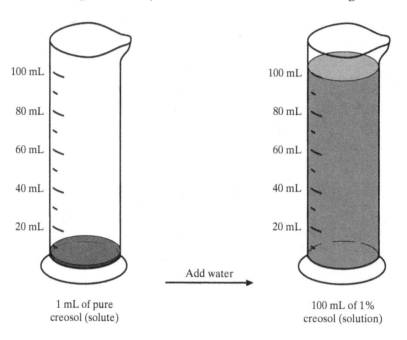

● **Figure 8.6**
**Preparing a 1% solution
from a liquid solute.**

1 mL of pure
creosol (solute)

Add water

100 mL of 1%
creosol (solution)

EXAMPLE 8.2

Suppose 40 *mL* of an iodine solution contains 10 *mL* of (solute) pure
iodine. Express the strength of this solution as a ratio, a fraction, and
a percentage.

The strength of a solution may be expressed as the ratio of the
*amount of pure drug in the solution to the total amount of the solu-
tion.* The amount of the solution is always expressed in milliliters, and
because iodine is a liquid in pure form, the amount of iodine is also
expressed in milliliters.

There are 10 *mL* of iodine (*solute*) in 40 *mL* of *solution*.

$$\text{Strength} = \frac{\text{Solute}}{\text{Solution}}$$

$$\text{Strength} = \frac{10\ mL}{40\ mL}$$

$$\text{Strength} = \frac{10\ mL}{40\ mL} = \frac{1}{4}$$

There are 10 *mL* of pure iodine in the 40 *mL* of the solution, so the strength of this iodine solution may be expressed as the ratio *1:4*, as the fraction $\frac{1}{4}$ *strength*, and as the percentage *25%*.

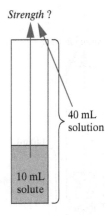

Strength ?

40 mL
solution

10 mL
solute

Dry Solutes

The ratio *1:20* means 1 part of the solute in 20 parts of solution, or 2 parts of the solute in 40 parts of solution, or 3 parts in 60, or 4 parts in 80, or 5 parts in 100, and so on. When a drug is in *dry* form, the ratio *1:20* means 1 g of drug in every 20 *mL* of solution. So 100 *mL* of a *1:20* potassium permanganate solution means 5 g of potassium permanganate dissolved in water to make a total of 100 *mL* of the solution. A *1:20* solution is the same as a *5%* solution. If each tablet is 5 g, then you would prepare this solution by placing 1 tablet of potassium permanganate in a graduated cylinder and adding some water to dissolve the tablet; then add more water until the level in the graduated cylinder reaches 100 *mL*.

Because a 5% potassium permanganate solution means 5 g of potassium permanganate in 100 *mL* of solution, the strength is also written as $\frac{5\ g}{100\ mL}$ or $\frac{1\ g}{20\ mL}$. See • **Figure 8.7**.

> **NOTE**
>
> For determining solution strength, you may want to think of *grams* as "equivalent" to *milliliters* because 1 *mL* of water weighs 1 gram. Thus, $\frac{1\ g}{20\ mL} = \frac{1\ mL}{20\ mL} = \frac{1}{20}$ strength.

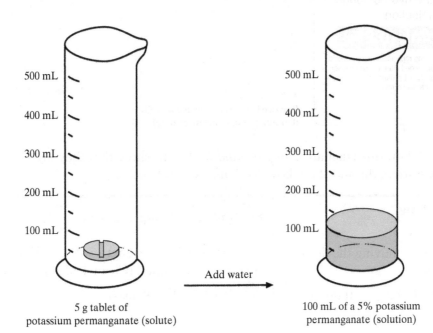

Add water →

5 g tablet of
potassium permanganate (solute)

100 mL of a 5% potassium
permanganate (solution)

• **Figure 8.7**
**Preparing a 5% solution
from a pure, dry drug.**

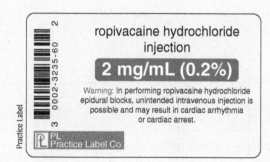

Strength = ?

140 mL
solution

70 g
solute

EXAMPLE 8.3

There are 70 *grams* of a drug dissolved in 140 *milliliters* of a solution. What is the strength of this solution expressed as a fraction, a ratio, and a percent?

$$Strength = \frac{Solute}{Solution}$$

There are 70 g of *solute* in 140 *mL* of *solution*.

$$Strength = \frac{70\ g}{140\ mL}$$

Because 1 *milliliter* of water weighs 1 *gram*, you may cancel *grams* with *milliliters*.

$$Strength = \frac{70\ \cancel{g}}{140\ \cancel{mL}} = \frac{70}{140} = \frac{1}{2}$$

So, the strength of this solution can be expressed as $\frac{1}{2}$ strength, as 1:2, or as 50%.

EXAMPLE 8.4

Read the label in • Figure 8.8 and verify that the two strengths stated on the label are equivalent.

Practice Label

2

0002-3235-60

3

ropivacaine hydrochloride
injection

2 mg/mL (0.2%)

Warning: In performing ropivacaine hydrochloride
epidural blocks, unintended intravenous injection is
possible and may result in cardiac arrhythmia
or cardiac arrest.

PL
Practice Label Co.

• **Figure 8.8**
Practice Label for ropivacaine HCl.
(For educational purposes only)

The two strengths stated on this label are *2 mg/mL and 0.2%*. To show that they are equivalent, take either one of these strengths and show how to change it to the other.

Method 1: Change $\frac{2\ mg}{mL} = ?\%$	**Method 2:** Change 0.2% to $?\ \frac{mg}{mL}$
Change 2 *mg* to grams by moving the decimal point 3 places to the left.	A solution whose strength is 0.2% has 0.2 g of solute (ropivacaine HCl) in 100 *mL* of solution. As a fraction, this is $\frac{0.2\ g}{100\ mL}$.
$2\ mg = 2.\ mg = .0\ 0\ 2\ g = 0.002\ g$	

So, *2 mg/mL* equals *0.002g/mL*. Now cancel the grams and milliliters and write the resulting number as a percent.

$$\frac{2\ mg}{1\ mL} = \frac{0.002\ \cancel{g}}{1\ \cancel{mL}} = \frac{0.002}{1} = 0.002 = 0.2\%$$

You need to change this fraction to *mg/mL*. That is,

$$\frac{0.2\ g}{100\ mL} = \frac{?\ mg}{mL}$$

One way to change $\frac{0.2\ g}{100\ mL}$ to $\frac{?\ mg}{mL}$ is to convert 0.2 g to *mg* by moving the decimal point three places to the right as follows:

$$0.2\ g = 0.200\ g = 0\ 2\ 0\ 0.\ mg = 200\ mg$$

Therefore,

$$\frac{0.2\ g}{100\ mL} = \frac{200\ mg}{100\ mL} = \frac{200\ mg}{100\ mL} = \frac{2\ mg}{1\ mL}$$

So, the two strengths (0.2% and 2 *mg/mL*) on the label are equivalent.

Determining the Amount of Solute in a Given Amount of Solution

Dimensional Analysis can be used to determine the amount of solute in a given amount of a solution of known strength.

The units of measurement for the amount of solution (volume), strength of solution, and amount of solute are listed as follows:

Amount of solution: Use *milliliters*.

Strength: Always write as a fraction for calculations.

For liquid solutes:
1:40 acetic acid solution is written as $\frac{1\ mL}{40\ mL}$
5% acetic acid solution is written as $\frac{5\ mL}{100\ mL}$

For dry or powder solutes:
1:20 potassium permanganate solution is written as $\frac{1\ g}{20\ mL}$

12% potassium permanganate solution is written as $\frac{12\ g}{100\ mL}$

Amount of solute: Use *milliliters* for liquids.

Use *grams* for tablets or powders.

To prepare a given amount of a solution of a given strength, you must first determine the amount of solute that will be in that solution. The amount of a given solution will be converted to the amount of solute by using the given strength as a unit fraction. Examples 8.5 through 8.7 illustrate the method for dry solutes, while examples 8.8 and 8.9 have liquid solutes.

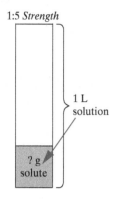

1:5 Strength

1 L
solution

? g
solute

EXAMPLE 8.5

How many grams of a solute would be needed to prepare 1 *liter* of a 1:5 *solution*? The solute is supplied in powdered form.

The diagram illustrates the problem.

You will change the single unit of measurement (1 *L*) to the single unit of measurement *(? g)* using the strength (1:5) as the unit fraction.

The strength of 1:5 can be written in fractional form as $\frac{1\,g}{5\,mL}$

You will have to do the following steps:

$$1\,L \rightarrow ?\,mL \rightarrow ?\,g$$

Use the fact that $1\,L = 1{,}000\,mL$, and then use the strength of the solution $\frac{1\,g}{5\,mL}$ as the unit fraction.

$$1\,L = \frac{1{,}000\,\cancel{mL}}{1} \times \frac{1\,g}{5\,\cancel{mL}} = 200\,g$$

So, 200 *g* of the solute would be needed to prepare 1 *liter* of a 1:5 solution.

EXAMPLE 8.6

Read the label in • Figure 8.9. How many grams of dextrose are contained in 30 *mL* of this solution?

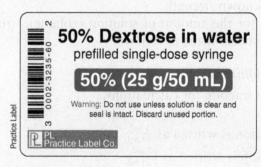

• **Figure 8.9**
Practice label for 50% Dextrose.
(For educational purposes only)

There are two equivalent strengths on the label: 50% and 25 g/50 *mL*. Either of them could be used to solve the problem. The percent will be used in this example.

The diagram illustrates the problem.

You will change the single unit of measurement (30 *mL*) to the single unit of measurement *(? g)* using the strength (50%) as the unit fraction.

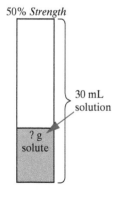

50% Strength

30 mL
solution

? g
solute

$$30\,mL \longrightarrow ?\,g$$

Use the strength of the solution $\frac{50\,g}{100\,mL}$ as the unit fraction.

$$\frac{30\,\cancel{mL}}{1} \times \frac{50\,g}{100\,\cancel{mL}} = 15\,g$$

So, 15 *grams* of dextrose are contained in 30 *mL* of a *50% dextrose* solution.

EXAMPLE 8.7

Determine the number of milligrams of lidocaine that are contained in 5 *mL* of a 4% lidocaine solution.

The diagram illustrates the problem.

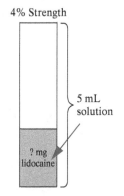

4% Strength

5 mL
solution

? mg
lidocaine

You will change the single unit of measurement (5 *mL*) to the single unit of measurement (? *mg*) using the strength (4%) as a unit fraction.

$$5 \text{ } mL = ? \text{ } mg$$

You will have to do the following steps:

$$5 \text{ } mL \longrightarrow ? \text{ } g \longrightarrow ? \text{ } mg$$

The strength of 4% can be written in fractional form as $\frac{4 \text{ } g}{100 \text{ } mL}$

Use the strength of the solution $\frac{4 \text{ } g}{100 \text{ } mL}$, and the fact that 1 *g* = 1,000 *mg* as the unit fractions.

$$\frac{5 \text{ } mL}{1} \times \frac{4 \text{ } g}{100 \text{ } mL} \times \frac{1,000 \text{ } mg}{1 \text{ } g} = 200 \text{ } mg$$

So, 200 *mg* of lidocaine are contained in 5 *mL* of a 4% *lidocaine* solution.

EXAMPLE 8.8

How would you prepare 2,000 *mL* of a *1:10* Clorox solution?

The diagram illustrates the problem.

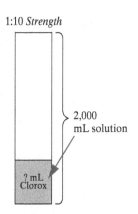

1:10 *Strength*

2,000
mL solution

? mL
Clorox

Because Clorox is a liquid in its pure form, it is measured in milliliters. So, a 1:10 strength means that 1 *mL* of Clorox is in each 10 *mL* of the solution.

You want to convert the amount of the solution (2,000 *mL*) to the amount of the pure Clorox.

$$2,000 \text{ } mL = ? \text{ } mL$$

The preceding expression contains *mL* on both sides. This can be confusing! To make it clearer, note that on the left side "*mL*" refers to the volume of the solution, whereas on the right side "*mL*" refers to the volume of the full-strength Clorox.

So, you have the following:

$$2{,}000 \; mL \; (\text{solution}) = ? \; mL \; (\text{Clorox})$$

The strength of the solution, 1:10, gives the unit fraction

$$\frac{1 \; mL \; (\text{Clorox})}{10 \; mL \; (\text{solution})}$$

$$2{,}000 \; \overline{mL \; (\text{solution})} \times \frac{1 \; mL \; (\text{Clorox})}{10 \; \overline{mL \; (\text{solution})}} = 200 \; mL \; (\text{Clorox})$$

So, you need 200 mL of Clorox to prepare 2,000 mL of a 1:10 solution. This means that 200 mL of Clorox is diluted with water to 2,000 mL of solution.

EXAMPLE 8.9

How would you prepare 250 mL of a $\frac{1}{2}$% Lysol solution?

The diagram illustrates the problem.

Because Lysol is a liquid in undiluted form, the amount of Lysol to be found is measured in milliliters.

$\frac{1}{2}$% can be written as 0.5% or as $\dfrac{0.5 \; mL \; (\text{Lysol})}{100 \; mL \; (\text{solution})}$

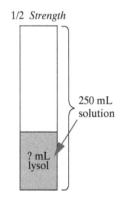

1/2 *Strength*

250 mL solution

? mL lysol

Convert the amount of the solution (250 mL) to the amount of Lysol.

$$250 \; mL \; (\text{solution}) = ? \; mL \; (\text{Lysol})$$

Use the strength of the solution $\dfrac{0.5 \; mL \; (\text{Lysol})}{100 \; mL \; (\text{solution})}$ as the unit fraction.

$$250 \; \overline{mL \; (\text{solution})} \times \frac{0.5 \; mL \; (\text{Lysol})}{100 \; \overline{mL \; (\text{solution})}} = 1.25 \; mL \; (\text{Lysol})$$

So, you need 1.25 mL of Lysol to prepare 250 mL of a $\frac{1}{2}$% Lysol solution. This means that 1.25 mL of Lysol is diluted with water to 250 mL of solution.

Determining the Amount of Solution that Contains a Given Amount of Solute

In the previous examples, you were given a volume of solution of known strength and had to find the amount of solute in that solution. Now, the process will be reversed. In the following examples, you will be given an amount of the solute in a solution of known strength and have to find the volume of that solution. The amount of given solute will be converted to the amount of solution by using the given strength as a unit fraction. Examples 8.10 and 8.11 illustrate the method for dry solutes, while examples 8.12 through 8.15 have liquid solutes.

EXAMPLE 8.10

How many milliliters of a 20% magnesium sulfate solution will contain 40 g of magnesium sulfate?

The diagram illustrates the problem.

   You want to convert the 40 g of solute to milliliters of solution.

$$40 \; g = ? \; mL$$

You want to cancel the grams and obtain the equivalent amount in milliliters.

$$40 \; g \times \frac{? \; mL}{? \; g} = ? \; mL$$

In a 20% solution there are 20 g of magnesium sulfate per 100 mL of solution. So, the unit fraction is

$$\frac{100 \; mL}{20 \; g}$$

$$\overset{2}{\cancel{40}} \; g \times \frac{100 \; mL}{\underset{1}{\cancel{20}} \; g} = 200 \; mL$$

So, 200 mL of a 20% magnesium sulfate solution contains 40 g of magnesium sulfate.

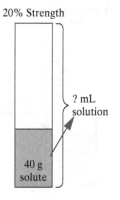

20% Strength

? mL solution

40 g solute

EXAMPLE 8.11

Calculate the number of milliliters of a 5% Mannitol solution that will contain 2 grams of Mannitol.

The diagram illustrates the problem.

   You will change the single unit of measurement (2 g) to the single unit of measurement (? mL) using the strength (5%) as the unit fraction.

$$2g \longrightarrow ? \; mL$$

Use the strength of the solution $\frac{100 \; mL}{5 \; g}$ as the unit fraction.

$$\frac{2 \; g}{1} \times \frac{100 \; mL}{5 \; g} = 40 \; mL$$

So, 40 *milliliters* of the 5% Mannitol solution contain 2 *grams* of Mannitol.

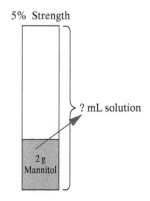

5% Strength

? mL solution

2 g Mannitol

EXAMPLE 8.12

How many milliliters of a *1:40* acetic acid solution will contain 25 *mL* of acetic acid?

The diagram illustrates the problem.

You want to convert the 25 *mL* of full-strength acetic acid to milliliters of solution.

$$25 \ mL \ (acid) = ? \ mL \ (solution)$$

There may be some confusion in the meaning of the previous line because there are milliliters on both sides of the equal sign. To aid your understanding, the parentheses are included to indicate whether "*mL*" refers to the amount of solute or to the amount of solution.

You want to cancel the milliliters of acid and obtain the equivalent amount in milliliters of solution.

$$25 \ mL \ (acid) \times \frac{? \ mL \ (solution)}{? \ mL \ (acid)} = ? \ mL \ (solution)$$

In a 1:40 acetic acid solution there is 1 *mL* of pure acetic acid in 40 *mL* of solution. So, the fraction is

$$\frac{40 \ mL \ (solution)}{1 \ mL \ (acid)}$$

$$25 \ \overline{mL \ (acid)} \times \frac{40 \ mL \ (solution)}{1 \ \overline{mL \ (acid)}} = 1{,}000 \ mL \ (solution)$$

So, 1,000 *mL* of a *1:40* acetic acid solution contain 25 *mL* of acetic acid.

1:40 Strength

? mL solution

25 mL acid

Irrigating Solutions, Soaks, and Oral Feedings

Sometimes healthcare professionals are required to prepare irrigating solutions, soaks, and nutritional feedings. These may be supplied in ready-to-use form, or they can be prepared from dry powders or from liquid concentrates.

Irrigating solutions and soaks are used for sterile irrigation of body cavities, wounds, and indwelling catheters; washing and rinsing purposes; or for soaking of surgical dressings, instruments, and laboratory specimens.

Enteral feedings are nutritional solutions that can be supplied in ready-to-use form, or they may be reconstituted from powders or from liquid concentrates. The nutritional solutions may be administered either orally or parenterally.

ALERT

Full-strength (ready-to-use) hydrogen peroxide is generally supplied as a 3% solution. This stock solution may be diluted to form weaker solutions depending on the application. These dilutions must be performed using aseptic techniques.

EXAMPLE 8.13

Using a full-strength hydrogen peroxide solution, how would you prepare 300 *mL* of $\frac{2}{3}$ strength hydrogen peroxide solution for a wound irrigation, using normal saline as the diluent?

The diagram illustrates the problem.
You want to convert *300 mL of solution* to *mL of solute* using the strength as the unit fraction.

$$300 \; mL \; (solution) = ? \; mL \; (solute)$$

Use the 2/3 strength as the unit fraction: $\dfrac{2 \; mL \; (solute)}{3 \; mL \; (solution)}$

$$\frac{300 \; \overline{mL(solution)}}{1} \times \frac{2 \; mL \; (solute)}{3 \; \overline{mL \; (solution)}} = 200 \; mL \; (solute)$$

So, 200 *mL* of full-strength hydrogen peroxide would be diluted with 100 *mL* of normal saline to make 300 *mL* of a 2/3 strength hydrogen peroxide solution.

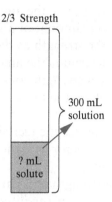

2/3 Strength

300 mL
solution

? mL
solute

EXAMPLE 8.14

How many ounces of $\frac{1}{4}$ strength Sustacal can be made from a 12-*ounce* can of full-strength Sustacal?

The diagram illustrates the problem.
You want to convert 12 *ounces of Sustacal* to ounces of solution using the strength as the unit fraction.

$$12 \; oz \; (Sustacal) = ? \; oz \; (solution)$$

The strength as a unit fraction is $\dfrac{1 \; oz \; (Sustacal)}{4 \; oz \; (solution)}$

$$\frac{12 \; \overline{oz \; (Sustacal)}}{1} \times \frac{4 \; oz \; (solution)}{1 \; \overline{oz \; (Sustacal)}} = 48 \; oz \; (solution)$$

So, 48 *ounces* of $\frac{1}{4}$ strength Sustacal can be made from a 12-*ounce* can of full-strength Sustacal by adding the 12-*ounce* can of Sustacal to 36 *ounces* (or three 12-*oz* cans) of water.

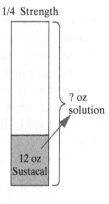

1/4 Strength

? oz
solution

12 oz
Sustacal

Summary

In this chapter, you learned that there are three important quantities associated with a solution: the *strength* of the solution, the *amount of solute* dissolved in the solution, and the total *volume of the solution*. If any two of these three quantities are known, the remaining quantity can be found.

- The *strength* of a solution is the ratio of the *amount of solute* dissolved in the solution to the total *volume of the solution*.
- The strength of a solution may be expressed in the form of a *ratio*, a *fraction*, or a *percentage*.

- A $\frac{1}{2}$ *strength* solution is a *1:2* or a *50%* solution and should not be confused with a $\frac{1}{2}$% solution.
- The amount of solute dissolved in the solution should be expressed in *milliliters* if the solute is a *liquid*.
- The amount of solute dissolved in the solution should be expressed in *grams* if the solute is a *solid* or a *powder*.
- The *volume of a solution* should be expressed in *milliliters*.

- $$\boxed{\text{Strength} = \frac{\text{Solute}}{\text{Solution}}}$$

- To determine the amount of solute contained in a given amount of a solution of known strength, use the strength as the unit fraction.
- To determine the amount of a solution of known strength containing a given amount of solute, use the strength as the unit fraction.
- Use the aseptic technique when diluting stock solutions for irrigations, soak, and nutritional liquids.
- The strength of a particular solution may be written in many different forms. The following strengths are all equivalent:

With stated units of measurement

$$Rates \begin{cases} 500 \text{ mg/mL} \\ 500 \text{ mg per mL} \\ \dfrac{500 \text{ mg}}{1 \text{ mL}} \end{cases}$$

Equivalence   500 *mg* = 1 *mL*

Without stated units of measurement

Fraction	$\frac{1}{2}$ strength
Ratio	1:2
Precentage	50%

Case Study 8.1

Read the Case Study and answer the questions. Answers can be found in Appendix A.

A 65-year-old male is admitted to a rehab facility, status post right-sided cerebral vascular accident (CVA). He has a past medical history of hypertension, hyperlipidemia, atrial fibrillation, osteoarthritis, and insulin-dependent diabetes mellitus. He is alert and oriented to person, place, time, and recent memory. He has left-sided weakness, needs assistance with activities of daily living (ADL), and has a 3 cm wound on his left heel. He rates his pain level as 8 on a scale of 0–10. Vital signs are: T 98.7° F; P 88; R 24; B/P 134/82.

His orders are as follows:

- diltiazem LA 120 *mg* po daily
- nabumetone 1,000 *mg* po at bedtime

- warfarin 2.5 *mg* po daily
- simvastatin 40 *mg* po at bedtime
- Sustacal 2 *oz* po with each oral medication administration
- Humulin R insulin 10 *units* and Humulin N insulin 34 *units* subcut 30 *minutes* ac breakfast
- Humulin R insulin 10 *units* and Humulin N insulin 28 *units* subcut 30 *minutes* ac dinner
- Pneumovax 0.5 *mL* IM stat for 1 dose
- Cleanse left heel with NS solution (0.9% Na Cl) and apply DSD daily

Refer to the labels below when necessary to answer the following questions.

1. Select the correct label for the diltiazem dose. How many tablets will you administer?
2. Select the correct label for the warfarin dose. How many tablets will you administer?
3. How many tablets of simvastatin will you administer?
4. How many tablets of nabumetone will you administer?
5. How many *mL* of Sustacal will the patient receive daily?

6. The pneumovax vial contains 2.5 *mL*. Choose the appropriate syringe below and place an arrow at the dose.

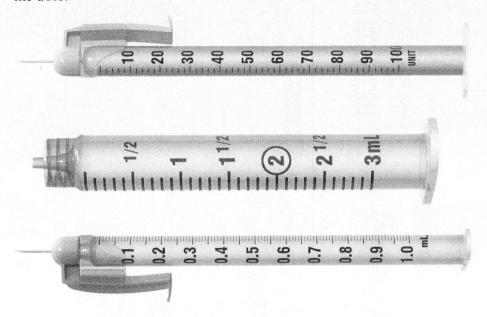

7. Describe how you will measure the morning insulin dose. Select the most appropriate syringe and mark the dose of Humulin R and Humulin N insulins.

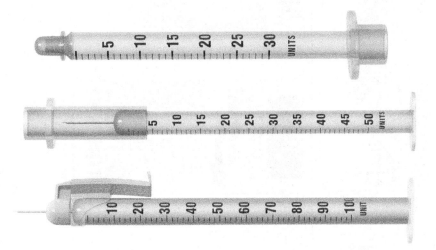

8. How many grams of sodium chloride are in 500 *mL* of the normal saline solution?

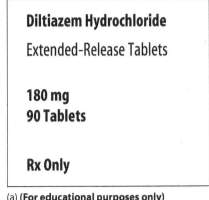

Diltiazem Hydrochloride

Extended-Release Tablets

180 mg
90 Tablets

Rx Only

(a) **(For educational purposes only)**

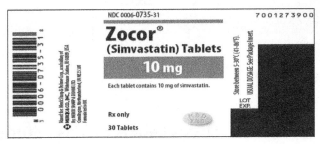

(b)

NDC 0006-0735-31   7001273900

Zocor®
(Simvastatin) Tablets
10 mg

Each tablet contains 10 mg of simvastatin.

Rx only

30 Tablets

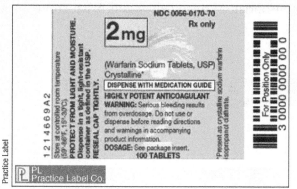

(c) **(For educational purposes only)**

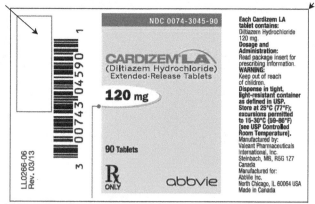

(d) **(For educational purposes only)**

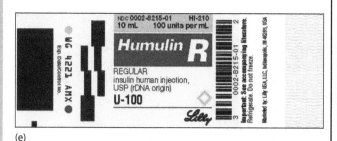

(e)

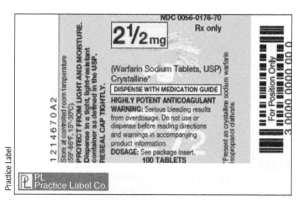

(f) **(For educational purposes only)**

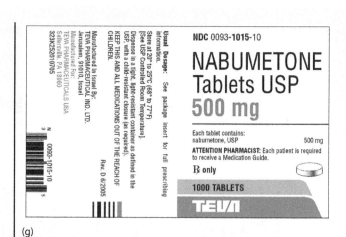

(g)

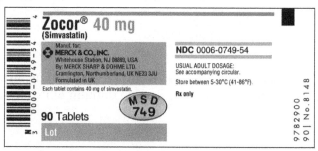

(h) **(For educational purposes only)**

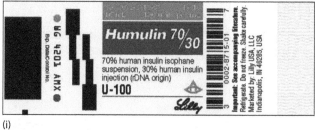

(i)

Drugs Labels for Case Study 8.1

Practice Sets

The answers to *Try These for Practice, Exercises,* and *Cumulative Review Exercises* are found in Appendix A. Ask your instructor for the answers to the *Additional Exercises.*

Try These for Practice

Test your comprehension after reading the chapter.

1. Express the strength of an iodine solution in the form of a fraction, a ratio, and a percent if 400 *mL* of the solution contain 80 *mL* of iodine.

2. Express the strength of a calcium chloride solution in the form of a fraction, a ratio, and a percent if 250 *mL* of the solution contain 100 *g* of calcium chloride.

3. How many grams of sodium chloride are contained in 400 *mL* of a 2% sodium chloride solution?

4. How many milliliters of a 2% lidocaine solution contain 10 grams of lidocaine?

5. How many milliliters of the cephalexin solution (• **Figure 8.10**) contain 100 *mg* of the pure drug?

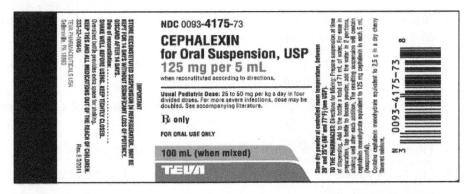

• **Figure 8.10**
Drug label for cephalexin.
(For educational purposes only)

Exercises

Reinforce your understanding in class or at home.

1. Express the strength of a solution in the form of a fraction, a ratio, and a percent if *200 mL* of the solution contain *50 mL* of a drug.

2. Express the strength of a solution in the form of a fraction, a ratio, and a percent if *8 mL* of the solution contain *3 g* of a drug.

3. Express the strength of a solution in the form of a fraction, a ratio, and a percent if *1 L* of the solution contains *60,000 mg* of a drug.

4. Express the strength of a solution of Isocal in the form of a fraction, a ratio, and a percent if *240 ounces* of the solution contain *80 ounces* of full-strength Isocal.

5. A vial of lidocaine solution has a strength of *0.5%*. A different vial of lidocaine solution has a strength of *40 mg/mL*. Which solution is stronger?

6. Which of the following could not be a solution strength?

   0.04%   *2:7*   *6 mL*   *4g/mL*   *balf strength*

7. Fill in the following chart of equivalent strengths.

Ratio	Fraction	Percent
1:5		
		10%
1:200		

8. Calculate the number of *grams* of dextrose in *500 mL* of a 5% dextrose solution.

9. How many *liters* of a normal saline (0.9% NaCl) solution will contain 18 *grams* of NaCl?

10. What is the strength of an Isocal solution made by adding 1 can of Isocal to 3 cans of water? Express as a fraction.

11. How many milligrams of sodium chloride are contained in 1 liter of 0.9% sodium chloride solution?

12. How many ounces of Sustacal are contained in 60 *ounces* of a 2/3 strength Sustacal solution?

13. How many milliliters of a 0.5% solution contain 4 *grams* of a drug?

14. How many grams of sodium chloride are contained in 2 *L* of a 4% sodium chloride solution?

15. How would 400 *mL* of a 20% solution be prepared using tablets that each contain 10 *grams* of the drug?

16. How many *mg* of NaCl are contained in 250 *mL* of a 0.45% NaCl solution?

17. The label on the vial of metoprolol tartrate indicates a strength of *5 mg/5 mL*. How many *mg* of metoprolol tartrate are contained in 87 *mL* of this solution?

18. Are the following two strengths equivalent: 2% and 20 *mg/mL*?

19. The label on a 20 *mL* aminophylline vial indicates a strength of 500 *mg*/20 *mL*.

    (a) How many *mL* of aminophylline would contain 200 *mg* of this drug?

    (b) How many *mg* of aminophylline would be contained in 1 *mL* of this solution?

20. One spray of a 0.06% solution of ipratropium bromide contains 42 mcg of the drug. Determine the number of milliliters that are in one spray.

Additional Exercises

Now, test yourself!

1. Express the strength of a solution both as a ratio and as a percentage if 500 *mL* of the solution contain 25 *mL* of solute.

2. Express the strength of a solution both as a ratio and as a percentage if 200 *mL* of the solution contain 40 *g* of solute.

3. Express the strength of a solution both as a ratio and as a percentage if 2 L of the solution contain 400 *mg* of solute.

4. Betadine solution is a 10% povidone-iodine solution. Express this strength both as a fraction and as a ratio.

5. Thorazine is available in a strength of 25 *mg/mL*. Express this strength as a percent.

6. Which of the following could be solution strengths?

   1:10,000   0.5%   25 *mL* $\frac{1}{3}$ 2 *mg/mL*   100 *g*

7. Read the label in • **Figure 8.11** and determine the number of milligrams of hydroxyzine pamoate that are contained in the vial of Vistaril.

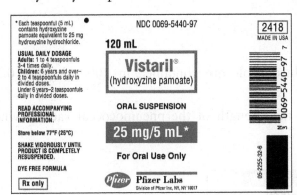

• **Figure 8.11**
Drug label for Vistaril.

(Reg. trademark of Pfizer Inc. Reproduced with permission.)

8. How many *mL* of a 10% magnesium sulfate solution will contain 14 *grams* of magnesium sulfate?

9. A pharmaceutical company sells ropivacaine HCl in various strengths as listed in the chart. Find the error in the "strength" column of the table by trying to verify that each of the four "concentrations" listed is equivalent to each of the corresponding "strengths."

Concentration	Strength	Vial Size
2 *mg/mL*	0.2%	100 *mL*
5 *mg/mL*	0.4%	30 *mL*
7.5 *mg/mL*	0.75%	20 *mL*
10 *mg/mL*	1%	20 *mL*

10. How many milliliters of 2% lidocaine viscous will contain 10 *mg* of lidocaine?

11. How many *mg* of fluconazole are contained in 200 *mL* of a 0.2% solution?

12. Express as a percent the strength of the pneumococcal vaccine whose label is in • **Figure 8.12**.

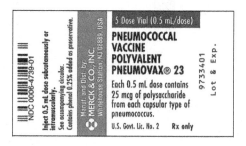

• **Figure 8.12**
Drug label for pneumococcal vaccine.

13. The nutritional formula Sustacal is supplied in 10-*ounce* cans. How would you prepare 40 *ounces* of a half-strength Sustacal solution?

14. How would you prepare 1 *liter* of a 25% boric acid solution from boric acid crystals?

15. Read the label in • **Figure 8.13** and determine the number of milligrams of erythromycin ethylsuccinate that are contained in 2 *mL* of the solution.

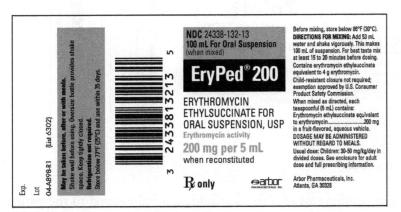

• **Figure 8.13**
Drug label for EryPed 200.

16. Read the label in Figure 8.13 and determine the number of milliliters of the solution that would contain 250 *mg* of erythromycin ethylsuccinate.

17. How would you prepare 1,200 *mL* of a 25% solution from a pure drug in solid form?

18. A drug label states that the strength of the solution is 10 *mg/mL* or 1%. Verify that the two stated strengths are equivalent.

19. A drug has a strength of 25 *mg/mL*. Write this strength in the form of a ratio, a fraction, and a percentage.

20. The nutritional formula Isomil is supplied in 4-, 8-, and 12-*ounce* cans. How would you prepare 6 *oz* of a 2/3 strength Isomil solution. What size can(s) would you use in order to minimize the amount of discarded Isomil?

Cumulative Review Exercises

Review your mastery of previous chapters.

1. 0.6 *g* = _____ *mg*

2. 3T = _____ *oz*

3. 110 *lb* = _____ *kg*

4. 45 *mm* = _____ *cm*

5. 1 *pt* = _____ *oz*

6. 8 *oz/day* = _____ *lb/wk*

7. A patient enters the ICU at 2230h on Tuesday and leaves 10 *hours* later. At what time (and day) does the patient leave the ICU?

Workspace

8. How many milliliters of Zoloft (sertraline HCl) contain 70 *mg* of Zoloft? See ● **Figure 8.14**.

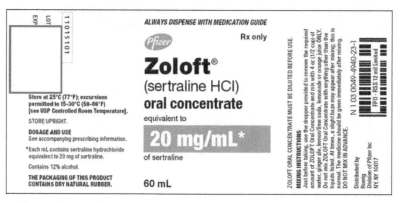

● **Figure 8.14**
Drug label for Zoloft.

9. How many milligrams of a drug should be administered to the patient if the order specifies 80 *mg* daily in 2 divided doses?

10. A 0.5 *mL* prefilled syringe contains 30 *mcg* of Avonex. How many mcg are contained in 0.25 *mL*?

11. A patient weighs 220 *lb*. Find the patient's weight in *kilograms*.

12. Order: *Provera (medroxyprogesterone acetate) 5 mg po daily for 5 days.* The tablets are supplied in 10 *mg* scored tablets. How many tablets of this hormone will you administer each day?

13. Order: *Zithromax (azithromycin) 500 mg po daily for 3 days.* It is supplied as an oral suspension with strength of 100 *mg/5 mL*. How many *mL* of this macrolide antibiotic will you administer?

14. How many *mg* of NaCl are contained in 200 *mL* of a 0.9% NaCl solution?

15. What is the weight in *grams* of an infant who weighs 6 *pounds*?

Parenteral Medications

Learning Outcomes

After completing this chapter, you will be able to

1. Calculate doses for parenteral medications in liquid form.
2. Interpret the directions on drug labels and package inserts for reconstituting medications supplied in powdered form.
3. Label reconstituted multidose medication containers with the necessary information.
4. Choose the most appropriate diluent volume when reconstituting a multiple-strength medication.
5. Calculate doses of parenteral medications measured in units.

This chapter introduces the calculations you will use to prepare and administer parenteral medications safely. Chapter 2 discussed the most common parenteral sites: intramuscular (IM), subcutaneous (subcut), and intravenous (IV). This chapter will focus on calculations for administering medications via the subcutaneous and intramuscular routes.

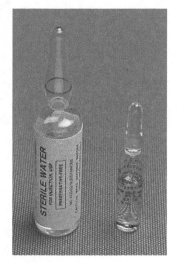

● **Figure 9.1**
Ampules.

Parenteral Medications

Parenteral medications are those that are injected into the body by various routes. Drugs for parenteral medications may be packaged in a variety of forms, including ampules, vials, and prefilled cartridges or syringes. Prefilled cartridges and syringes were discussed in Chapter 7.

An **ampule** is a glass container that holds a single dose of medication. It has a narrowed neck that is designed to snap open. The medication is aspirated into a syringe by gently pulling back on the plunger, which creates a negative pressure and allows the liquid to be pulled into the syringe (● **Figure 9.1**).

A **vial** is a glass or plastic container that has a rubber membrane on the top. This membrane is covered with a lid that maintains the sterility of the membrane until the vial is used for the first time. Multidose vials contain more than one dose of a medication. Single-dose vials contain one dose of medication, and many drugs are now prepared in single-dose format to reduce the chance of error. The medication in a vial may be supplied in liquid or powdered form (● **Figure 9.2**).

The CDC's guidelines state that medications labeled "single dose" or "single use" are to be used only once. Because single-dose vials (SDVs) typically lack antimicrobial preservatives, this practice protects patients from life-threatening infections that occur when medications get contaminated from unsafe use.

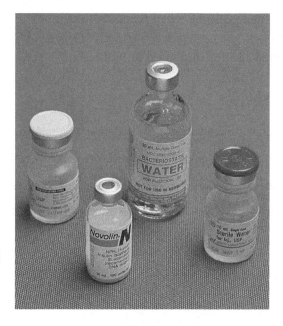

● **Figure 9.2**
Vials.

Parenteral Medications Supplied as Liquids

When parenteral medications are in liquid form, you must calculate the volume of the solution that contains the prescribed amount of the medication. To perform this calculation, you also need to know the strength of the solution. You will use Dimensional Analysis to calculate the volume that will be administered.

The following rough guidelines for the volumes generally administered subcutaneously or intramuscularly can be used to test the reasonableness of your calculated dosages.

Subcut:	Infant:	less than 0.1 *mL*
	Child:	less than 0.5 *mL*
	Adult:	from 0.5 *mL* to 1 *mL*
IM:	Infant:	less than 1 *mL*
	Child:	less than 2 *mL*
	Adult:	less than 3 *mL* (in the deltoid less than 2 *mL*)

EXAMPLE 9.1

The prescriber ordered *Sandostatin (octreotide acetate)* 50 *mcg subcut q8h*. Read the label in • Figure 9.3a and determine how many milliliters of this hormone suppressant you will administer. Indicate the dose on the syringe shown in • Figure 9.3b.

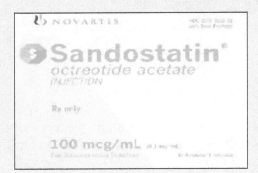

• Figure 9.3a
Drug label for Sandostatin.

Begin by determining how many milliliters contain the prescribed quantity of the medication. That is, you want to convert 50 *mcg* to an equivalent in milliliters.

$$50 \ mcg = ? \ mL$$

You cancel the micrograms and obtain the equivalent quantity in milliliters.

$$50 \ mcg \times \frac{? \ ml}{? \ mcg} = ? \ mL$$

The label reads "100 micrograms per 1 milliliter." Therefore, the unit fraction is $\dfrac{1 \ mL}{50 \ mcg}$

$$50 \ \cancel{mcg} \times \frac{1 \ mL}{100 \ \cancel{mcg}} = 0.5 \ mL$$

So, you would administer 0.5 *mL* of Sandostatin.

ALERT

In Example 9.1, the strength indicates that 100 *mcg* = 1 *mL*. Because the order (50 *mcg*) is less than 100 *mcg*, you would administer less than 1 *mL*. Always check to see whether the amount of drug prescribed is smaller (or larger) than the amount of drug stated in the strength available.

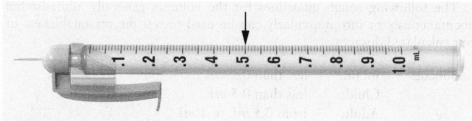

● Figure 9.3b
Syringe with 50 *mcg* of Sandostatin

EXAMPLE 9.2

The prescriber ordered *Cleocin (clindamycin)* 600 *mg IM q12h*.
Read the label in ● Figure 9.4 and calculate how many milliliters of
this lincosamide antibiotic you will administer.

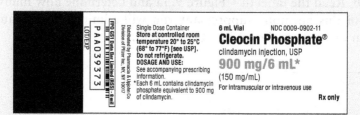

● Figure 9.4
Drug label for Cleocin.

Begin by determining how many milliliters contain the prescribed
quantity of the medication (600 *mg*). That is, you want to convert
600 *mg* to an equivalent in milliliters.

$$600 \ mg = ? \ mL$$

You cancel the milligrams and obtain the equivalent quantity in
milliliters.

$$600 \ mg \times \frac{? \ ml}{? \ mg} = ? \ mL$$

The label reads 900 *milligrams per 6 milliliters*. So, the unit fraction
is $\dfrac{6 \ mL}{900 \ mg}$

$$600 \ \cancel{mg} \times \frac{6 \ mL}{900 \ \cancel{mg}} = 4 \ mL$$

So, you would administer 4 *mL* of Cleocin.

EXAMPLE 9.3

The prescriber ordered *amikacin sulfate IM loading dose* for an adult patient who weighs 110 *pounds* and has a severe infection. Read the Drug Guide information in • Figure 9.5. The strength is 250 *mg/mL*.

(a) How many *mg/kg* will the prescriber order for the maximum loading dose?

(b) Calculate the number of milliliters of this aminoglycoside antibiotic you would administer.

	ROUTE & DOSAGE
	Moderate to Severe Infections
AMIKACIN SULFATE (am-i-kay'sin) Amikin **Classification:** AMINOGLYCOSIDE ANTIBIOTIC Therapeutic: ANTIBIOTIC **Prototype:** Gentamicin **Pregnancy Category:** C	*Adult:* **IV/IM** 5–7.5 mg/kg loading dose, then 7.5 mg/kg q12h (max: 15 mg/kg/day) for 7–10 days *Child:* **IV/IM** 5–7.5 mg/kg loading dose, then 5 mg/kg q8h or 7.5 mg/kg q12h for 7–10 days (max: 1.5 g/day) *Neonate:* **IV/IM** 10 mg/kg loading dose, then 7.5 mg/kg q12h for 7–10 days

• **Figure 9.5**
Drug vial and information for amikacin sulfate.

(a) First read the information in the Drug Guide, and you will see that the maximum loading dose should be 7.5 *mg/kg*.

(b) You must first convert the patient's weight to kilograms using the unit fraction $\dfrac{1\ kg}{2.2\ lb}$

$$110\ \cancel{lb} \times \frac{1\ kg}{2.2\ \cancel{lb}}$$

Then, multiply the patient's weight (in kg) by the order (7.5 *mg/kg*) to obtain the dose in milligrams.

$$110\ \cancel{lb} \times \frac{1\ kg}{2.2\ \cancel{lb}} \times \frac{7.5\ mg}{kg} = ?\ mL$$

Finally, use the strength to obtain the unit fraction $\dfrac{1\ mL}{250\ mg}$ to change the *mg* to *mL*.

$$110\ \cancel{lb} \times \frac{1\ kg}{2.2\ \cancel{lb}} \times \frac{7.5\ \cancel{mg}}{kg} \times \frac{1\ mL}{250\ \cancel{mg}} = 1.5\ mL$$

So, you would administer 1.5 *mL* IM to the patient.

EXAMPLE 9.4

The prescriber ordered *haloperidol 3 mg IM q4h prn.* • Figure 9.6 and determine how many milliliters of this antipsychotic drug you will prepare. Indicate the dose on the syringe below.

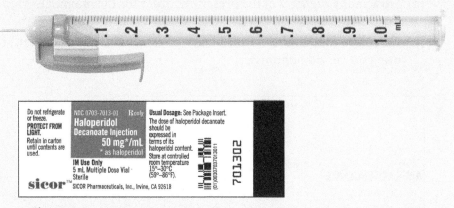

• **Figure 9.6**
Drug label for haloperidol.

You have a 5 *mL* multiple-dose vial, and the label indicates that the strength is 50 *mg/mL*. Begin by determining how many milliliters of the solution in the vial contain the prescribed quantity of the medication. That is, you want to convert 3 *mg* to an equivalent in milliliters.

$$3 \; mg = ? \; mL$$

You cancel the milligrams and obtain the equivalent in milliliters.

$$3 \; mg \times \frac{? \; mL}{? \; mg} = ? \; mL$$

The label indicates a strength of 50 *mg* per milliliter.

So, the unit fraction is $\dfrac{1 \; mL}{50 \; mg}$

$$3 \; \cancel{mg} \times \frac{1 \; mL}{50 \; \cancel{mg}} = 0.06 \; mL$$

So, you would use a 1-*mL* syringe and give the patient 0.06 *mL*.

0.06 mL

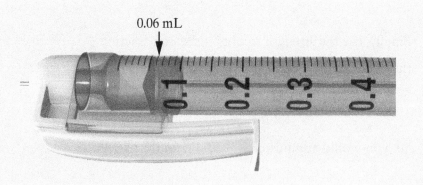

EXAMPLE 9.5

Prescriber's order: *Tobramycin* 120 *mg IM q8h, draw peak and trough levels after second dose. Notify MD if above 2 mcg/mL.* Read the label in • Figure 9.7 and calculate how many milliliters of this aminoglycoside you will administer.

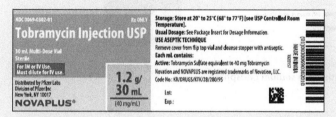

• **Figure 9.7**
Drug label for Tobramycin.

Determine how many milliliters of the solution in the vial contain the prescribed quantity of the medication. That is, you want to convert 120 *mg* to an equivalent in milliliters.

$$120 \ mg = ? \ mL$$

You cancel the milligrams and obtain the equivalent quantity in milliliters.

$$120 \ mg \times \frac{? \ mL}{? \ mg} = ? \ mL$$

The label indicates that the strength is 40 *mg per milliliter*.

Therefore, the unit fraction is $\dfrac{1 \ mL}{40 \ mg}$

$$120 \ mg \times \frac{1 \ mL}{40 \ mg} = 3 \ mL$$

So, you would administer 3 *mL* of Tobramycin to the patient.

EXAMPLE 9.6

The order for an adult who has adrenal insufficiency is *dexamethasone sodium phosphate* 5 *mg IM q12h.* The patient weighs 100 *kg.* Read the label in • Figure 9.8.

(a) If the recommended daily dosage is 0.03–0.15 *mg/kg,* is the prescribed dosage safe?

(b) How many milliliters will you administer?

(a) Using the recommended daily dosage, calculate the minimum and maximum number of milligrams the patient could receive each day.

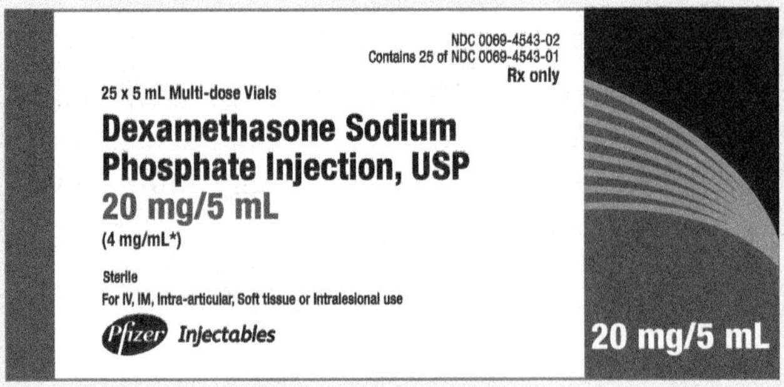

● **Figure 9.8**
Label for dexamethasone sodium phosphate.

Minimum Daily Dosage

Because the *minimum* recommended daily dosage (0.03 *mg/kg*) is based on the size of the patient (100 *kg*), multiply these as follows:

$$100 \ kg \times \frac{0.03 \ mg}{kg} = 3 \ mg$$

Maximum Daily Dosage

Because the *maximum* recommended daily dosage (0.15 *mg/kg*) is based on the size of the patient (100 *kg*), multiply these as follows:

$$100 \ kg \times \frac{0.15 \ mg}{kg} = 15 \ mg$$

So, the safe dose range for this patient is 3–15 *mg* daily.

The prescribed dosage is safe because the prescribed dosage of 5 *mg* q12h means the patient would receive 10 *mg* per day, which is in the safe dose range of 3–15 *mg* per day.

(b) Determine how many milliliters of liquid in the vial contain the prescribed quantity of the medication. That is, you want to convert 5 *mg* to an equivalent in milliliters.

$$5 \ mg = ? \ mL$$

You cancel the milligrams and obtain the equivalent quantity in milliliters.

$$5 \ mg \times \frac{? \ mL}{? \ mg} = ? \ mL$$

The label reads 4 *milligrams* per milliliter; therefore, the unit fraction is $\frac{1 \ mL}{4 \ mg}$

$$5 \ \overline{mg} \times \frac{1 \ mL}{4 \ \overline{mg}} = 1.25 \ mL$$

So, you would administer 1.3 *mL*.

Parenteral Medications Supplied in Powdered Form

Some parenteral medications are unstable when stored in liquid form, so they are packaged in powdered form. Before they can be administered, the powder in the vial must be diluted with a liquid (*diluent* or *solvent*). This process is referred to as *reconstitution.*

Sterile water for injection (SW) and 0.9% sodium chloride (NS) are the most commonly used *diluents.* Using the wrong diluent may result in an incompatability resulting in crystallization and/or clumping of the drug in solution form. This can cause problems in the tissue or circulation of the patient. Bacteriostatic water for injection is another type of diluent that may NOT be used in place of sterile water for injection. Both the type and the amount of diluent to be used must be determined when reconstituting parenteral medications. This information is found on the medication label or package insert. Because many reconstituted parenteral medications can be administered intramuscularly or intravenously, it is essential to verify the route ordered **before** reconstituting the medication—different routes may require different strengths.

Drugs dissolve completely in the diluent. Some drugs do not add any volume to the amount of diluent added, whereas other drugs increase the amount of total volume. This increase in volume is called the *displacement factor.* For example, directions for a 1 g powdered medication may state to add 2 *mL* of diluent to provide an approximate volume of *2.5 mL*. When the 2 *mL* of diluent is added, the 1 g of powdered drug displaces an additional 0.5 *mL* for a total volume of *2.5 mL*. The available strength after reconstitution is 1 g in *2.5 mL* or 400 *mg/mL*.

To reconstitute a powdered medication:

- Follow the directions on the label or package insert exactly as specified.
- Check the expiration dates of the drug and the diluent.
- Add the diluent to the vial.
- Shake, roll, or invert the vial as directed.
- Make sure that the powder is fully dissolved.

NOTE

If there are no directions for reconstitution on the label or package insert, consult appropriate resources such as the *PDR*, the pharmacist, DailyMed, or the prescribing information on the manufacturer's Web site before reconstituting.

ALERT

Reconstitution directions on vial labels may be very small and difficult to read. Use great care in identifying both the type and volume of the diluent to be used.

EXAMPLE 9.7

The prescriber ordered *ceftriaxone* 250 *mg IM stat* to treat a patient who has gonorrhea.

Read the label and the directions for reconstitution in • Figure 9.9 to determine how to prepare and administer this cephalosporin antibiotic.

Directions for Use

Intramuscular Administration

Reconstitute ceftriaxone for injection powder with sterile water for injection. Inject diluent into vial, and shake vial thoroughly to form solution.

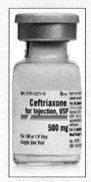

Vial Dosage Size	Amount of Diluent to Be Added	
	250 *mg/mL*	350 *mg/mL*
250 mg	0.9 *mL*	—
500 mg	1.8 *mL*	1.0 *mL*
1 g	3.6 *mL*	2.1 *mL*
2 g	7.2 *mL*	4.2 *mL*

● **Figure 9.9**
Ceftriaxone vial and portion of reconstitution directions.

After reconstitution, each 1 *mL* of solution contains approximately 250 *mg* or 350 *mg* equivalent of ceftriaxone, according to the amount of diluent indicated.

As with all intramuscular preparations, ceftriaxone for injection, USP, should be injected well within the body of a relatively large muscle; aspiration helps to avoid unintentional injection into a blood vessel.

To prepare the solution, inject 1.8 *mL* of air into the vial of sterile water for injection and withdraw 1.8 *mL* of sterile water. Then inject the 1.8 *mL* of sterile water into the 500 *mg* ceftriaxone vial and shake well to form a solution. ● **Figure 9.10**.

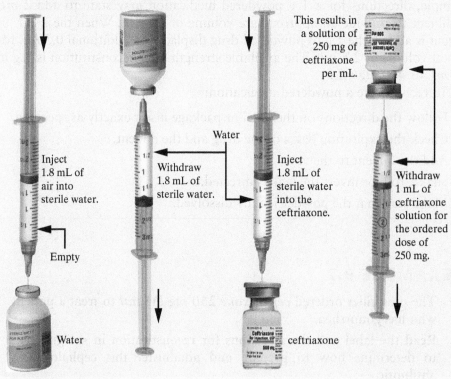

Inject 1.8 mL of air into sterile water.

Empty

Water

Withdraw 1.8 mL of sterile water.

Water

Inject 1.8 mL of sterile water into the ceftriaxone.

This results in a solution of 250 mg of ceftriaxone per mL.

Withdraw 1 mL of ceftriaxone solution for the ordered dose of 250 mg.

ceftriaxone

● **Figure 9.10**
Reconstitution of ceftriaxone.

Now the vial contains a reconstituted solution in which 1 *mL* = 250 *mg*.

So, you would withdraw 1 *mL* of ceftriaxone from the vial and administer it to the patient.

NOTE

The label in Example 9.7 states that when 1.8 *mL* of diluent is added, the resulting solution has a strength of 250 *mg/mL*. There is an approximate volume of 2 *mL* as a result of the displacement factor of 0.2 *mL*, which adds 0.2 *mL* to the 1.8 *mL* of diluent, to yield a total solution of 2 *mL*.

When you reconstitute a multiple-dose vial of powdered medication, it is important that you clearly label the vial with the following:

1. date and time of preparation
2. strength of the solution
3. date and time the reconstituted solution will expire
4. storage directions
5. your initials

Suppose that at 6 P.M. on January 23, 2016, Marie Colon, R.N., reconstitutes a drug to a strength of *50 mg/mL*, which will retain its potency for one week if kept refrigerated. Nurse Colon would write the following information on the label:

> *1/23/2016, 1800h, 50 mg/mL,*
> *Expires 1/30/2016, 1800h,*
> *Keep refrigerated. MC*

EXAMPLE 9.8

Order:*Unasyn (ampicillin sodium/sulbactam sodium) 1,700 mg IM q6h*. Read the drug label and portion of the package insert in • Figure 9.11. The package insert indicates that the solution must be used within one hour of preparation.

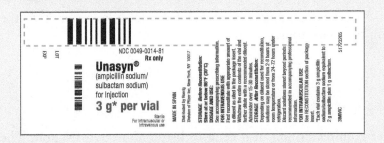

Preparation for Intramuscular Injection

1.5 g and 3.0 g Standard Vials: Vials for intramuscular use may be reconstituted with Sterile Water for Injection USP, 0.5% Lidocaine Hydrochloride Injection USP or 2% Lidocaine Hydrochloride Injection USP. Consult the following table for recommended volumes to be added to obtain solutions containing 375 *mg* UNASYN per *mL* (250 *mg* ampicillin/125 *mg* sulbactam per *mL*). Note: Use only freshly prepared solutions and administer within one hour after preparation.

UNASYN Vial Size	Volume of Diluent to Be Added	Withdrawal Volume*
There is sufficient excess present to allow withdrawal and administration of the stated volumes.		
1.5 g	3.2 *mL*	4.0 *mL*
3.0 g	6.4 *mL*	8.0 *mL*

• **Figure 9.11**
Drug label and portion of package insert for Unasyn.

(a) How much diluent must be added to the vial?

(b) If Nurse Susan Green reconstitutes the Unasyn at 0600h on February 1, 2016, complete the label she will place on the vial.

(c) Determine how many milliliters of this antibiotic Nurse Green will give the patient.

(a) First, prepare the solution. Because the vial contains 3 g, inject 6.4 *mL* of air into a vial of Sterile Water for Injection and withdraw 6.4 *mL* of sterile water. Add the sterile water to the Unasyn 3 g vial and be sure the solution is completely mixed.

(b) Nurse Green would write the following on the label:

> *2/1/2016, 0600h, reconstituted strength 375 mg/mL. Expires 2/1/2016, 0700h. SG*

(c) To calculate the amount of this solution, you need to convert the milligrams to milliliters.

$$1{,}700 \; mg \times \frac{?\; mL}{?\; mg} = ?\; mL$$

The vial contains 3,000 *mg* in a volume of 8 *mL* or 375 *mg* per 1 *mL*, so the unit fraction is $\dfrac{1\; mL}{375\; mg}$

$$1{,}700\; mg \times \frac{1\; mL}{375\; mg} = 4.533\; mL$$

So, Nurse Green would withdraw 4.5 *mL* and administer it to the patient in two injections.

EXAMPLE 9.9

An order requires 80 *mg* of a drug to be administered IM stat. The vial has the following three choices of strength after reconstitution:

> 10 *mg/mL*
> 20 *mg/mL*
> 40 *mg/mL*

For each of the three strengths:

(a) Determine the required volume of the solution to be administered.

(b) Choose the most appropriate strength.

(a) To calculate the amount of the 10 *mg/mL* solution (weakest strength), you need to convert the milligrams prescribed to milliliters.

$$80\; mg \times \frac{?\; mL}{?\; mg} = ?\; mL$$

- The vial contains 10 *mg* per 1 *mL*, so the unit fraction is $\dfrac{1\ mL}{10\ mg}$

$$80\ \cancel{mg} \times \frac{1\ mL}{10\ \cancel{mg}} = 8\ mL$$

- Using the 20 *mg/mL* solution (moderate strength), the unit fraction is $\dfrac{1\ mL}{20\ mg}$

$$80\ \cancel{mg} \times \frac{1\ mL}{20\ \cancel{mg}} = 4\ mL$$

- Using the 40 *mg/mL* solution (strongest strength), the unit fraction is $\dfrac{1\ mL}{40\ mg}$

$$80\ \cancel{mg} \times \frac{1\ mL}{40\ \cancel{mg}} = 2\ mL$$

In summary:

(Weakest)   10 *mg/mL* requires 8 *mL*
(Moderate)   20 *mg/mL* requires 4 *mL*
(Strongest)   40 *mg/mL* requires 2 *mL*

(b) **Weakest: 10 *mg/mL*** requires 8 *mL* to be administered. However, IM volumes are generally less that 3 *mL*. Therefore, this strength *should not be selected*.

Moderate: 20 *mg/mL* requires 4 *mL* to be administered. However, IM volumes are generally less that 3 *mL*. Therefore, this strength is a *poor choice*. However, the 4 *mL* could be divided into two syringes and administered at two different sites.

Strongest: 40 *mg/mL* requires 2 *mL* to be administered. This is less than 3 *mL* and is the *best choice*.

EXAMPLE 9.10

A prescriber ordered *Pfizerpen (penicillin potassium)* 200,000 *units* IM *stat and q6h*. Read the label in • Figure 9.12 and calculate how many milliliters of this penicillin antibiotic you will administer to the patient.

First, reconstitute the solution. The label lists three options: 250,000 *units/mL*; 500,000 *units/mL*; and 1,000,000 *units/mL*. If you

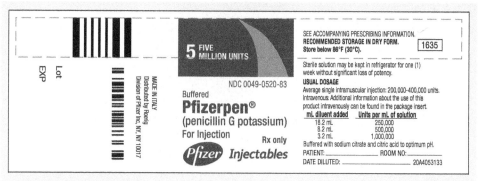

● **Figure 9.12**
Drug label for Pfizerpen.

From Daily Med (Reg. trademark of Pfizer Inc. Reproduced with permission.)

choose the first option, 18.2 *mL* of diluent must be added to obtain a dosage strength of 250,000 *units/mL*.

Now, inject 18.2 *mL* of air into a vial of sterile water for injection and then withdraw 18.2 *mL* of sterile water. Add the sterile water to the Pfizerpen vial and shake well. Now the vial contains a solution in which 1 *mL* = 250,000 *units*.

To calculate the amount of this solution to be administered, you need to convert units to milliliters.

$$200{,}000 \ units \times \frac{? \ mL}{? \ units} = ? \ mL$$

The vial contains 250,000 *units* per 1 *milliliter*, so the unit fraction is

$$\frac{1 \ mL}{250{,}000 \ units}$$

$$200{,}000 \ units \times \frac{1 \ mL}{250{,}000 \ units} = \frac{20 \ mL}{25} = 0.8 \ mL$$

So, you would withdraw 0.8 *mL* from the vial and administer it to the patient.

In Example 9.10, if a *stronger concentration* had been chosen for the reconstitution, then a *smaller volume* of the solution would be administered. The calculations would be similar to those just completed. The bottom two lines of the following table show the volumes for the other two options.

Concentration	Amount of diluent	Strength of the solution	Volume to administer
Weakest	18.2 *mL*	250,000 *units/mL*	0.8 *mL*
Moderate	8.2 *mL*	500,000 *units/mL*	0.4 *mL*
Strongest	3.2 *mL*	1,000,000 *units/mL*	0.2 *mL*

EXAMPLE 9.11

Order: *ampicillin* 300 *mg IM q6h*. Read the label in • Figure 9.13 and determine:

Some medications must be reconstituted immediately before administering them because they lose potency rapidly. Ampicillin, for example, must be used within one hour of being reconstituted.

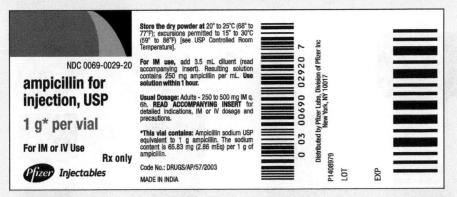

• **Figure 9.13**
Drug label for ampicillin.

(a) the number of milliliters of diluent needed to reconstitute the medication.

(b) whether the prescribed dose is safe or unsafe.

(c) the number of milliliters you will administer if the dose is safe.

(a) The label indicates that 3.5 *mL* of diluent must be added to the vial.

(b) From the label, we know that the usual dose for this medication ranges from a minimum of 250 *mg* (q6h) to a maximum of 500 *mg* (q6h). The order prescribes 300 *mg* (q6h). Because 300 *mg* is in the safe dose range of 250–500 *mg*, the prescribed dose is safe.

(c) The strength of the reconstituted ampicillin shown on the label is 250 *mg* per *mL*.

To calculate the amount of solution to be administered, you need to convert 300 *mg* to milliliters.

$$300 \ mg \times \frac{? \ mL}{? \ mg} = ? \ mL$$

The vial has a concentration of 250 *mg* per *mL*, so the unit fraction is $\dfrac{1 \ mL}{250 \ mg}$

$$300 \ \cancel{mg} \times \frac{1 \ mL}{250 \ \cancel{mg}} = 1.2 \ mL$$

So, you would administer 1.2 *mL* of the reconstituted ampicillin to the patient.

How to Use a Mix-O-Vial

Some medications are manufactured in a vial that contains a single dose of medication in which the vial has two compartments, separated by a rubber stopper. The top portion contains a sterile liquid (diluent), and the bottom portion contains the medication in powder form. When pressure is applied to the top of the vial, the rubber stopper that separates the medication from the diluent is released. This allows the diluent and powder to mix. • Figure 9.14.

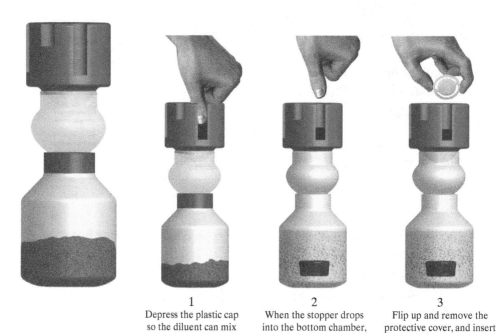

1
Depress the plastic cap so the diluent can mix into the bottom chamber.

2
When the stopper drops into the bottom chamber, it allows the diluent to mix with the drug.

3
Flip up and remove the protective cover, and insert needle squarely through the center to aspirate medication.

• **Figure 9.14**
How to prepare a Mix-O-Vial.

EXAMPLE 9.12

The prescriber ordered *Solu-Cortef (hydrocortisone sodium succinate)* 200 *mg IM q6h.* Read the label in • Figure 9.15 and determine how many milliliters of this glucocorticoid you will administer.

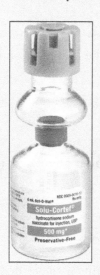

• **Figure 9.15**
Solu-Cortef Act-O-Vial and drug label.

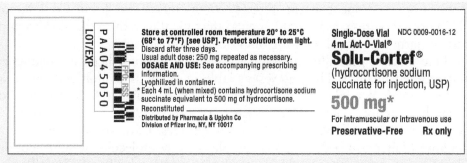

● **Figure 9.15**
(Continued)

First, reconstitute the solution:

1. Press down on the plastic activator to force diluent into the lower compartment.
2. Gently agitate to effect solution.

Now the vial contains a solution with the strength of $4\ mL = 500\ mg$.

To calculate the amount of this solution to be administered, you need to convert the dose of 200 *mg* to milliliters.

$$200\ mg \times \frac{?\ mL}{?\ mg} = ?\ mL$$

The vial contains 500 *mg per* 4 *mL*, so the unit fraction is $\dfrac{4\ mL}{500\ mg}$

$$200\ \overline{mg} \times \frac{4\ mL}{500\ \overline{mg}} = 1.6\ mL$$

So, you would administer 1.6 *mL* of Solu-Cortef.

3. Remove the protective cap.
4. Insert needle squarely through center of stopper until tip is just visible. Invert vial and withdraw dose.

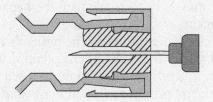

Heparin

Heparin sodium is a potent anticoagulant that inhibits clot formation and blood coagulation. Heparin is a high-alert drug and can be administered subcutaneously or intravenously. It is *never given intramuscularly because of the danger of hematomas.* According to the ISMP, anticoagulant medications are more likely to cause harm resulting from complex dosing, insufficient monitoring, and inconsistent patient compliance. The Joint Commission (TJC) now requires a National Patient Safety Goal to reduce the likelihood of patient harm associated with use of anticoagulant therapy.

Like insulin, penicillin, and some other medications, heparin is supplied and ordered in units. Heparin is available in single and multidose vials, as well as in commercially prepared IV solutions. It is available in a variety of strengths, ranging from 10 units/mL to 50,000 units/mL. See • **Figure 9.16**. Heparin is also available in prepackaged syringes. Lovenox (enoxaprin) and Fragmin (dalteparin sodium) are examples of low molecular weight heparin. They are used to prevent and treat deep vein thrombosis (DVT) following abdominal surgery, hip or knee replacement, unstable angina, and acute coronary syndromes.

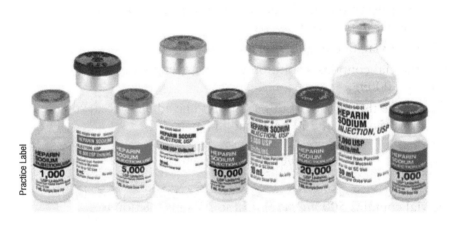

Practice Label

• **Figure 9.16**
Heparin vials.

When administered as a continuous IV infusion (see Chapter 11), the heparin dosage rate may be ordered as units per hour (units/h) or individualized by weight as units per kilogram per hour (units/kg/h). Initially, a bolus dose is administered to achieve a therapeutic blood level. This is followed by a continuous IV infusion. To maintain a constant rate, heparin is always administered by an electronic infusion pump. Dosage rates are adjusted according to lab results. The nurse may have to recalculate the heparin dosage to meet the patient's new requirements.

Heparin requires close monitoring of the patient's blood work because of the bleeding potential associated with anticoagulant drugs. To assure accuracy of dose measurement, a 1 *mL* syringe should be used to administer heparin subcutaneously. Healthcare providers should know and follow agency policies when administering heparin.

Heparin flush solutions (e.g., Hep-Flush or Hep-Lock) are used for maintaining the patency of indwelling IV catheters. These solutions are available in strengths of 10 *units/mL* and 100 *units/mL* see • **Figure 9.17**. Heparin sodium injections and heparin flush solutions are different and cannot be used interchangeably. Note the large differences in dosage strength between heparin sodium (1,000 to 50,000 *units/mL*) and heparin flush solutions (10 to 100 *units/mL*). Thus, the healthcare provider must be careful when preparing heparin.

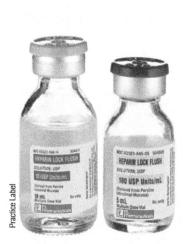

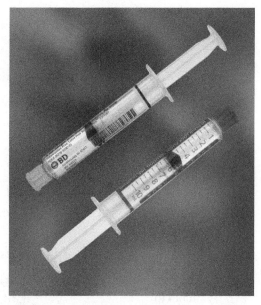

Heparin flush syringes.

• Figure 9.17
Heparin flush. (For educational purposes only)

EXAMPLE 9.13

The prescriber ordered *heparin 4,000 units subcut q12h*. Read the drug label in • Figure 9.18.

(a) Calculate the number of milliliters you will administer to the patient.

(b) Indicate the dose on the syringe below.

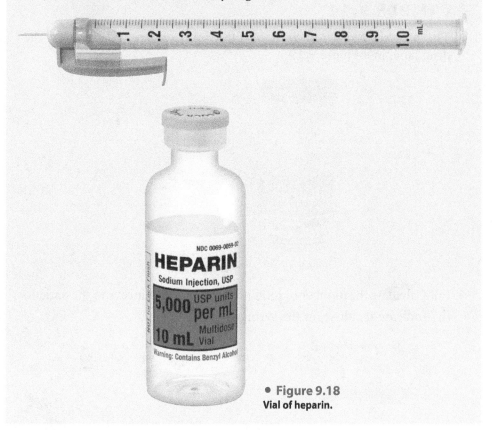

• Figure 9.18
Vial of heparin.

(a) You want to convert units to milliliters.

$$4,000 \ units = ? \ mL$$

You cancel the units and obtain the equivalent amount in milliliters.

$$4,000 \ units \times \frac{? \ mL}{? \ units} = ? \ mL$$

The strength on the vial is 5,000 *units* per milliliter, so the unit fraction is

$$\frac{1 \ mL}{5,000 \ units}$$

$$4,000 \ \cancel{units} \times \frac{1 \ mL}{5,000 \ \cancel{units}} = \frac{4 \ mL}{5} = 0.8 \ mL$$

So, you would use a 1 *mL* syringe and administer 0.8 *mL* of heparin.

(b)

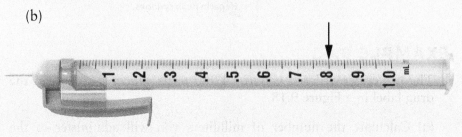

ALERT

Observe that, in Examples 9.13 and 9.14, the order for heparin is exactly the same (4,000 *units* subcutaneously *q12h*). However, the available dosage strengths are different. In Example 9.14 the strength (10,000 *units/ mL*) is twice the strength of that in Example 9.13 (5,000 *units/mL*). Therefore, only half the amount of the stronger solution is needed.

EXAMPLE 9.14

The prescriber ordered *heparin* 4,000 *units subcut q12h*. Read the drug label in • Figure 9.19.

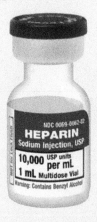

• **Figure 9.19**
Vial of heparin.

(a) Calculate the number of milliliters you will administer to the patient.

(b) Indicate the dose on the syringe below.

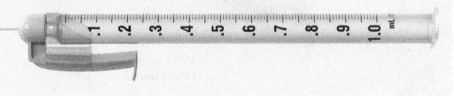

(a) You want to convert units to milliliters.

$$4,000 \ units = ? \ mL$$

You cancel the units and obtain the equivalent amount in milliliters.

$$4,000 \ units \times \frac{? \ mL}{? \ units} = ? \ mL$$

The strength on the vial is 10,000 *units* per milliliter, so the unit fraction is

$$\frac{1 \ mL}{10,000 \ units}$$

$$4,000 \ \cancel{units} \times \frac{1 \ mL}{10,000 \ \cancel{units}} = \frac{4 \ mL}{10} = 0.4 \ mL$$

So, you would use a 1 *mL* syringe and administer 0.4 *mL* of heparin.

(b)

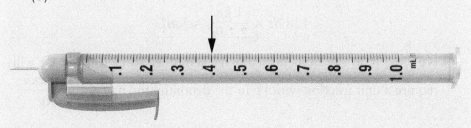

EXAMPLE 9.15

The prescriber ordered *Fragmin (dalteparin sodium)* 120 *units/ kg subcutaneously q12h* for a patient who weighs 138 *pounds*. See • Figure 9.20 and determine how many milliliters of this low molecular weight heparin you will need to administer the dose.

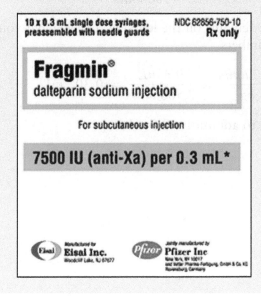

• **Figure 9.20**
Box label for Fragmin single-dose syringes.

Because this example contains a lot of information, it is useful to summarize it as follows:

Patient: 138 *lb* (single unit of measurement)
Known equivalences: 1 *kg* = 2.2 *lb* (needed to convert lb to kg)
                                    120 *units/kg* (order)
                                    7,500 *units*/0.3 *mL* (strength on
                                    the drug label)
Administer: ? *mL*

You want to convert a single unit of measurement (138 *lb*) to another single unit of measurement (*mL*).

$$138 \ lb = ? \ mL$$

You want to cancel *lb*. To do this you must use a unit fraction containing lb in the denominator. Using the equivalence 1 *kg* = 2.2 *lb*, this fraction will be $\dfrac{1 \ kg}{2.2 \ lb}$

$$138 \ \cancel{lb} \times \frac{1 \ \boxed{kg}}{2.2 \ \cancel{lb}} = ? \ mL$$

Now, kg is in the numerator on the left side. To cancel the kg will require a unit fraction with kg in the denominator, namely, $\dfrac{120 \ units}{kg}$

$$138 \ \cancel{lb} \times \frac{1 \ kg}{2.2 \ \cancel{lb}} \times \frac{120 \ \boxed{units}}{kg} = ? \ mL$$

Now, units is in the numerator on the left side. To cancel the units will require a fraction with units in the denominator, namely, $\dfrac{0.3 \ mL}{7,500 \ units}$

$$138 \ \cancel{lb} \times \frac{1 \ kg}{2.2 \ \cancel{lb}} \times \frac{120 \ \cancel{units}}{kg} \times \frac{0.3 \ \boxed{mL}}{7500 \ \cancel{units}} = ? \ mL$$

After cancelation, only *mL* remains on the left side. This is what you want. Now multiply the numbers.

$$138 \ \cancel{lb} \times \frac{kg}{2.2 \ \cancel{lb}} \times \frac{120 \ \cancel{units}}{kg} \times \frac{0.3 \ mL}{7,500 \ \cancel{units}} = 0.301 \ mL$$

Therefore, you would need to administer 0.3 *mL*.

Summary

In this chapter, you learned how to calculate doses for administering parenteral medications in liquid form, the procedure for reconstituting medications in powdered form, and how to calculate dosages for medications supplied in units.

- Medications supplied in powdered form must be reconstituted following the manufacturer's directions.
- You must determine the best dosage strength when there are several options for reconstituting the medication.
- After reconstituting a multiple-dose vial, label the medication vial with the dates and times of both preparation and expiration, storage directions, your initials, and the strength.

- When directions on the label are provided for both IM and IV reconstitution, be sure to read the order and the label carefully to determine the necessary type and amount of diluent to use.
- Heparin is measured in USP units.
- It is especially important that heparin orders be carefully checked with the available dosage strength before calculating the amount to be administered.
- A tuberculin 1 *mL* or a 0.5 *mL* syringe should be used when administering heparin.
- Heparin sodium and heparin flush solutions are different and should never be used interchangeably.

Case Study 9.1

Read the Case Study and answer the questions. Answers can be found in Appendix A.

A 69-year-old male is admitted to the ambulatory surgery unit for a laproscopic repair of a torn meniscus. He reports a past medical history of hypertension, hypercholesterolemia, osteoarthritis, and atrial fibrillation. He has a past surgical history of bilateral repair of rotator cuffs and a right total hip replacement. He is 6 *feet* tall and weighs 175 *pounds*. He denies any allergies to food or drugs. His vital signs are: T 98.9° F; B/P 138/90; P 96; R 18.

Pre-op orders:

- NPO
- IV RL @ 125 *mL/h*
- ondansetron hydrochloride 4 *mg* IM stat before anesthesia induction
- fentanyl 75 mcg IVP stat
- Transfer to OR

Post-op orders:

- NPO, progress to clear liquids as tolerated
- IV D5NS @ 125 *mL/h* until tolerating liquids
- Nexium (esomeprazole magnesium) 20 *mg* IVP stat

- Morphine sulfate 5 *mg* IM once if needed for pain
- V/S q15 *min* × 4, then q30 *min* × 2h, then q1h × 2h
- Cold compresses to right leg q1h × 20 *minutes*
- Discharge when stable

Discharge orders:

- losartan potassium-hydrochlorathiazide 100/12.5 *mg* PO daily
- lovastatin 20 *mg* PO daily
- escitalopram oxalate 15 *mg* PO daily
- warfarin 3.75 *mg* PO daily
- Nexium (esomeprazole magnesium) 20 *mg* PO 1h ac meals
- hydrocodone 5 *mg* PO q6h prn pain
- Cold compresses to right leg q1h × 20 *minutes*
- Make appointment for follow-up in one week

Refer to the labels in • **Figure 9.21** when necessary to answer the following questions.

1. The ondansetron hydrochloride is supplied in vials labeled 32 mg/5 *mL*.
   (a) How many milliliters are needed for the prescribed dose?
   (b) What type of syringe is needed to administer the dose?

2. The fentanyl is supplied in vials labeled 0.05 *mg/mL*.
   (a) How many milliliters are needed for the prescribed dose?
   (b) What type of syringe is needed to administer the dose?

3. The anesthetist will be administering propofol 2 *mg/kg* IV q 10 *seconds* until induction onset.
   (a) How many milliliters will the anesthetist prepare?
   (b) What type of syringe will be used to draw up the propofol?

4. The esomeprazole magnesium is supplied in 40 *mg* vials, and the label states to reconstitute the powder with 5 *mL* of Normal Saline. Calculate how many milliliters the patient will receive.

5. During your discharge teaching, you are reviewing the patient's medication vials and dosages.
   (a) Select the correct label for the losartan potassium-hydrochlorathiazide order.
   (b) How many tablets should you instruct the patient to take?

6. (a) Select the correct label for the lovastatin dose.
   (b) How many tablets should you instruct the patient to take?

7. (a) Select the correct label for the escitalopram oxalate dose.
   (b) How many milliliters should you instruct the patient to take?

8. (a) Select the correct label for the hydrocodone dose.
   (b) How many tablets may the patient take in a 24-*hour* period?

9. How many tablets of warfarin should you instruct the patient to take each day?

10. How many milligrams of esomeprazole magnesium may the patient take each day?

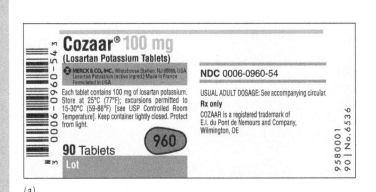

(a)

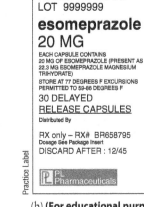

(b) **(For educational purposes only)**

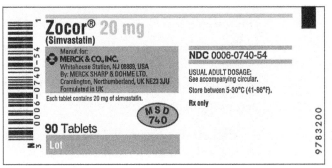

(c)

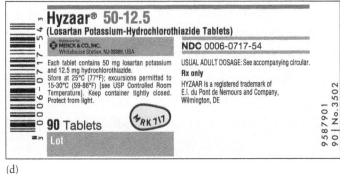

(d)

● **Figure 9.21**
Drug labels for Case Study.

(e) **(For educational purposes only)**

NDC 51672-4034-3

Warfarin Sodium

Tablets, USP Crystalline

7.5 mg

PROTECT FROM LIGHT.   HIGHLY POTENT ANTICOAGULANT.
WARNING: Serious bleeding results from overdosage. Do not use or dispense before reading directions and warnings in accompanying product information.

Rx only

1000 Tablets

Usual adult dosage: Read accompanying product information.
Store at 20-25C (68-77F) [see USP Controlled Room Temperature].
Dispense in a tight, light-resistant container as defined in the USP.
RESEAL CAP TIGHTLY.

Dispense with Medication Guide

TARO

Practice Label

PL Pharmaceuticals

(f)

NDC 0074-1973-14   100 Tablets

vicodin ES®

**hydrocodone bitartrate
and acetaminophen
tablets, USP**

Each tablet contains:
hydrocodone bitartrate   7.5 mg
acetaminophen   750 mg

Rx only   Abbott

Lot
Exp.

3
00741 97314 5
L0W11-R3 Rev 07/0708
04-4245-R3

Usual adult dosage:
See package insert.

Storage: Store at 25°C (77°F);
excursions permitted to
15°-30°C (59°-86°F). [See USP
Controlled Room Temperature].

Dispense in tight, light-resistant
container as defined in the USP.

Do not accept if seal over bottle
opening is broken or missing.

©Abbott

Manufactured for
Abbott Laboratories
North Chicago, IL 60064 U.S.A.

by Mallinckrodt Inc.
Hazelwood, MO 63042 U.S.A.

(g)

Keep this and all drugs out
of the reach of children.

Dispense in tight container
as described in the USP.

NDC 0456-2101-08

Lexapro
escitalopram oxalate

Oral Solution • 5mg/5mL

Equivalent to **1mg** escitalopram/mL

8 fl oz (240 mL)

Rx only

LOT NO. 189462

EXP. DATE Aug. 2014

3 04562 10108 4

FP FOREST PHARMACEUTICALS, INC.
Subsidiary of Forest Laboratories, Inc.
St. Louis, Missouri 63045

**Pharmacist: Must be dispensed
with Medication Guide**

Store at 25°C (77°F)–
Excursions permitted to
15° to 30°C (59° to 86°F)

See package insert for full
prescribing information.

Licensed from H. Lundbeck A/S

RMC 5372
Rev. 10/04

(h)

Mevacor® 20 mg
(Lovastatin)

MERCK & CO., INC.
Whitehouse Station, NJ 08889, USA

Store between 5-30°C (41-86°F).
Protect from light.

60 Tablets

Mevacor® 20 mg
(Lovastatin)

NDC 0006-0731-61

USUAL ADULT DOSAGE:
See accompanying circular.
Rx only

60 Tablets

3 0006-0731-617

LIFT HERE

9541400
60 | No. 3561

(i)

NDC 0074-1949-14   100 Tablets

vicodin®

**hydrocodone bitartrate
and acetaminophen
tablets, USP**

Each tablet contains:
hydrocodone bitartrate   5 mg
acetaminophen   500 mg

Rx only   Abbott

Lot
Exp.

3
00741 94914 0
L0W008-R3 Rev 07/0708
04-4243-R3

Usual adult dosage:
See package insert.

Storage: Store at 25°C (77°F);
excursions permitted to
15°-30°C (59°-86°F). [See USP
Controlled Room Temperature].

Dispense in tight,
light-resistant container as
defined in the USP.

Do not accept if seal over bottle
opening is broken or missing.

©Abbott

Manufactured for
Abbott Laboratories
North Chicago, IL 60064 U.S.A.

by Mallinckrodt Inc.
Hazelwood, MO 63042 U.S.A.

(j)

Hyzaar® 100-12.5
(Losartan Potassium-Hydrochlorothiazide Tablets)

Manufactured for
MERCK & CO., INC.
Whitehouse Station, NJ 08889, USA

Each tablet contains 100 mg losartan potassium
and 12.5 mg hydrochlorothiazide.
Store at 25°C (77°F); excursions permitted to
15-30°C (59-86°F) [see USP Controlled Room
Temperature]. Keep container tightly closed.
Protect from light.

90 Tablets   745

Lot

NDC 0006-0745-54

USUAL ADULT DOSAGE: See accompanying circular.

Rx only

HYZAAR is a registered trademark of
E.I. du Pont de Nemours and Company,
Wilmington, DE

3 0006-0745-546

9637300
90 | No. 6729

(k)

Cozaar® 25 mg
(Losartan Potassium Tablets)

Manufactured for:
MERCK & CO., INC. Whitehouse Station, NJ 08889, USA
Losartan Potassium (active ingred.) Made in France
Formulated in UK
By: MERCK SHARP & DOHME LTD.
Cramlington, Northumberland, UK NE23 3JU

Each tablet contains 25 mg of losartan potassium.
Store at 25°C (77°F); excursions permitted to
15-30°C (59-86°F) [see USP Controlled Room
Temperature]. Keep container tightly closed. Protect
from light.

90 Tablets   951

Lot

NDC 0006-0951-54

USUAL ADULT DOSAGE: See accompanying circular.

Rx only

COZAAR is a registered trademark of
E.I. du Pont de Nemours and Company,
Wilmington, DE

3 0006-0951-541

9721700
90 | No. 3612

(l)

Store between 4-25°C (40-77°F).
Do not freeze.
Protect from light.
SHAKE WELL BEFORE USE.
Discard unused portion within
six hours.
A0-0065/R2

LOT
EXP.

PropoFlo™
(propofol) Intravenous Anesthetic
Injection for Use in Dogs

200 mg/20 mL (10 mg/mL)

Each mL contains
10 mg of propofol
Single Dose Vial

Abbott

5206-04-03

CAUTION: Federal law restricts
this drug to use by or on the
order of a licensed veterinarian.

IMPORTANT: Read accompanying
product information for directions
pertaining to use of PropoFlo™
(propofol).

NADA No. 141-098. Approved by FDA
PropoFlo™ is a trademark of Abbott
Laboratories.

Product of Sweden

Manufactured for:
Abbott Laboratories.
North Chicago, IL 60064 USA

333.756

● **Figure 9.21**
(Continued)

Practice Sets

The answers to *Try These for Practice*, *Exercises*, and *Cumulative Review Exercises* are found in Appendix A. Ask your instructor for the answers to the *Additional Exercises*.

Try These for Practice

Test your comprehension after reading the chapter.

1. Order: *ceftriaxone 1 g IM daily in 2 equally divided doses.*

   Read the label in • **Figure 9.22**. How many *mL* will you administer?

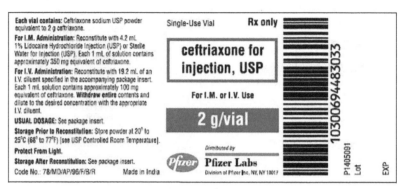

• **Figure 9.22**
Drug label for ceftriaxone.

2. Order: *ampicillin 400 mg IM q6h.*

   Read the label in • **Figure 9.23**. How many milliliters will you administer?

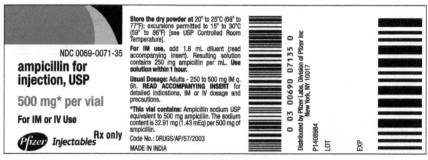

• **Figure 9.23**
Drug label for ampicillin.

3. Order: *Cleocin Phosphate (clindamycin) 600 mg IM q12h.*

   Read the label in • **Figure 9.24** and calculate how many milliliters of this antibiotic you will administer.

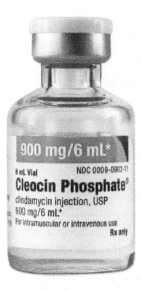

• Figure 9.24
Vial of Cleocin phosphate.

4. Order: *Neumega (oprelvekin) 50 mcg/kg subcut once daily.*

Calculate the number of milliliters of this platelet-stimulating drug you will administer to a patient who weighs 150 *pounds*. Note that this drug is supplied as a kit containing a vial of the drug and a prefilled syringe of the diluent, whose labels are shown in • **Figure 9.25**.

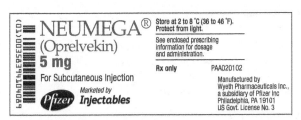

• **Figure 9.25(a)**
Drug label for Neumega.

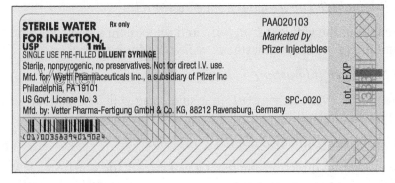

• **Figure 9.25(b)**
Drug label for diluent syringe for reconstituting and administering Neumega.

5. Order: Claforan (cefotaxime) 1.5g IM q12h

Use the portion of the package insert in • **Figure 9.26**.

Workspace

(a) What vial would you use for reconstitution?
(b) How much diluent must be added to the vial?
(c) What is the reconstituted volume in the vial?
(d) What is the strength of the reconstituted solution?
(e) How many milliliters would you administer?
(f) How many full doses are in the vial?

Cefotaxime for injection for IM or IV administration should be reconstituted as follows:

Strength	Diluent (mL)	Withdrawable Volume (mL)	Approximate Concentration (mg/mL)
(*) in conventional vials			
500 mg vial* (IM)	2	2.2	230
1 g vial* (IM)	3	3.4	300
2 g vial* (IM)	5	6	330
500 mg vial* (IV)	10	10.2	50
1 g vial* (IV)	10	10.4	95
2 g vial* (IV)	10	11	180

• **Figure 9.26**
A portion of package insert instructions for cefotaxime.

Exercises

Reinforce your understanding in class or at home.

1. Order: *hydralazine hydrochloride* 10 *mg IM q.i.d.*

   The strength in the vial is 20 *mg/mL*. How many milliliters of this antihypertensive will you administer?

2. Order: *Robinul (glycopyrrolate)* 4 *mcg/kg IM q3h.*

   The strength in the vial is 0.2 *mg/mL*, and the patient weighs 46 *kg*. How many milliliters of this preanesthetic will you administer?

3. Order: *Neupogen (filgrastim)* 5 *mcg/kg subcut daily.*

   The strength is 300 *mcg* = 1 *mL* in a single-use vial. The patient weighs 39 kg. How many milliliters of this drug will you administer?

4. Order: *Ticar (ticarcillin disodium)* 1 *g IM q6h.*

   The reconstitution directions on the 3 *g* vial state, "add 6 *mL* Sterile Water for Injection to the vial yielding a concentration of 385 *mg/mL*." How many milliliters of this antibiotic drug will you administer?

5. Order: *heparin* 4,000 *units subcut q12h.*

   Read the label in • **Figure 9.27**. How many milliliters will you administer?

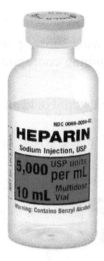

● **Figure 9.27**
**Vial of heparin. (For educational
purposes only)**

6. Order: *penicillin G potassium 250,000 units IM q6h*. Read the label in
   ● **Figure 9.28**.

   (a) Calculate the number of milliliters of this antibiotic you would admin-
       ister to the patient if you use the 8.2 *mL* of diluent to reconstitute the
       drug.

   (b) Indicate the dose by placing an arrow on the most appropriate syringe
       below.

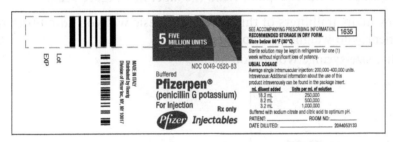

● **Figure 9.28**
Drug label for penicillin G potassium.

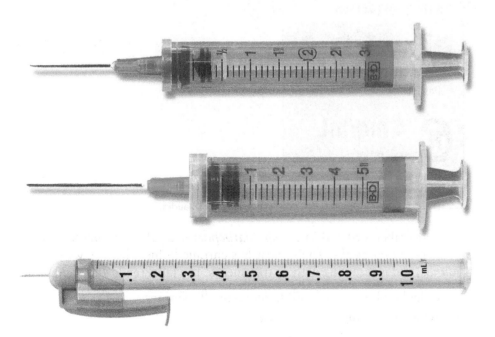

Workspace

7. Order: *ticarcillin disodium* 1 g IM q6h

   The label reads, "reconstitute each 1 g of ticarcillin with 2 *mL* of Sterile Water for Injection or NS and use promptly. The resulting concentration is 1g/2.6 *mL*."

   (a) Calculate the number of milliliters of this antibiotic you would administer to the patient.
   (b) Indicate which size syringe you would use and place arrow at the dosage.

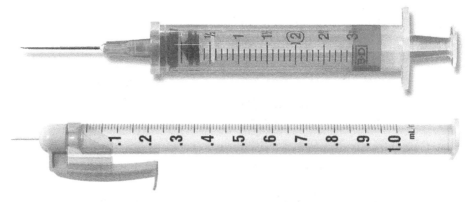

8. The prescriber ordered Dilaudid (HYDROmorphone HCl) 0.01 *mg/kg* subcut q3h prn moderate pain. Read the label in • **Figure 9.29**.

   (a) How many milliliters of this opioid analgesic will you administer to a patient who weighs 154 *pounds*?
   (b) What size syringe would you use?

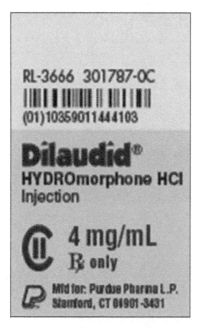

• Figure 9.29
Drug label for Dilaudid.

9. The prescriber ordered *Aranesp (darbepoetin alfa)* 0.75 *mcg/kg subcut once every two weeks*. The patient has chronic kidney disease, weighs 110 *pounds*, and is receiving dialysis treatments. The label reads 40 *mcg/0.4 mL*.

   (a) Calculate how many milliliters you will administer.
   (b) What size syringe will you use?

10. The prescriber ordered *ZYPREXA (olanzapine for injection) 7.5 mg IM stat*. Read the information on the drug package in • **Figure 9.30**.

    (a) How much diluent will you add to the vial?
    (b) What type of diluent will you use?
    (c) How many milliliters will you administer?
    (d) What size syringe will you use?

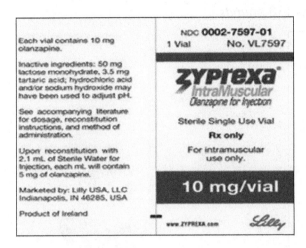

• **Figure 9.30**
Drug information for ZyPREXA.

11. The prescriber ordered *Pitocin (oxytocin) 20 units IM stat*. Read the label in • **Figure 9.31**.

    (a) Calculate how many milliliters you will prepare.
    (b) What size syringe will you use?

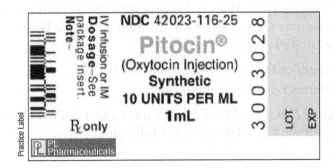

• **Figure 9.31**
Drug label for Pitocin.
(For educational purposes only)

12. Order: *Epogen (epoetin alfa) 100 units/kg subcut three times a week*. The label reads 10,000 *units* per *mL*, and the patient weighs 200 *pounds*.

    (a) How many milliliters will you administer?
    (b) What size syringe will you use?

13. Order: *Tigan (trimethobenzamide HCl) 200 mg IM q3h prn nausea and vomiting*. The 20 *mL* multiple-dose vial is labeled 100 *mg* per *mL*.

    (a) How many milliliters will you administer?
    (b) What is the maximum number of milliliters the patient may receive in 24 *hours*?

14. Order: *Neupogen 5 mcg/kg subcut daily*. The patient weighs 200 *pounds*. There are two vials; the strength of one vial is 480 mcg per 0.8 *mL*, and the strength of the other is 300 *mcg* per *mL*.

    (a) What strength vial will you use?

    (b) How many milliliters will you administer?

15. The prescriber ordered *streptomycin 15 mg/kg IM stat*. Use the label in • **Figure 9.32** to calculate the number of milliliters you would administer to a patient who weighs 150 *pounds*.

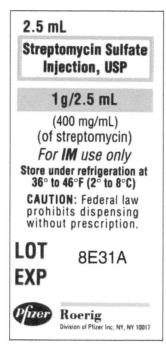

• **Figure 9.32**
Drug label for streptomycin.

16. The prescriber ordered *oxacillin 500 mg IM q6h*. The instructions on the 2 *g* vial state to reconstitute the powder with "11.5 *mL* of Sterile Water for Injection, yielding 250 *mg*/1.5 *mL*."

    (a) What is the strength of the reconstituted solution?

    (b) How many milliliters would you administer?

17. The prescriber ordered *Humalog Mix 75/25 15 units subcut ac breakfast*. Use the label in • **Figure 9.33** to determine the following:

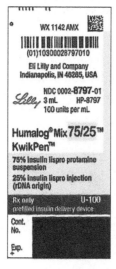

• **Figure 9.33**
Drug label for Humalog Mix 75/25.

(a) How many units will you administer?

(b) How many units are contained in the pen?

18. Use the insulin "sliding scale" below to determine how much insulin you would give to a patient whose blood glucose is 244.

The prescriber ordered *Humulin R Unit 100 insulin subcutaneously for blood-glucose levels as follows:*

Glucose less than 160   no insulin
Glucose 160–220   give 2 *units*
Glucose 221–280   give 4 *units*
Glucose 281–340   give 6 *units*
Glucose 341–400   give 8 *units*
Glucose more than 400   hold insulin and call MD stat

19. A patient weighs 110 *pounds*. The daily recommended safe dose range for a certain drug is 0.03−0.04 *mg/kg.*

(a) What is the minimum number of milligrams of this drug that this patient should receive each day?

(b) What is the maximum number of milligrams of this drug that this patient should receive each day?

20. The prescriber ordered *terbutaline 0.25 mg subcut q15 to 30 minutes, no more than 0.5 mg in 4 h.* Read the label in • **Figure 9.34** to answer the following:

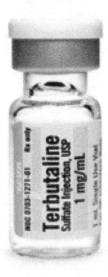

• **Figure 9.34**
Drug label for terbutaline.

(a) How many milliliters would you administer?

(b) What size syringe would you use?

(c) What is the maximum number of milliliters of this bronchodilator the patient may receive in 30 *minutes*?

Additional Exercises

Now, test yourself!

1. The prescriber ordered *Navane (thiothixene hydrochloride) 4 mg IM B.I.D.* The label on the vial reads *5 mg/mL.* Calculate how many milliliters of this antipsychotic drug you would administer.

Workspace

2. The prescriber ordered *Amevive (alefacept) 15 mg IM once per week for 12 weeks.*

   The instructions on the 15 *mg* vial states "reconstitute with 0.4 *mL* of the supplied diluent to yield 15 *mg/0.5 mL*." How many milliliters of this biologic response modifier would you administer?

3. The prescriber ordered *heparin 8,000 units subcut q8h.* Read the label in
   • **Figure 9.35.**

   (a) How many milliliters of this anticoagulant will you administer?
   (b) What size syringe will you use?

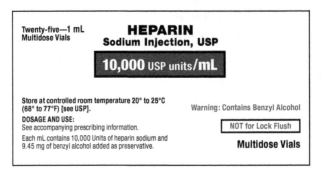

• **Figure 9.35**
Drug label for heparin.

4. The prescriber ordered *Unasyn (ampicillin sodium/sublactam sodium) 2g IM q6h.* Use the information from the package insert in • **Figure 9.36.**

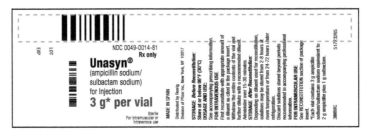

Unasyn Vial Size	Volume of Diluent to Be Added	Withdrawal Volume
1.5 g	3.2 mL	4 mL
3 g	6.4 mL	8 mL

• **Figure 9.36**
Drug label for and portion of package insert for Unasyn.

   (a) How much diluent must be added to the vial?
   (b) What is the reconstituted volume in the vial?
   (c) What is the strength of the reconstituted solution?
   (d) How many milliliters of this antibiotic will you administer?

5. The prescriber ordered *lincomycin hydrochloride 600 mg IM q12h.* Read the label in • **Figure 9.37.** Calculate how many milliliters of this lincos-amide antibiotic you would administer.

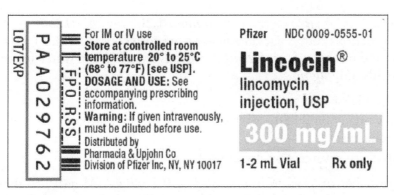

● **Figure 9.37**
Drug label for Lincocin.

6. The prescriber ordered *Benadryl (diphenhydramine hydrochloride) 45 mg IM q4h*. Read the label in ● **Figure 9.38**. The manufacturer states not to exceed 400 *mg/day*.

   (a) Is this a safe dose?

   (b) How many milliliters of this antihistamine would you administer?

   (c) What size syringe would you use?

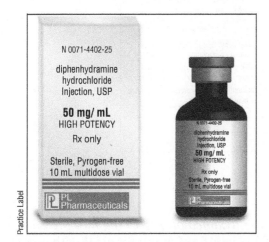

● **Figure 9.38**
Drug box and vial for diphenhydramine hydrochloride.
(For educational purposes only)

7. The prescriber ordered *fentanyl citrate 55 mcg IM prn pain*. Read the label in ● **Figure 9.39**.

   (a) How many milliliters of this narcotic analgesic would you administer?

   (b) Which size syringe would you use?

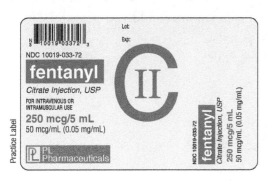

● **Figure 9.39**
Drug label for fentanyl citrate.
(For educational purposes only)

Workspace

8. The prescriber ordered *ceftriaxone sodium 1,200 mg IM q12h for 4 days*. The instructions in the package insert state to reconstitute the 1 g or 2 g vial by adding 2.1 *mL* or 4.2 *mL*, respectively, of sterile water for injection, yields 350 *mg/mL*.

   (a) What vial would you use?
   (b) How many milliliters of this cephalosporin antibiotic would you administer?
   (c) What size syringe would you use?

9. The prescriber ordered *morphine sulfate 0.2 mg/kg IM q4h prn moderate-severe pain*. Read the label in • **Figure 9.40.**

   (a) How many milliliters of this narcotic analgesic would you administer to a patient who weighs 154 *pounds*?
   (b) What size syringe would you use?
   (c) The package insert states that the maximum dose is 10 *mg*/24h. Is the patient receiving a safe dose?

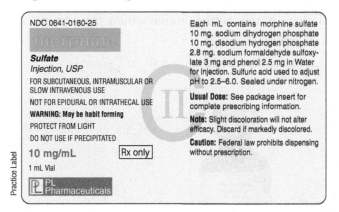

NDC 0641-0180-25

morphine

Sulfate
Injection, USP

FOR SUBCUTANEOUS, INTRAMUSCULAR OR
SLOW INTRAVENOUS USE

NOT FOR EPIDURAL OR INTRATHECAL USE

WARNING: May be habit forming

PROTECT FROM LIGHT

DO NOT USE IF PRECIPITATED

10 mg/mL   Rx only

1 mL Vial

Practice Label

PL Pharmaceuticals

Each mL contains morphine sulfate 10 mg, sodium dihydrogen phosphate 10 mg, disodium hydrogen phosphate 2.8 mg, sodium formaldehyde sulfoxylate 3 mg and phenol 2.5 mg in Water for Injection. Sulfuric acid used to adjust pH to 2.5–6.0. Sealed under nitrogen.

Usual Dose: See package insert for complete prescribing information.

Note: Slight discoloration will not alter efficacy. Discard if markedly discolored.

Caution: Federal law prohibits dispensing without prescription.

• **Figure 9.40**
Drug label for morphine sulfate.
(For educational purposes only)

10. The prescriber ordered *Kenalog (triamcinolone) 15 mg into the knee joint stat*. The medication is available in a *5 mL* multidose vial with a strength of 10 *mg/mL*.

    (a) How many milliliters of this synthetic glucocorticoid will the patient receive?
    (b) How many doses of 15 *mg* are contained in the vial?

11. The prescriber ordered *leuprolide acetate injection 1 mg subcut now*. The 2.8 *mL* multiple dose vial has a strength of 1 *mg/0.2 mL*.

    (a) How many milliliters of this hormone would you prepare?
    (b) What size syringe would you use?
    (c) How many doses are in the vial?

12. Use the label in • **Figure 9.42** to answer the following:

    (a) How much diluent must be added to the vial to prepare 500,000 *units/ mL* strength?
    (b) What strength would be available if you added 18.2 *mL* of diluent?
    (c) What is the total dose of penicillin G potassium in the vial?
    (d) The prescriber ordered *penicillin G potassium 2 million units IM q4h*. Which dosage strength would you use?
    (e) How many milliliters of this antibiotic would you administer?

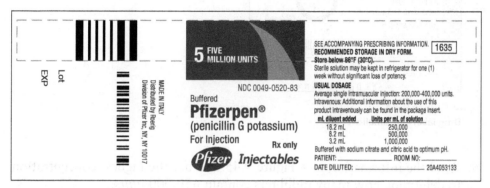

• **Figure 9.42**
Drug label for Pfizerpen.

13. The prescriber ordered *Ancef (cefazolin sodium) 250 mg IM q8h*. The directions for the 1 *g* vial state "for IM administration add 2.5 *mL* of Sterile Water for Injection. Provides an approximate volume of 3 *mL*."

    (a) What is the total amount of Ancef in the vial?
    (b) How many milliliters of this cephalosporin antibiotic would you administer?

14. The prescriber ordered *furosemide 30 mg IM B.I.D*. Read the label in • **Figure 9.43**.

    (a) How many milliliters of this loop diuretic would you administer?
    (b) What size syringe would you use?

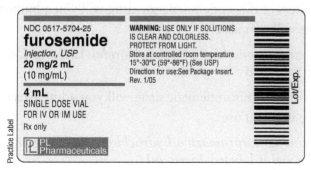

• **Figure 9.43**
Drug label for furosemide.
(For educational purposes only)

15. The prescriber ordered *NPH human insulin 15 units subcut ac breakfast.* Read the label in • **Figure 9.44** and determine how many doses are contained in the pen.

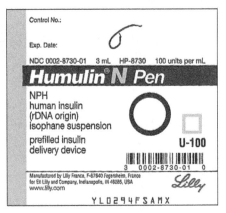

• **Figure 9.44**
Drug label for Humulin N Pen.

16. Read the information in • **Figure 9.45** and use the highest concentration to determine how many milliliters contain 650,000 *units.*

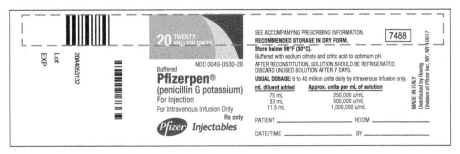

• **Figure 9.45**
Drug label for Pfizerpen.

(Reg. Trademark of Pfizer Inc. Reproduced with permission.)

17. A patient is to receive *atropine sulfate 0.2 mg IM 30 minutes before surgery.* The vial is labeled 0.4 *mg/mL.*

    (a) How many milliliters of this anticholenergic drug will you administer?

    (b) What size syringe will you use?

18. The order is *Phenergan (promethazine hydrochloride) 12.5 mg IM q4h prn nausea.* The vial is labeled 50 *mg/mL.*

    (a) How many milliliters of this antiemetic drug will you administer?

    (b) What size syringe will you use?

19. The order is *Thorazine (chlorpromazine hydrochloride) 40 mg IM q6h prn for agitation.* The vial is labeled 25 *mg/mL.*

    (a) How many milliliters of this antipsychotic drug will you administer?

    (b) What size syringe will you use?

20. Use the information in • **Figure 9.46** and answer the following:

    (a) How much diluent must be added to the vial to prepare a 250,000 *units/mL* strength?

    (b) How much diluent must be added to the vial to prepare a 500,000 *units/mL* strength?

    (c) What is the total dose of this vial?

    (d) The order is *penicillin G 2,000,000 units IM stat*. How will you prepare this dose?

Workspace

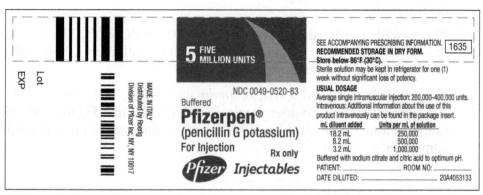

• **Figure 9.46**
Drug label for Pfizerpen.
(Reg. Trademark of Pfizer Inc. Reproduced with permission.)

Cumulative Review Exercises

Review your mastery of previous chapters.

1. 330 *lb* = ? *kg*

2. How many grams of sodium chloride are contained in 500 *mL* of normal saline (0.9% NaCl)?

3. A patient is receiving 10 *mg* of a drug q4h. If the safe dose range for the drug is 20–40 *mg/d*, is the patient receiving a safe dose?

4. Estimate the body surface area of a patient who weighs 200 *pounds* and is 6 *feet* tall.

5. Order: *Oxycontin (oxycodone hydrochloride) 10 mg po q6h prn moderate to severe pain*. The strength available is 20 *mg/mL*.

    How many milliliters of this analgesic will you administer?

    Read the label in • **Figure 9.47** to answer questions 6 through 10.

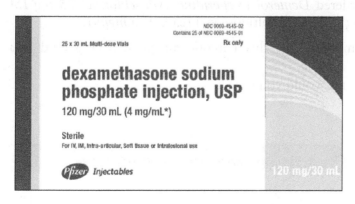

• **Figure 9.47**
Drug label for dexamethasone.

Workspace

6. What is the generic name of this drug?

7. What is the dosage strength?

8. What is the route of administration?

9. A patient is to receive 3 *mg* injected into the knee joint. How many milliliters will be injected?

10. What is the total volume in the vial?

11. How many grams of dextrose are contained in 2,000 *mL* of a 10% dextrose solution?

12. The prescriber ordered *Suprax (cefixime)* 400 *mg PO daily.* The label on the 75 *mL* bottle reads 100 *mg/5 mL.* How many milliliters of this cephalosporin antibiotic would the patient receive?

13. The prescriber ordered *Crixivan (indinavir sulfate)* 800 *mg PO q8h,* 1 *h before meals or 2 h after meals.* Read the label in • **Figure 9.48** and calculate how many capsules of this protease inhibitor drug you would administer.

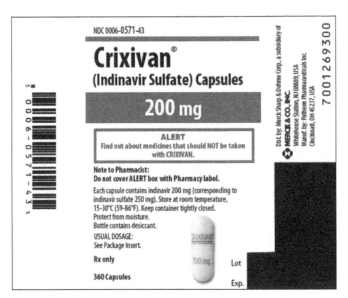

• **Figure 9.48**
Drug label for Crixivan.

14. The prescriber ordered 240 *mL* of *2/3 strength Sustacal PO B.I.D.* How will you prepare this solution using a 240 *mL* can of Sustacal?

15. The prescriber ordered *Demerol (meperidine hydrochloride)* 75 *mg IM stat.* The label on the 20 *mL* multidose vial reads 100 *mg/mL.*

    (a) How many milliliters of this narcotic analgesic drug would you administer?

    (b) What size syringe would you use?

Unit

4

Infusions and Pediatric Dosages

Flow Rates and Durations of Enteral and Intravenous Infusions

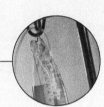

Learning Outcomes

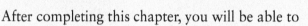

After completing this chapter, you will be able to

1. Describe the basic concepts and standard equipment used in administering enteral and intravenous (IV) infusions.
2. Quickly convert flow rates between *gtt/min* and *mL/h*.
3. Calculate the flow rates of enteral and IV infusions.
4. Calculate the durations of enteral and IV infusions.
5. Determine fluid replacement volumes.

This chapter introduces the basic concepts and standard equipment used in enteral and intravenous (IV) therapy. You will also learn how to calculate flow rates for these infusions and to determine how long it will take for a given amount of solution to infuse (its duration).

Introduction to Enteral and Intravenous Solutions

Fluids can be given to a patient slowly—over a period of time—through a vein (*intravenous*) or through a tube inserted into the alimentary tract (*enteral*). The rate at which these fluids flow (flow rate) into the patient is important and must be controlled precisely.

Enteral Feedings

When a patient cannot ingest food or if the upper gastrointestinal tract is not functioning properly, the prescriber may write an order for an *enteral* feeding (*tube feeding*). Enteral feedings provide nutrients and other fluids by way of a tube inserted directly into the gastrointestinal system (alimentary tract).

There are various types of tube feedings. A gastric tube may be inserted into the stomach through the nares (**nasogastric**, as shown in • **Figure 10.1**) or through the mouth (**orogastric**). A longer tube may be similarly inserted, but would extend beyond the stomach into the upper small intestine, the jejunum (a **nasojejunum** or **orojejunum**).

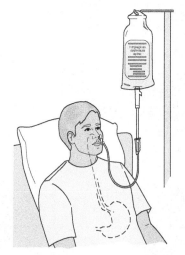

• **Figure 10.1**
A patient with a nasogastric tube.

For long-term feedings, tubes can be inserted surgically or laproscopically through the wall of the abdomen and directly into either the stomach (gastrostomy) or through the stomach and on to the jejunum (jejunostomy). These tubes are sutured in place and are referred to as *percutaneous endoscopic gastrostomy (PEG)* tubes and *percutaneous endoscopic jejunostomy (PEJ)* tubes, respectively (• **Figure 10.2**).

Enteral feedings may be given *continuously* (over a 24-*hour* period) or *intermittently* (over shorter periods, perhaps several times a day). There are many enteral feeding solutions, including Boost, Compleat, Ensure, Isocal, Resource, and Sustacal. Enteral feedings are generally administered via pump. See • **Figure 10.3**.

Orders for enteral solutions always indicate a volume of fluid to be infused over a period of time—that is, a flow rate. For example, a tube feeding order might read *Isocal 50 mL/h via nasogastric tube for 6 hours beginning 6 A.M.* This order is for an intermittent feeding in which the name of the solution is Isocal, the rate of flow is *50 mL/h*, the route of administration is via nasogastric tube, and the duration is 6 *hours*.

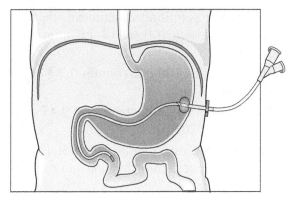

• **Figure 10.2**
A percutaneous endoscopic jejunostomy (PEJ) tube.

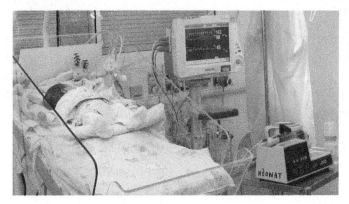

• **Figure 10.3**
Enteral feeding via pump.

(Photographer: Elena Dorfman)

Intravenous Infusions

Intravenous (IV) means "through the vein." Fluids are administered intravenously to provide to the patient a variety of fluids, including blood, water containing nutrients, electrolytes, minerals, and specific medications. IV fluids can replace lost fluids, maintain fluid and electrolyte balance, or serve as a medium to introduce medications directly into the bloodstream.

Replacement fluids are ordered for a patient who has lost fluids through hemorrhage, vomiting, or diarrhea. *Maintenance fluids* help sustain normal levels of fluids and electrolytes. They are ordered for patients who are at risk of becoming depleted—for example, patients who are ordered to have nothing by mouth (NPO).

Intravenous infusions may be *continuous* or *intermittent*. Continuous IV infusions are used to replace or maintain fluids or electrolytes. Intermittent IV infusions—for example, IV piggyback (IVPB) and IV push (IVP)—are used to administer drugs and supplemental fluids. *Intermittent peripheral infusion devices* (saline locks or heparin locks) are used to maintain venous access without continuous fluid infusion. Intermittent IV infusions are discussed in Chapter 11.

A healthcare professional must be able to perform the calculations to determine the correct rate at which an enteral or intravenous solution will enter the body (*flow rate*). Infusion flow rates usually are measured in drops per minute (*gtt/min*) or milliliters per hour (*mL/h*). It is important to be able to convert each of these rates to the other and to determine how long a given amount of solution will take to infuse.

For example, a continuous IV order might read *IV fluids: D5W 125 mL/h for 8h*. In this case, the order is for an IV infusion in which the name of the solution is 5% dextrose in water, the rate of flow is 125 *mL/h*, the route of administration is intravenous, and the duration is 8 *hours*.

Intravenous Solutions

A **saline solution**, which is a solution of *sodium chloride (NaCl)* in sterile water, is commonly used for intravenous infusion. Sodium chloride is ordinary table salt. Saline solutions are available in various concentrations for different purposes. A 0.9% NaCl solution is also referred to as **normal saline (NS)**. Other saline solutions commonly used include **half-normal saline** (0.45% NaCl), written as $\frac{1}{2}$ NS; and **quarter-normal saline** (0.225% NaCl), written as $\frac{1}{4}$ NS.

Intravenous fluids generally contain dextrose, sodium chloride, or electrolytes:

- D5W, D5/W, or 5% D/W is a 5% dextrose solution, which means that 5 *g* of dextrose are dissolved in water to make each 100 *mL* of this solution. See • **Figures 10.4a** and **10.4b**.

- NS or 0.9% NaCl is a solution in which each 100 *mL* contain 0.9 *g* of sodium chloride. See • **Figures 10.4c** and **10.4d**.

- 5% D/0.45% NaCl is a solution containing 5 *g* of dextrose and 0.45 *g* of NaCl in each 100 *mL* of solution (• **Figure 10.5b**).

- Ringer's Lactate (RL), also called Lactated Ringer's solution (LRS), is a solution containing electrolytes, including potassium chloride and calcium chloride. See • **Figure 10.5c**.

Additional information on the many other IV fluids can be found in nursing and pharmacology textbooks.

NOTE

Pay close attention to the abbreviations of the names of the IV solutions. *Letters* indicate the solution compounds, whereas *numbers* indicate the solution strength (e.g., D5W).

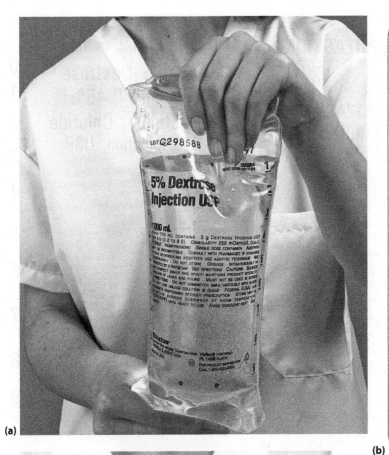

(a)

(b)

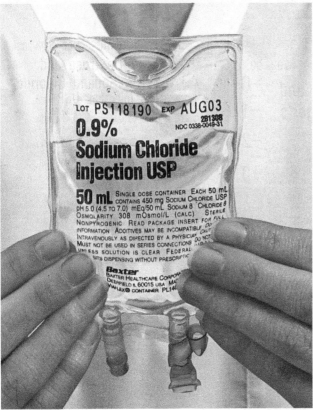

(c)

(d)

● **Figure 10.4**
Examples of IV bags and labels.

• **Figure 10.5**
Examples of intravenous fluids.
(Reproduced with permission of Abbott Laboratories.)

ALERT

In Figure 10.5, solutions (a) and (b) both contain 5% dextrose and $\frac{1}{2}$ NS. However, solution (a) also contains 20 *mEq* of potassium chloride, which is a high-alert medication. Do not confuse these two solutions.

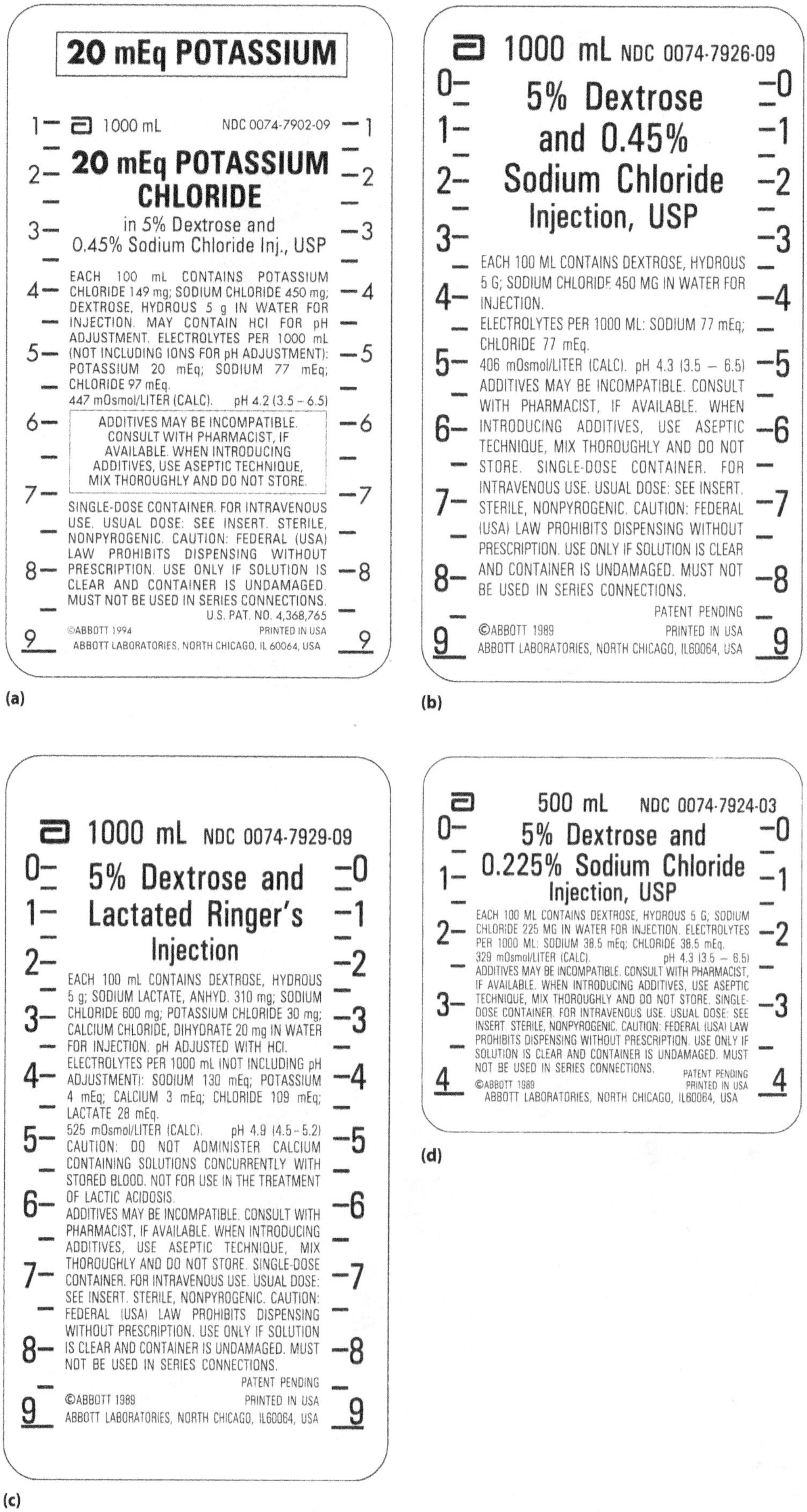

20 mEq POTASSIUM

⌐∂ 1000 mL   NDC 0074-7902-09

20 mEq POTASSIUM CHLORIDE

in 5% Dextrose and
0.45% Sodium Chloride Inj., USP

EACH 100 mL CONTAINS POTASSIUM CHLORIDE 149 mg; SODIUM CHLORIDE 450 mg; DEXTROSE, HYDROUS 5 g IN WATER FOR INJECTION. MAY CONTAIN HCl FOR pH ADJUSTMENT. ELECTROLYTES PER 1000 mL (NOT INCLUDING IONS FOR pH ADJUSTMENT): POTASSIUM 20 mEq; SODIUM 77 mEq; CHLORIDE 97 mEq.
447 mOsmol/LITER (CALC).   pH 4.2 (3.5 – 6.5)

ADDITIVES MAY BE INCOMPATIBLE. CONSULT WITH PHARMACIST, IF AVAILABLE. WHEN INTRODUCING ADDITIVES, USE ASEPTIC TECHNIQUE, MIX THOROUGHLY AND DO NOT STORE.

SINGLE-DOSE CONTAINER. FOR INTRAVENOUS USE. USUAL DOSE: SEE INSERT. STERILE, NONPYROGENIC. CAUTION: FEDERAL (USA) LAW PROHIBITS DISPENSING WITHOUT PRESCRIPTION. USE ONLY IF SOLUTION IS CLEAR AND CONTAINER IS UNDAMAGED. MUST NOT BE USED IN SERIES CONNECTIONS.
U.S. PAT. NO. 4,368,765
©ABBOTT 1994   PRINTED IN USA
ABBOTT LABORATORIES, NORTH CHICAGO, IL 60064, USA

(a)

∂ 1000 mL NDC 0074-7926-09

5% Dextrose and 0.45% Sodium Chloride Injection, USP

EACH 100 ML CONTAINS DEXTROSE, HYDROUS 5 G; SODIUM CHLORIDE 450 MG IN WATER FOR INJECTION.
ELECTROLYTES PER 1000 ML: SODIUM 77 mEq; CHLORIDE 77 mEq.
406 mOsmol/LITER (CALC). pH 4.3 (3.5 – 6.5) ADDITIVES MAY BE INCOMPATIBLE. CONSULT WITH PHARMACIST, IF AVAILABLE. WHEN INTRODUCING ADDITIVES, USE ASEPTIC TECHNIQUE, MIX THOROUGHLY AND DO NOT STORE. SINGLE-DOSE CONTAINER. FOR INTRAVENOUS USE. USUAL DOSE: SEE INSERT. STERILE, NONPYROGENIC. CAUTION: FEDERAL (USA) LAW PROHIBITS DISPENSING WITHOUT PRESCRIPTION. USE ONLY IF SOLUTION IS CLEAR AND CONTAINER IS UNDAMAGED. MUST NOT BE USED IN SERIES CONNECTIONS.
PATENT PENDING
©ABBOTT 1989   PRINTED IN USA
ABBOTT LABORATORIES, NORTH CHICAGO, IL60064, USA

(b)

∂ 1000 mL NDC 0074-7929-09

5% Dextrose and Lactated Ringer's Injection

EACH 100 mL CONTAINS DEXTROSE, HYDROUS 5 g; SODIUM LACTATE, ANHYD. 310 mg; SODIUM CHLORIDE 600 mg; POTASSIUM CHLORIDE 30 mg; CALCIUM CHLORIDE, DIHYDRATE 20 mg IN WATER FOR INJECTION. pH ADJUSTED WITH HCl. ELECTROLYTES PER 1000 mL (NOT INCLUDING pH ADJUSTMENT): SODIUM 130 mEq; POTASSIUM 4 mEq; CALCIUM 3 mEq; CHLORIDE 109 mEq; LACTATE 28 mEq.
525 mOsmol/LITER (CALC).   pH 4.9 (4.5 – 5.2) CAUTION: DO NOT ADMINISTER CALCIUM CONTAINING SOLUTIONS CONCURRENTLY WITH STORED BLOOD. NOT FOR USE IN THE TREATMENT OF LACTIC ACIDOSIS.
ADDITIVES MAY BE INCOMPATIBLE. CONSULT WITH PHARMACIST, IF AVAILABLE. WHEN INTRODUCING ADDITIVES, USE ASEPTIC TECHNIQUE, MIX THOROUGHLY AND DO NOT STORE. SINGLE-DOSE CONTAINER. FOR INTRAVENOUS USE. USUAL DOSE: SEE INSERT. STERILE, NONPYROGENIC. CAUTION: FEDERAL (USA) LAW PROHIBITS DISPENSING WITHOUT PRESCRIPTION. USE ONLY IF SOLUTION IS CLEAR AND CONTAINER IS UNDAMAGED. MUST NOT BE USED IN SERIES CONNECTIONS.
PATENT PENDING
©ABBOTT 1989   PRINTED IN USA
ABBOTT LABORATORIES, NORTH CHICAGO, IL60064, USA

(c)

∂ 500 mL NDC 0074-7924-03

5% Dextrose and 0.225% Sodium Chloride Injection, USP

EACH 100 ML CONTAINS DEXTROSE, HYDROUS 5 G; SODIUM CHLORIDE 225 MG IN WATER FOR INJECTION. ELECTROLYTES PER 1000 ML: SODIUM 38.5 mEq; CHLORIDE 38.5 mEq.
329 mOsmol/LITER (CALC).   pH 4.3 (3.5 – 6.5) ADDITIVES MAY BE INCOMPATIBLE. CONSULT WITH PHARMACIST, IF AVAILABLE. WHEN INTRODUCING ADDITIVES, USE ASEPTIC TECHNIQUE, MIX THOROUGHLY AND DO NOT STORE. SINGLE-DOSE CONTAINER. FOR INTRAVENOUS USE. USUAL DOSE: SEE INSERT. STERILE, NONPYROGENIC. CAUTION: FEDERAL (USA) LAW PROHIBITS DISPENSING WITHOUT PRESCRIPTION. USE ONLY IF SOLUTION IS CLEAR AND CONTAINER IS UNDAMAGED. MUST NOT BE USED IN SERIES CONNECTIONS.
PATENT PENDING
©ABBOTT 1989   PRINTED IN USA
ABBOTT LABORATORIES, NORTH CHICAGO, IL60064, USA

(d)

Gravity Systems and Pumps

Equipment used for the administration of continuous IV infusions includes the IV solution and IV tubing, a drip chamber, at least one injection port, and a roller clamp. The tubing connects the IV solution to the hub of an IV catheter at the infusion site. The rate of flow of the infusion is regulated by an electronic infusion device (pump or controller) or by gravity. See • **Figures 10.6** and **10.9**.

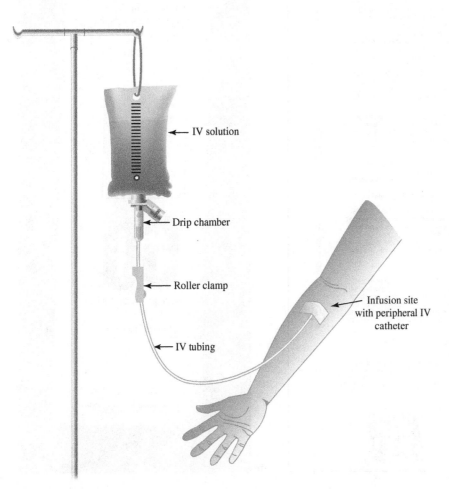

• **Figure 10.6**
Primary IV line (gravity flow).

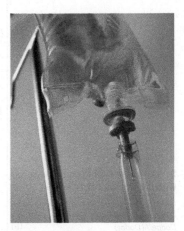

• **Figure 10.7**
Tubing with drip chamber.
(Photodisc/Getty Images)

The drip chamber (Figure 10.6) is located at the site of the entrance of the tubing into the container of intravenous solution. It allows you to count the number of drops per minute that the client is receiving (flow rate).

A roll valve clamp or clip is connected to the tubing and can be manipulated to increase or decrease the flow rate.

The size of the drop that IV tubing delivers is not standard; it depends on the way the tubing is designed (• **Figure 10.7**). Manufacturers specify the number of drops that equal 1 *mL* for their particular tubing. This equivalent is called the tubing's drop factor (• **Figure 10.8** and Table 10.1). You must know the tubing's **drop factor** when calculating the flow rate of solutions in drops per minute (*gtt/min*) or microdrops per minute (*mcgtt/min*).

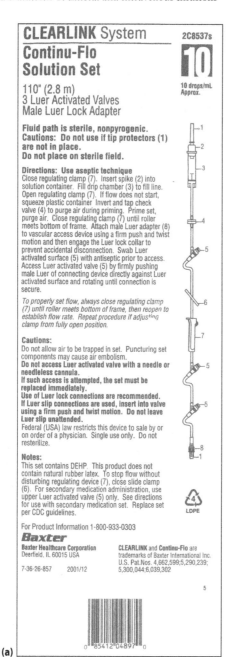

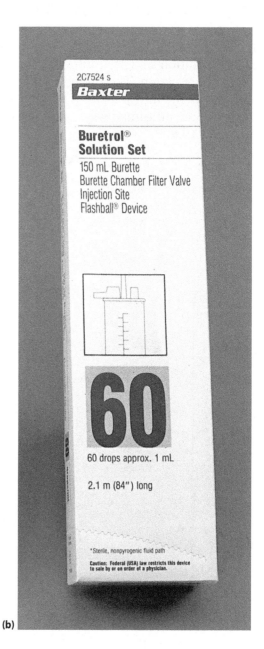

• **Figure 10.8**
Samples of IV tubing containers with drop factors of 10 and 60.

(10-8a Courtesy of Baxter Healthcare Corporation. All rights reserved. 10-8b Al Dodge/Al Dodge)

(a)

(b)

It is difficult to visually make an accurate count of the drops falling per minute when setting the flow rate on a gravity system infusion. In addition, the flow rate of a gravity system infusion depends on the *relative heights* of the IV bag and the infusion site; changes in the relative position of either may cause flow rate changes. Electric IV pumps and controllers now make up the majority of infusion systems in use in health facilities.

Table 10.1 **Common Drop Factors**	
$10\ gtt = 1\ mL$	
$15\ gtt = 1\ mL$	macrodrops
$20\ gtt = 1\ mL$	
$60\ mcgtt = 1\ mL$	microdrops

NOTE

The universal drop factor for IV tubing calibrated in microdrops is 60 microdrops = 1 *mL*.

An intravenous infusion can flow solely by the force of gravity or by an electronic infusion pump. There are many different types of electronic infusion pumps. See • **Figure 10.9.**

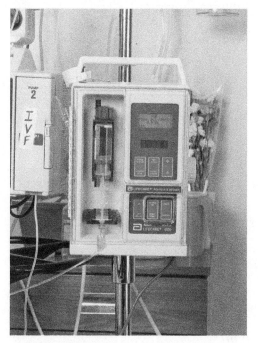

• **Figure 10.9**
Volumetric infusion pump.

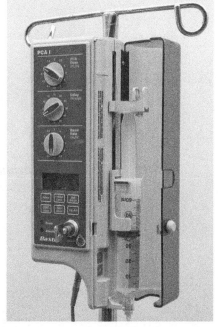

(a)

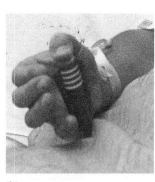

(b)

• **Figure 10.10**
Patient-controlled analgesia (PCA) (a) pump (b) control button.

These electrically operated devices allow the rate of flow (usually specified in *mL/h*) to be simply keyed into the device by the user. The pumps can more precisely regulate the flow rate than can the gravity systems. For example, pumps detect an interruption in the flow (constriction) and sound an alarm to alert the nursing staff and the patient, sound an alarm when the infusion finishes, indicate the volume of fluid already infused, and indicate the time remaining for the infusion to finish. "Smart" pumps may contain libraries of safe dosage ranges that will help prevent the user from keying in an unsafe dosage.

A *patient-controlled analgesia (PCA) pump* (See • **Figure 10.10**) allows a patient to self-administer pain-relieving drugs. The dose is predetermined by the physician, and the pump is programmed accordingly. To receive the drug when pain relief is needed, the patient presses the button on the handset, which is connected to the PCA pump. A lockout device in the pump prevents patient overdose.

Calculations for Infusions

Infusions involve three quantitative components: flow rate, volume of fluid infused, and duration of the IV. For most of the calculations involving infusions, two of these three major components are known, and you are asked to find the missing third component. Most intravenous or enteral solutions are administered by using a pump that measures flow rates in *milliliters per hour*. Examples 10.1 through 10.6 illustrate problems where pumps are used.

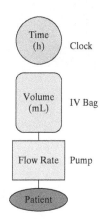

Finding the Flow Rate on a Pump

The **flow rate** of an infusion is the *volume of fluid* that enters the patient over a *period of time*. For example, 25 *mL/h* and 15 *gtt/min* are flow rates. The following formula may be used to determine a flow rate.

$$Flow\ Rate = \frac{Volume}{Time}$$

Examples 10.1 and 10.2 will use the above formula to find flow rates.

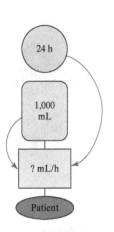

EXAMPLE 10.1

Order: *NS* 1,000 *mL continuous IV for 24 hours*. Find the pump setting in milliliters per hour.

To find the flow rate, use the formula

$$Flow\ Rate = \frac{Volume}{Time}$$

Substitute 1,000 *mL* for the volume in the bag, and 24 *h* for the time.

$$Flow\ Rate = \frac{1,000\ mL}{24\ h} = 41.67 mL/h$$

So, the pump setting is 42 *mL/h*.

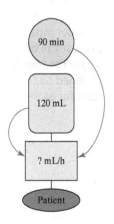

EXAMPLE 10.2

A patient must receive a tube-feeding of *Ensure* 120 *milliliters in* 90 *minutes*. Calculate the flow rate in *milliliters per hour*.

To find the flow rate, use the formula

$$Flow\ Rate = \frac{Volume}{Time}$$

Substitute 120 *mL* for the volume in the bag, and 90 *min* for the time.

$$Flow\ Rate = \frac{120\ mL}{90\ min}$$

$$\frac{120\ mL}{90\ min} = ?\ \frac{mL}{h}$$

You want to change one flow rate (*mL/min*) to another flow rate (*mL/h*). Each flow rate has *mL* in the numerator, which is what you want. You want to cancel *min*, which is in the denominator. To do this, you must use a unit fraction containing *min* in the numerator.

Because 1 h = 60 min, this fraction will be $\dfrac{60\ min}{1\ h}$

$$\dfrac{120\ mL}{90\ min} \times \dfrac{60\ min}{1\ h} = \dfrac{80\ mL}{1\ h}$$

So, the flow rate is 80 *milliliters per hour*.

Finding the Volume Infused Using a Pump

In Examples 10.3 and 10.4, you are asked to find the infused volume. This will be done by converting the time (h) to volume (mL) by using the flow rate (mL/h) as the unit fraction.

EXAMPLE 10.3

Order: *Lactated Ringer's at 167 mL/h IV for 6 h*. How many milliliters will the patient receive in 6 *hours*?

In this example, you change 6 h to ? mL, using 167 mL/h as the unit fraction.

$$6\ h = ?\ mL$$

$$\dfrac{6\ h}{1} \times \dfrac{167\ mL}{h} = 1{,}002\ mL$$

So, the patient will receive 1,002 mL of Lactated Ringer's.

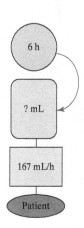

EXAMPLE 10.4

D5/W has been infusing at 30 mL/h IV for 8 hours. How many milliliters have infused?

In this example, you change 8 h to ? mL, using 30 mL/h as the unit fraction.

$$8\ h = ?\ mL$$

$$\dfrac{8\ h}{1} \times \dfrac{30\ mL}{h} = 240\ mL$$

So, 240 mL of D5/W have infused.

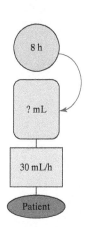

Finding the Duration of an Infusion Using a Pump

In Examples 10.5 and 10.6, you are asked to find the duration of an infusion. This will be done by converting the volume (mL) to time (h) by using the flow rate (mL/h) as the unit fraction.

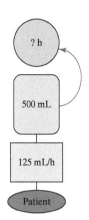

EXAMPLE 10.5

Order: 0.9% NaCl 500 mL IV at 125 mL/h. How long will this infusion take?

In this example, you change 500 mL to ? h, using 125 mL/h as the unit fraction.

$$500 \ mL = ? \ h$$

$$\frac{500 \ mL}{1} \times \frac{1 \ h}{125 \ mL} = 4 \ h$$

So, the infusion will take 4 *hours*.

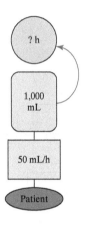

EXAMPLE 10.6

Order: $\frac{1}{2}$ NS 1,000 mL IV at 50 mL/h. If the IV starts at 1200h on Monday, at what time will it finish?

In this example, you change 1,000 mL to ? h, using 50 mL/h as the unit fraction.

$$1,000 \ mL = ? \ h$$

$$\frac{1,000 \ mL}{1} \times \frac{1 \ h}{50 \ mL} = 20 \ h$$

One way to continue is to add

$$
\begin{array}{r}
1200 \ h \\
+ \ 2000 \ h \\
\hline
3200 \ h
\end{array}
$$

Because military time has a 24-hour clock, you must now subtract 2400 h.

$$
\begin{array}{r}
3200 \ h \\
- \ 2400 \ h \\
\hline
0800 \ h
\end{array}
$$

So, the infusion will finish at 0800 h on *Tuesday*.

Finding the Flow Rate (Drip Rate) Using a Gravity System

Solutions also are infused using gravity systems that measure flow rates in *drops per minute*. Calculations for gravity systems will be similar to those for pumps, except that the *drop factor* will be used as a unit fraction. Examples 10.7 through 10.13 illustrate problems in which gravity systems are used.

Examples 10.7 through 10.9 involve finding drip rates of gravity systems.

EXAMPLE 10.7

The prescriber ordered $\frac{1}{4}$ NS 850 *mL IV in 8 hours.* The label on the box containing the IV set to used for this infusion is shown in • Figure 10.11. Calculate the flow rate in drops per minute.

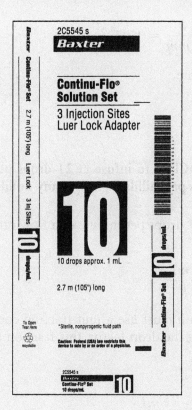

• **Figure 10.11**
Continu-Flo Solution Set box label.
(Courtesy of Baxter Healthcare Corporation. All rights reserved.)

To find the flow rate, use the formula

$$Flow\ Rate = \frac{Volume}{Time}$$

Substitute 850 *mL* for the volume in the bag, and 8 *h* for the time.

$$Flow\ Rate = \frac{850\ mL}{8\ h}$$

You want to convert the flow rate from milliliters per hour to drops per minute.

$$\frac{850\ mL}{8\ h} = \frac{?\ gtt}{min}$$

You want to cancel *mL*. To do this you must use a unit fraction containing *mL* in the denominator. Using the drop factor, this fraction will be $\frac{10\ gtt}{1\ mL}$

$$\frac{850\ \cancel{mL}}{8\ h} \times \frac{10\ gtt}{1\ \cancel{mL}} = \frac{?\ gtt}{min}$$

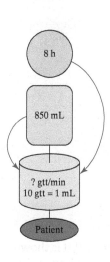

Now, on the left side *gtt* is in the numerator, which is what you want. But *h* is in the denominator and it must be cancelled. This will require a unit fraction with *h* in the numerator—namely, $\dfrac{1\ h}{60\ min}$

Now cancel and multiply the numbers

$$\frac{850\ \cancel{mL}}{8\ \cancel{h}} \times \frac{10\ \cancel{gtt}}{1\ \cancel{mL}} \times \frac{1\ \cancel{h}}{60\ \cancel{min}} = 17.7\ \frac{gtt}{min}$$

So, the flow rate is 18 drops per minute.

EXAMPLE 10.8

The prescriber orders D5/0.45% NaCl IV to infuse at 21 drops per minute. If the drop factor is 20 drops per milliliter, how many milliliters per hour will the patient receive?

You want to convert a flow rate of 21 drops per minute to a flow rate in milliliters per hour.

$$\frac{21\ gtt}{min} = \frac{?\ mL}{h}$$

You want to cancel *gtt*. To do this you must use a unit fraction containing *gtt* in the denominator. Using the drop factor, this fraction is $\dfrac{1\ mL}{20\ gtt}$

$$\frac{21\ \cancel{gtt}}{min} \times \frac{1\ mL}{20\ \cancel{gtt}} = \frac{?\ mL}{h}$$

Now, on the left side *mL* is in the numerator, which is what you want. But *min* is in the denominator, and it must be cancelled. This will require a unit fraction with *min* in the numerator—namely, $\dfrac{60\ min}{1\ h}$

Now cancel and multiply the numbers

$$\frac{21\ \cancel{gtt}}{\cancel{min}} \times \frac{1\ \cancel{mL}}{20\ \cancel{gtt}} \times \frac{60\ \cancel{min}}{1\ \cancel{h}} = 63\ \frac{mL}{h}$$

So, the flow rate is 63 *mL* per hour.

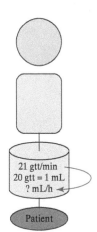

21 gtt/min
20 gtt = 1 mL
? mL/h

Patient

NOTE

In Example 10.9, it is shown that 125 *mL* per hour is the same flow rate as 125 microdrops per minute because the 60s always cancel. The flow rates of *milliliters per hour* and *microdrops per minute* are equivalent. Therefore, calculations are not necessary to change *mL/h* to *mcgtt/min*.

EXAMPLE 10.9

The order reads 125 *mL* 5% D/W IV in 1 *hour.* What is the flow rate in microdrops per minute?

To find the flow rate, use the formula

$$Flow\ Rate = \frac{Volume}{Time}$$

Substitute 125 *mL* for the volume in the bag, and 1 *h* for the time.

$$Flow\ Rate = \frac{125\ mL}{1\ h} = 125\ mL/h$$

You want to change the flow rate from 125 *mL* per hour to micro-drops per minute.

$$\frac{125\ mL}{h} = \frac{?\ mcgtt}{min}$$

You want to cancel *mL*. To do this you must use a unit fraction containing *mL* in the denominator. Using the drop factor, this fraction will be $\frac{60\ mcgtt}{1\ mL}$

$$\frac{125\ mL}{h} \times \frac{60\ mcgtt}{1\ mL} = \frac{?\ mcgtt}{min}$$

Now, on the left side *mcgtt* is in the numerator, which is what you want. But *h* is in the denominator, and it must be cancelled. This will require a unit fraction with *h* in the numerator—namely, $\frac{1\ h}{60\ min}$

Now cancel and multiply the numbers

$$\frac{125\ mL}{h} \times \frac{60\ mcgtt}{1\ mL} \times \frac{1\ h}{60\ min} = 125\ \frac{mcgtt}{min}$$

So, 125 *mL* per hour is the same rate of flow as 125 microdrops per minute.

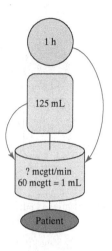

Finding the Volume Infused Using a Gravity System

EXAMPLE 10.10

How many milliliters of D5W will infuse intravenously in 10 *hours* at the rate of 13 *gtt/min*? The drop factor is 15 *gtt/mL*.

In this example, you change 10 *h* to ? *mL*, using both the flow rate of 13 *gtt/min* and the drop factor of 15 *gtt/mL* as unit fractions.

$$10\ h = ?\ mL$$

Now, you will have to do the following:

$$10\ h \longrightarrow ?\ min \longrightarrow ?\ gtt \longrightarrow ?\ mL$$

$$\frac{10\ h}{1} \times \frac{60\ min}{h} \times \frac{13\ gtt}{min} \times \frac{mL}{15\ gtt} = 520\ mL$$

So, 520 *mL* will infuse in 10 *hours*.

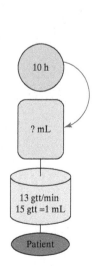

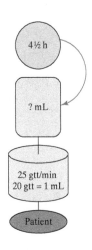

EXAMPLE 10.11

An IV of 1,000 *mL D5 and* $\frac{1}{2}$ *NS* has been ordered to infuse at **25** *gtt/min*. The drop factor is **20** *gtt/mL*. If the IV was hung at **10** P.M. on Tuesday, how many milliliters will have infused by **2:30** A.M. on Wednesday?

From 10 P.M. Tuesday until 2:30 A.M. Wednesday is $4\frac{1}{2}$ *hours*.

In this example you change $4\frac{1}{2}$ *h* to ? *mL*, using both the flow rate of 25 *gtt/min* and the drop factor of 20 *gtt/mL* as unit fractions.

$$4\tfrac{1}{2}\,h = ?\ mL$$

Now, you will have to do the following:

$$4\tfrac{1}{2}\,h \longrightarrow ?\ min \longrightarrow ?\ gtt \longrightarrow ?\ mL$$

$$\frac{9\,h}{2} \times \frac{60\,min}{h} \times \frac{25\,gtt}{min} \times \frac{mL}{20\,gtt} = 337.5\ mL$$

So, 338 *mL* will have infused by 2:30 A.M. Wednesday.

Finding the Duration of an IV Using a Gravity System

EXAMPLE 10.12

An IV of 5% D/W is infusing at a rate of 20 *drops* per minute. If the drop factor is 15 *drops* per milliliter, how many hours will it take for the remaining solution in the bag to infuse (• Figure 10.12)?

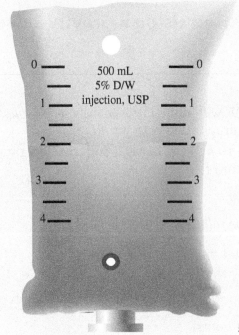

• **Figure 10.12**
5% D/W IV solution.

In Figure 10.12 you can see that 500 *mL* of solution were originally in the bag and that the patient has received 200 *mL*. Therefore, 300 *mL* remain to be infused.

In this example, you change 300 *mL* to ? *h*, using both the flow rate of 20 *gtt/min* and the drop factor of 15 *gtt/mL* as unit fractions.

$$300 \ mL = ? \ h$$

Now, you will have to do the following:

$$300 \ mL \longrightarrow ? \ gtt \longrightarrow ? \ min \longrightarrow ? \ h$$

$$\frac{300 \ \cancel{mL}}{1} \times \frac{15 \ \cancel{gtt}}{\cancel{mL}} \times \frac{\cancel{min}}{20 \ \cancel{gtt}} \times \frac{h}{60 \ \cancel{min}} = 3.75 \ h$$

So, it will take $3\frac{3}{4}$ *hours* for the remaining solution to infuse.

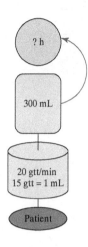

EXAMPLE 10.13

An IV of 1,000 *mL* of 5% D/0.9% NaCl is started at 8 P.M. The flow rate is 38 drops per minute, and the drop factor is 10 drops per milliliter. At what time will this infusion finish?

In this example, you change 1,000 *mL*? to *h*, using both the flow rate of 38 *gtt/min* and the drop factor of 10 *gtt/mL* as unit fractions.

$$1,000 \ mL = ? \ h$$

In this example, you will have to do the following:

$$1,000 \ mL \longrightarrow ? \ gtt \longrightarrow ? \ min \longrightarrow ? \ h$$

$$\frac{1,000 \ \cancel{mL}}{1} \times \frac{10 \ \cancel{gtt}}{\cancel{mL}} \times \frac{\cancel{min}}{38 \ \cancel{gtt}} \times \frac{h}{60 \ \cancel{min}} = 4.386 \ h$$

Now, change 0.386 *h* to minutes.

$$\frac{0.386 \ \cancel{h}}{1} \times \frac{60 \ min}{\cancel{h}} = 23.16 \ min \approx 23 \ min$$

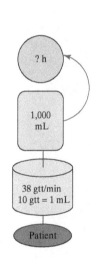

So, the infusion will take 4 *hours* and 23 *minutes*. Because the infusion began at 8 P.M., it will finish at 12:23 A.M. the next day.

Adjusting the Flow Rate of an IV

Example 10.14 will illustrate how to adjust a flow rate on a gravity system, and Example 10.15 will do the same for a pump.

EXAMPLE 10.14

The order reads 1,000 *mL D5W IV over 8 hours*. The drop factor is 10 *gtt/mL*.

(a) Calculate the initial flow rate in *gtt/*min for this infusion.

(b) After 5 *hours*, 700 *mL* remain to be infused. How must the flow rate be adjusted so that the infusion will finish on time?

(c) If the facility has a policy that flow rate adjustments must not exceed 25% of the original rate, is the required adjustment within the guidelines?

(a) At the Start

To find the initial flow rate, use the formula

$$Flow\ Rate = \frac{Volume}{Time}$$

Substitute 1,000 *mL* for the volume in the bag, and 8 *h* for the time.

$$Flow\ Rate = \frac{1,000\ mL}{8\ h}$$

Now, convert this flow rate to *gtt/min*, using the drop factor of 10 *gtt/mL* and 1 *h/60 min* as unit fractions.

$$\frac{1,000\ \cancel{mL}}{8\ \cancel{h}} \times \frac{10\ gtt}{1\ \cancel{mL}} \times \frac{1\ \cancel{h}}{60\ min} = 20.83\ \frac{gtt}{min}$$

So, the initial flow rate is 21 *gtt/min*.

(b) After 5 *hours*, 700 *mL* must infuse in the remaining 3 *hours*.

To find the new flow rate, use the formula

$$Flow\ Rate = \frac{Volume}{Time}$$

Substitute 700 *mL* for the volume in the bag, and *3 h* for the time.

$$Flow\ Rate = \frac{700\ mL}{3\ h}$$

Now convert this flow rate to *gtt/min*, using the drop factor of *10 gtt/mL* as a unit fraction.

$$\frac{700\ \cancel{mL}}{3\ \cancel{h}} \times \frac{10\ gtt}{1\ \cancel{mL}} \times \frac{1\ \cancel{h}}{60\ min} = 38.89\ \frac{gtt}{min}$$

So, the new flow rate is 39 *gtt/min*.

(a)

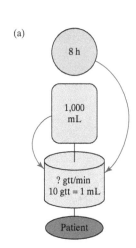

8 h

1,000 mL

? gtt/min
10 gtt = 1 mL

Patient

(b)

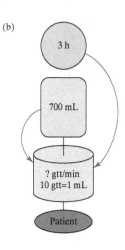

3 h

700 mL

? gtt/min
10 gtt=1 mL

Patient

(c) Calculate the percent of increase when the flow rate is changed from 21 *gtt/min* to 39 *gtt/min*. To find the fraction of increase, use the formula *Fraction of Change* $= \dfrac{Change}{Original}$

$$\frac{Change}{Original} = \frac{39 - 21}{21} = \frac{18}{21} \approx 0.86 = 86\%$$

Because 86% exceeds the 25% maximum allowable change, the change is not within the guidelines, and the adjustment may not be made. You must contact the prescriber.

EXAMPLE 10.15

Order: *NS 600 mL IV infuse in 5 hours stat.*

(a) Calculate the initial pump setting in *mL/h*.

(b) When the nurse checks this infusion 2 *hours* later, 330 *mL* are LIB (left in the bag). Recalculate the pump setting for the remaining 330 *mL*.

(c) If the facility protocols indicate that flow rate adjustments must not exceed 20% of the original rate, may the adjustment be made?

(a) At the Start

To find the initial flow rate, use the formula

$$Flow\ Rate = \frac{Volume}{Time}$$

Substitute 600 *mL* for the volume in the bag, and 5 *h* for the time.

$$Flow\ Rate = \frac{600\ mL}{5\ h} = 120\ \frac{mL}{h}$$

So, the initial flow rate is 120 *mL/h*.

(b) After 2 *hours*

Now there are 330 *mL* in the bag and there are 3 *hours* left for the infusion.

To find the new flow rate, use the formula

$$Flow\ Rate = \frac{Volume}{Time}$$

Substitute 330 *mL* for the volume in the bag, and 3 *h* for the time.

$$Flow\ Rate = \frac{330\ mL}{3\ h} = 110\ \frac{mL}{h}$$

So, the new adjusted flow rate is 110 *mL/h*.

(a)

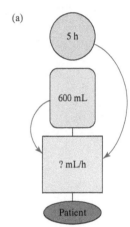

(b)

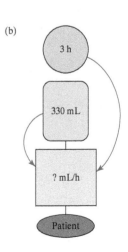

(c) Calculate the percent of decrease when the flow rate is changed from 120 *mL/h* to 110 *mL/h*. To find the fraction of decrease, use the formula *Fraction of Change* $= \dfrac{Change}{Original}$

$$\frac{Change}{Original} = \frac{120 - 110}{120} = \frac{10}{120} = \frac{10}{120} \approx 0.08 = 8\%$$

Because 8% does not exceed the 20% maximum allowable change, the change is within the guidelines, and the adjustment may be made.

Fluid Balance: Intake/Output

To work well, the various body systems need a stable environment in which their tissues and cells can function properly. For example, the body requires somewhat constant levels of temperature, salts, glucose, and, in particular, adequate hydration to maintain homeostasis.

Part of hydration management involves the monitoring of a patient's fluid intake and output. This is especially important with pediatric, geriatric, and critical care patients.

Fluid intake is the amount of fluid that enters the body (oral and parenteral fluids), while **fluid output** is the amount of fluid that leaves the body (urine, sweat, liquid stool, emesis, and drainage).

Fluid replacement is sometimes necessary to avoid dehydration. If (as in Example 10.16) a physician provides an order with a specific ratio comparing the necessary replacement fluid with the patient's fluid output and if the patient's fluid output is known, then *Dimensional Analysis* could be used to determine the volume of replacement fluid to give the patient.

EXAMPLE 10.16

Order: *For every* 100 *mL of urine output, replace with* 40 *mL of water via PEG tube q4h.* **The patient's urine output is 300 *mL*. What is the replacement volume?**

Think of the problem as:

Output:	300 *mL* (out)	[single unit of measurement]
Replacement:	100 *mL* (out)/40 *mL* (in)	[equivalence]
Input:	? *mL* (in)	[single unit of measurement]

In this example, you want to change the single unit of measurement [300 *mL(out)*] to another single unit of measurement [*mL(in)*].

$$300 \, mL(out) = ? \, mL(in)$$

The order provides the equivalence [100 *mL(out)*/40 *mL(in)*] for the unit fraction.

$$300 \; \cancel{mL(out)} \times \frac{40 \, mL(in)}{100 \; \cancel{mL(out)}} = 120 \, mL(in)$$

So, the replacement volume is 120 *mL*.

Summary

In this chapter, the basic concepts and standard equipment used in enteral and intravenous therapy were introduced.

- Fluids can be given to a patient slowly over a period of time through a vein (*intravenous*) or through a tube inserted into the alimentary tract (*enteral*).
- Enteral and IV fluids can be administered continuously or intermittently.
- There is a wide variety of commercially prepared enteral and IV solutions.
- In IV solutions, *letters* indicate solution compounds, whereas *numbers* indicate solution concentration.
- Care must be taken to eliminate the air from, and maintain the sterility of, IV tubing.
- An IV infusion can flow solely by the force of gravity or by an electronic infusion pump.
- Use the following formula to determine flow rate:

$$Flow\ Rate = \frac{Volume}{Time}$$

- Flow rates usually are given as either *mL/h* or *gtt/min*.
- The drop factor of the IV administration set must be known in order to calculate flow rates.

- *Microdrops/minute* are equivalent to *milliliters/hour*.
- For microdrops, the drop factor is 60 microdrops per milliliter.
- For macrodrops, the usual drop factors are 10, 15, or 20 drops per milliliter.
- To find the *duration* of an IV using a *pump*, change the *volume infused (mL)* to *time (hours)* using the *flow rate (mL/h)* as the unit fraction.
- To find the *duration* of an IV using a *gravity system*, change the *volume infused (mL)* to *time (hours)* using the *flow rate (gtt/min)*, 60 *min/1 h*, and the *drop factor (gtt/mL)* as the unit fractions.
- To find the *volume infused* of an IV using a *pump*, change the *duration (hours)* to *volume (mL)* using the *flow rate (mL/h)* as the unit fraction.
- To find the *volume infused* of an IV using a *gravity system*, change the *duration (hours)* to *volume (mL)* using the *flow rate (gtt/min)*, 60 *min/1 h*, and the *drop factor (gtt/mL)* as the unit fractions.
- Know the policy of the facility regarding readjustment of flow rates.

Case Study 10.1

Read the Case Study and answer the questions. Answers can be found in Appendix A.

A 68-yr-old male is brought by ambulance to the hospital from home. He is clammy, has tachypnea, and decreased level of responsiveness. He has no known allergies to food, but is allergic to aspirin and penicillin. He has a history of HTN, DM, COPD, osteoarthritis, and congestive heart failure. He had a right sided CVA 10 yrs ago, is aphasic, and has right sided hemiplegia. He is 6 *foot* 3 *inches* and weighs 140 *pounds*, and has a PEG feeding tube. His vitals are: T 102°F, B/P 100/60, P 100, R 26 and shallow. His admitting diagnosis is dehydration, R/O pneumonia, UTI, and sepsis.

   His orders include:

- Chest X-ray stat
- Blood cultures stat

- Urine culture stat
- CBC and SMA 12 stat
- Hbg and Hct stat
- NPO
- IV: NS infuse at 90 *mL/h*
- Perative (1,300 cal/L) via PEG 480 *mL* over 6 *h*, flush with 50 *mL* water after feeding and after medication administration
- Check gastric residual every 4 *h*, hold feeding if residual greater than 200 *mL*. Reinfuse residual and recheck in 2 *h*
- O_2 via nasal cannula at 2 *L/min*
- Suprax (cefixime) 400 *mg* via PEG daily

- Cleocin (clindamycin) 360 *mg* via PEG q12h
- enoxaparin 1 *mg/kg* subcut q12h
- Humalog 50/50 *mix* 35 *units* subcut before tube feeding
- cimetidine HCl 400 *mg* via PEG at bedtime

1. The label on the Suprax reads 500 *mg/mL*. How many milliliters will you administer?

2. The IV is infusing via gravity flow. Calculate the rate in *mcgtt/min*.

3. The strength on the enoxaparin label is 300 *mg/mL*. How many milliliters will you administer?

4. Place an arrow at the correct measurement on the most appropriate syringe to indicate the amount of enoxaparin to be administered.

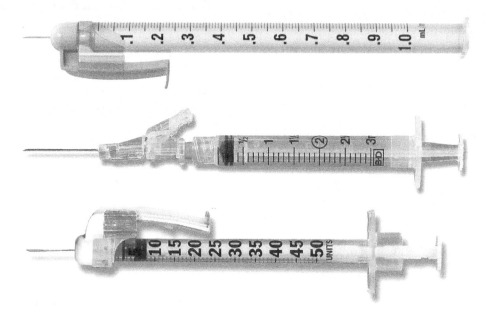

5. How many milligrams of enoxaparin is the patient receiving each day?

6. Calculate the flow rate of the Perative in *mL/h*.

7. How many milliliters of IV fluid is the patient receiving in 24 hours?

8. The label on the Cleocin reads 75 *mg/5 mL*. How many milliliters will you administer?

9. The label on the cimetidine reads 300 *mg/5 mL*. How many milliliters will you administer?

10. Calculate the total amount of enteral fluid the patient will receive in 24 *hours*.

Practice Sets

Workspace

The answers to *Try These for Practice*, *Exercises*, and *Cumulative Review Exercises* are found in Appendix A. Ask your instructor for the answers to the *Additional Exercises*.

Try These for Practice

Test your comprehension after reading the chapter.

1. Order: D_5W 500 *mL* IV infuse over 12 *hours*. Find the pump setting in *mL/h*. _____

2. Order: NS 1,000 *mL* IV infuse over 24 *h*. Find the drip rate in *drops per minute* if the drop factor is 15 *gtt/mL*. _____

3. A continuous IV is infusing at 120 *mL/h*. How many milliliters will infuse in *two hours and thirty minutes?* _____

4. An IV starts at 1500*h* and runs at 24 *gtt/min* with a drop factor of 10 *gtt/mL*. What time will it be when 300 *mL* have infused into the patient? _____

5. Order: *For every* 200 *mL of urine output, replace with* 50 *mL of water via nasogastric tube q4h.* If the patient's urine output for the past 4 *hours* is 300 *mL*, what is the replacement volume of water needed?

_____

Exercises

Reinforce your understanding in class or at home.

1. Order: *RL* 1,000 *mL IV infuse over* 16 *hours.* What is the pump setting in *mL/h?*

_____

2. Normal saline is infusing intravenously at 125 *mL/h*. What is the flow rate measured in *mcgtt/min?*

_____

3. Order: *D5/W* 2,000 *mL IV infuse over* 12 *h.* The drop factor is 10 *gtt/mL.* Calculate the flow rate in *gtt/min.*

_____

4. Order: *3/4 strength Ensure* 240 *mL via NG tube over* 8 *h.* What is the pump setting in *mL/h?*

_____

5. How many *mL* of solution will be infused in 4 *hours* if the flow rate is 20 *mL/h?*

_____

6. Order: *NS* 1,000 *mL IV infuse over* 24 *h.* Find the pump setting in *milliliters per hour.*

_____

7. Order: *D$_5$W* 1,000 *mL IV infuse over* 12 *h.* Find the flow rate in *drops per minute* if the drop factor is 20 *gtt/mL.*

_____

8. Order: *NS* 800 *mL IV infuse in* 6 *hours.*

   (a) Calculate the initial pump setting in *mL/h.*
   (b) When the nurse checks this infusion 4 *hours* later, 500 *mL* are LIB (left in the bag). Recalculate the pump setting for the remaining 500 *mL.*
   (c) If the facility protocols indicate that flow rate adjustments must not exceed 25% of the original rate, may the adjustment be made?

_____

9. A 500 *mL* IV starts at 9 P.M. and runs at 33 *gtt/min* with a drop factor of 10 *gtt/mL*. At what time will it finish?

_____

Workspace

10. How long will it take 1,000 *mL* to infuse if the flow rate is 125 *mL/h*?

_____

11. How many milliliters will infuse in 2 *hours* at the rate of 30 *gtt/min* with a drop factor of 15 *gtt/mL*?

_____

12. A continuous IV is infusing at 120 *mcgtt/min*. How many milliliters will infuse in 4 *hours*?

_____

13. Order: *NS 1,000 mL IV infuse in 12 hours.* The drop factor is 20 *gtt/mL*.

    (a) Calculate the initial drip rate in *gtt/min*.
    (b) When the nurse checks this infusion 7 *hours* later, 500 *mL* are LIB (left in the bag). Recalculate the drip rate for the remaining 500 *mL*.
    (c) If the facility protocols indicate that flow rate adjustments must not exceed 20% of the original rate, may the adjustment be made?

_____

14. A continuous IV is infusing at 40 *mL/h*. How many milliliters will infuse in 30 *minutes*?

_____

15. Order: *NS 750 mL IV infuse at 75 mL/h.* If the IV started at 11 P.M. on Wednesday, at what time will it finish?

_____

16. Order: *1,000 mL D5 $\frac{1}{2}$ NS to run at 90 mL/h.* Find the drip rate for 15 *gtt/mL* tubing.

_____

17. Order: *NS 1,000 mL intravenous over 10 h.* At 0700h, 400 *mL* has infused. At what time will the infusion finish?

_____

18. Order: *RL 1,000 mL IV 8 A.M.–8 P.M.* What is the pump setting in *mL/h*?

_____

19. Order: *150 mL NS IV over 3 hours.* At how many *mcgtt/min* would you run this infusion?

_____

20. For every 200 *mL of urine output, replace with* 40 *mL of H$_2$O through the jejunostomy tube (J-tube) q8h.* If urine output for the past 8 *hours* is 700 *mL*, find the replacement fluid volume.

_____

Additional Exercises

Now, test yourself!

1. Order: *5%D 0.45% NaCl 500 mL IV over 3 hours.* Find the pump setting in *milliliters per hour*.

_____

2. Order: *Ringer's Lactate* 500 *mL* IV over 12 *h*. Find the flow rate in *drops per minute* if the drop factor is 15 *gtt/mL*.

_____

3. D5/W is infusing at 90 *mL/h* using an electronic controler. How much D5/W will infuse in 90 minutes?

_____

4. NS is infusing intravenously at 75 *mL/h*. How long will it take for 500 *mL* to infuse?

_____

5. Order: 1,000 *mL* NS *infuse at* 75 *mL/h*. The infusion starts at 7 A.M. on Tuesday. When is the infusion scheduled to be completed?

_____

6. Order: 500 *mL* NS *IV run* 75 *mL/h*. How many milliliters will infuse in 3 *hours*?

_____

7. Order: *NS* 1,500 *mL* over 12 *h*. After 3 *hours* 1,200 *mL* remain in the bag. The facility policy indicates that flow rate adjustments may not exceed 25% of the original rate. Recalculate the flow rate so that the infusion will finish on time, and decide if the adjustment is within the guidelines.

_____

8. Find the flow rate in *drops per minute* that is equivalent to a flow rate of 75 *mL/h* when you are using 20 *gtt/mL* macrodrip tubing.

_____

9. A pump is set at 200 *mL/h*. Find the flow rate in *gtt/min* if the drop factor is 10 *gtt/mL*.

_____

10. Find the flow rate in *microdrops per minute* that is equivalent to a rate of 35 *mL/h*.

_____

11. Order: *For every* 100 *mL of urine output, replace with* 30 *mL of* H_2O *through the persutaneous endoscopic gastrostomy (PEG) tube q4h*. If urine output for the last 4 *hours* is 500 *mL*, find the replacement fluid volume.

_____

12. Determine the completion time of 200 *mL* packed blood cells that ran at 50 *mL/h*. The bag was hung at 3:15 P.M. on Monday.

_____

13. Order: *RL* 375 *mL* IV over 3 *h*. The tubing has a drop factor of 10 *gtt/mL*.

    (a) Calculate the initial flow rate in *gtt/min*.
    (b) After 1 *hour*, 175 *mL* have infused. Determine the adjusted flow rate so that the infusion will finish on time.

Workspace

(c) If flow rate adjustments cannot exceed 25% of the original rate, is the adjustment in part (b) within the guidelines?

_____

14. An infusion is running at 50 *mL/h*. Find the equivalent flow rate in *gtt/min* when the drop factor is 15 *gtt/mL*.

_____

15. The order reads 1,000 *mL D₅W IV in 8 hours start at 10* A.M. The IV was stopped at 4:30 P.M. for 45 *minutes* with 90 *mL* of fluid remaining. Determine the new flow rate setting for the infusion pump in *mL/h* so that the infusion finishes on time.

_____

16. An IV bag has 350 *mL* remaining. It is infusing at 35 *gtt/min*, and a 15 *gtt/mL* set is being used. How long will it take to finish?

_____

17. An IV solution is infusing at 32 microdrops per minute. How many milliliters of this solution will the patient receive in 6 *hours*?

_____

18. A patient must have a tube-feeding of 1,000 *mL* Ensure for 10 *hours*. The drop factor is 15 *gtt/mL*. After 5 *hours*, a total of 650 *mL* has infused. Recalculate the new *gtt/min* flow rate to complete the infusion on schedule.

_____

19. An IV is infusing at a rate of 30 *drops* per minute. The drop factor is 15 *gtt/mL*. Calculate the flow rate in milliliters per hour.

_____

20. A patient is to receive 1 *unit* (500 *mL*) of packed red blood cells over 4 *hours*. For the first 15 *minutes*, infuse at 50 *mL/h*. At what rate would you set the pump to complete the infusion?

_____

Cumulative Review Exercises

Review your mastery of previous chapters.

1. Find the height in centimeters of a woman who is 5 *feet* 6 *inches* tall.

2. 120 *mL* = ? *oz*

3. Find the weight in kilograms of a man who weighs 187 *pounds*.

4. 5.6 *cm* = ? *mm*

5. Write 4:55 P.M. in military time.

6. How many milligrams of sodium chloride are contained in 500 *mL* of a 0.9% NaCl solution?

_____

Workspace

7. What is the strength expressed as a percent of a 400 *mL* solution that contains 10 *grams* of magnesium sulfate?

8. Calculate the BSA of a patient who is 150 *cm* tall and weighs 88 *kg*.

9. The drug in a vial has a concentration of 40 *mg* per *mL*. If 3 *mL* are withdrawn from this vial into a syringe, what is the concentration of the solution in the syringe?

10. A patient weighs 100 *lb*. The order calls for 0.6 *mg/kg po daily*. How many *mg* of the drug will the patient receive?

11. Order: *interferon beta-1a 0.25 mg subcut every other day*. The strength available is 0.25 *mg/mL*. How many *mL* will you administer?

12. Order: *Clarinex (desloratadine) 5 mg po daily*. How many 2.5 *mg* tablets of this antihistamine would you administer?

13. How many grams of a drug are contained in a bottle of 100 *tablets* if each tablet contains 50 *mg* of the drug?

14. How many *mL* of 2% lidocaine contain 3 *grams* of lidocaine?

15. If an IV starts at 2300h on Wednesday and lasts for 13 *hours*, when does it finish?

Chapter

11

Flow Rates and Dosage Rates for Intravenous Medications

Learning Outcomes

After completing this chapter, you will be able to

1. Describe intravenous (IV) medication administration.
2. Convert from dosage rates (drug/time) to IV rates (volume/time).
3. Convert from IV rates (volume/time) to dosage rates (drug/time).
4. Calculate infusion rates when medication must be added to the intravenous piggyback (IVPB) bag.
5. Calculate infusion rates based on the size (weight or body surface area [BSA]) of the patient.
6. Calculate flow rates for IV push medications.
7. Calculate the duration of an IVPB infusion.
8. Calculate flow rates for medication requiring titration.
9. Construct a titration table.

T his chapter extends the discussion of infusions to include the administration of intravenous (IV) *medications*.

In the previous chapter, the focus was on **flow rates** (*volume of fluid per time* [e.g., *mL/h* or *gtt/min*]). However, in this chapter, the infusing solutions will contain medication, so you will also calculate **dosage rates** (*amount of drug per time* [e.g., *mg/min* or *unit/hr*]).

This chapter also introduces orders that indicate the dosage rate based on the size of the patient—namely, **compound rates** (*amount of drug per size of the patient per time* [e.g., *mg/kg/min* or *mcg/m²/min*]).

The calculations involved in medication administered by *IV push* and *titration* are also introduced.

Intravenous Administration of Medications

Intravenous (IV) administration of medications provides rapid access to a patient's circulatory system, thereby presenting potential hazards. Errors in medications, dose, or dosage strength can prove fatal. Therefore, *caution must be taken in the calculation, preparation, and administration of IV medications.*

Typically, a **primary** IV line provides continuous fluid to the patient. **Secondary** lines can be attached to the primary line at injection ports, and these lines are often used to deliver *continuous or intermittent* medication intravenously. A secondary line is referred to as a **piggyback** or **intravenous piggyback (IVPB)**. With intermittent IVPB infusions, the bags generally hold 50–250 *mL* of fluid containing dissolved medication and usually require 20–60 *minutes* to infuse. Like a primary line, an IVPB infusion may use a manually controlled gravity system or an electronic infusion device.

A **heplock,** or **saline lock,** is an infusion port attached to an indwelling needle or cannula in a peripheral vein. Intermittent IV infusions can be administered through these ports via IV lines connected to the ports. An **IV push** (IVP), or **bolus,** is a direct injection of medication either into the heplock/saline lock or directly into the vein.

Syringe pumps also can be used for intermittent infusions. A syringe with the medication is inserted into the pump. The medication is delivered at a set rate over a short period of time.

A **volume-control set** is a small container, called a *burette*, that is connected to the IV line. Burettes are often used in pediatric or geriatric care, where accurate volume control is critical. The danger of overdose is limited because of the small volume of solution in the burette. Burettes will be discussed in Chapter 12.

Intravenous Piggyback Infusions

Patients can receive a medication through a port in an existing IV line. This is called **intravenous piggyback (IVPB)** (• **Figure 11.1**). The medication is in a secondary bag. Notice in Figure 11.1 that the secondary bag is higher than the primary bag so that the pressure in the secondary line will be greater than the pressure in the primary line. Therefore, the secondary medication infuses first. Once the secondary infusion is completed, the primary line begins to flow. Be sure to keep both lines open. If you close the primary line, the primary line will not flow into the vein when the secondary IVPB is completed.

A typical IVPB order might read: *cimetidine 300 mg IVPB q6h in 50 mL NS infuse over 20 min.* This is an order for an IV piggyback infusion in which 300 *mg* of the drug cimetidine diluted in 50 *mL* of a normal saline solution must infuse in 20 *minutes.* So, the patient receives 300 *mg* of cimetidine in 20 *minutes* via a secondary line, and this dose is repeated every 6 *hours.*

In this chapter, you will encounter both flow rates and dosage rates. The following formulas will apply:

$$Flow\ Rate = \frac{Volume}{Time}$$

$$Dosage\ Rate = \frac{Drug}{Time}$$

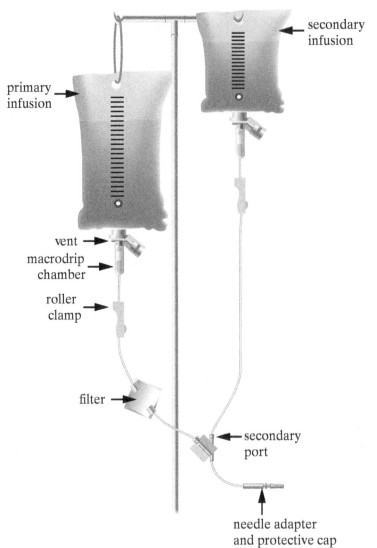

● **Figure 11.1**
Primary and secondary (IVPB) infusion setup.

secondary infusion

primary infusion

vent
macrodrip chamber

roller clamp

filter

secondary port

needle adapter and protective cap

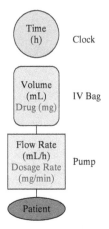

Time (h) — Clock

Volume (mL) Drug (mg) — IV Bag

Flow Rate (mL/h) Dosage Rate (mg/min) — Pump

Patient

The setup shown in Figure 11.1 may look intimidating. However, the mathematics involved in IVPB infusions is simplified by the fact that when the IVPB bag is infusing, the primary bag is not running and may therefore be ignored. In the examples for this chapter, the following diagram will be used to show the structure of the IVPB infusion.

Finding the Dosage Rate

Dosage rates are calculated in Examples 11.1 and 11.2.

EXAMPLE 11.1

Order: *cimetidine* 300 *mg IVPB q6h in 50 mL NS infuse in 20 min.*
Find the

(a) **IV flow rate measured in milliliters/min.**
(b) **Dosage rate measured in milligrams/min.**

(a) To find the flow rate, use the formula

$$Flow\ Rate = \frac{Volume}{Time}$$

Substitute 50 mL for the volume in the bag, and 20 min for the time.

$$Flow\ Rate = \frac{50\ mL}{20\ min} = 2.5\ mL/min$$

So, the IV flow rate is 2.5 mL/min, which means that the patient receives a volume of 2.5 mL of solution every minute.

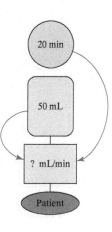

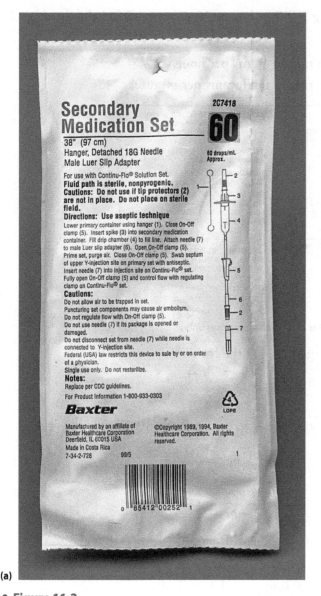

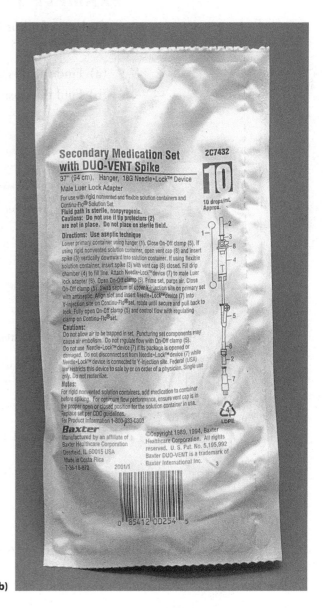

(a)   (b)

● **Figure 11.2**
Packages of secondary IV tubing: (a) 60 drops per *mL*, (b) 10 drops per *mL*.

(Courtesy of Baxter Healthcare Corporation. All rights reserved. Photos by Al Dodge.)

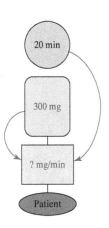

(b) To find the dosage rate, use the formula

$$Dosage\ Rate = \frac{Drug}{Time}$$

Substitute 300 *mg* for the drug in the bag, and 20 *min* for the time.

$$Dosage\ Rate = \frac{300\ mg}{20\ min} = 15\ mg/min$$

So, the dosage rate is 15 *mg/min*, which means that the patient receives 15 *mg* of cimetidine every *minute*.

EXAMPLE 11.2

Order: *cefoxitin 1 g IVPB q6h over 30 minutes*. Read the drug label in • Figure 11.3

(a) **Find the dosage rate in grams per hour.**

(b) **Find the dosage rate in milligrams per minute.**

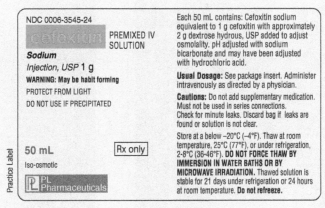

• **Figure 11.3**
Drug label for cefoxitin. (For educational purposes only)

(a) To find the dosage rate, use the formula

$$Dosage\ Rate = \frac{Drug}{Time}$$

Substitute 1 *g* for the drug in the bag, and 30 *min* for the time.

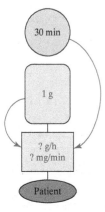

$$Dosage\ Rate = \frac{1\ g}{30\ min}$$

$$\frac{1\ g}{30\ min} = ?\ \frac{g}{h}$$

Use 1 *h* = 60 *min* as the unit fraction.

$$\frac{1\ g}{30\ \cancel{min}} \times \frac{60\ \cancel{min}}{1\ h} = \frac{2\ g}{h}$$

So, the dosage rate is 2 *g/h*.

(b) To find the dosage rate, use the formula

$$Dosage\ Rate = \frac{Drug}{Time}$$

Substitute 1 *g* for the drug in the bag, and 30 *min* for the time.

$$Dosage\ Rate = \frac{1\ g}{30\ min}$$

$$\frac{1\ g}{30\ min} = ?\ \frac{mg}{min}$$

Use 1 *g* = 1,000 *mg* as the unit fraction.

$$\frac{1\ \cancel{g}}{30\ min} \times \frac{1,000\ mg}{1\ \cancel{g}} = 33.33\ \frac{mg}{min}$$

So, the dosage rate is 33 *mg/min*.

Converting IV Dosage Rates to Flow Rates

The next two examples illustrate how to convert rates from dosage rates (*amount of medication per time*) to IV flow rates (*volume of solution per time*).

EXAMPLE 11.3

The medication order reads: *heparin* 1,250 *units/hour IV*. See • Figure 11.4a. Calculate the infusion rate in *mL/h*.

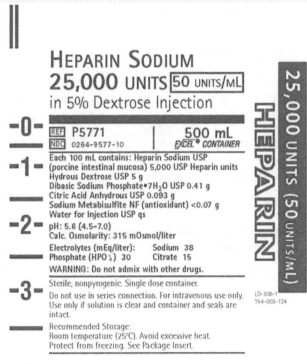

• **Figure 11.4a**
IV heparin solution.
(For educational purposes only)

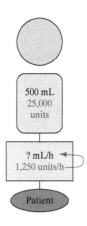

You want to convert the prescribed dosage rate of 1,250 *units/hour* to a flow rate in *milliliters/hour*.

$$\frac{1,250 \; units}{h} = ? \; \frac{mL}{h}$$

Use the concentration in the bag of 25,000 *units* = 500 *mL* as the unit fraction.

$$\frac{1,250 \; \cancel{units}}{h} \times \frac{500 \; mL}{25,000 \; \cancel{units}} = \frac{25 \; mL}{h}$$

So, the flow rate is 25 *mL/h.*

EXAMPLE 11.4

The prescriber writes an order for 1,000 *mL* of 5% D/W with 10 *units* of Pitocin (oxytocin). Your patient must receive 3 *mU* of this drug per minute. Calculate the flow rate in microdrops per minute.

You want to convert the prescribed dosage rate of 3 *mU/min* to a flow rate of *microdrops per minute.*

$$\frac{3 \; mU}{min} = ? \; \frac{mcgtt}{min}$$

You want to cancel mU. To do this, you must use a unit fraction containing mU in the denominator. Using the equivalence 1 *mU* = 1,000 *units*, this fraction will be $\frac{1 \; unit}{1,000 \; mU}$.

$$\frac{3 \; mU}{min} \times \frac{1 \; \text{(unit)}}{1,000 \; mU} = ? \; \frac{mcgtt}{min}$$

Now, on the left side unit is in the numerator, and it must be cancelled. This will require a unit fraction with unit in the denominator. Using the strength, this fraction will be $\frac{1,000 \; mL}{10 \; units}$.

$$\frac{3 \; mU}{min} \times \frac{1 \; \cancel{unit}}{1,000 \; mU} \times \frac{1,000 \; \text{(mL)}}{10 \; \cancel{units}} = ? \; \frac{mcgtt}{min}$$

Now, *mL* is in the numerator on the left side, and it must be cancelled. This will require a unit fraction with *mL* in the denominator. Using the drop factor, this fraction will be $\frac{60 \; mcgtt}{mL}$.

Now, cancel and multiply the numbers

$$\frac{3 \; mU}{min} \times \frac{1 \; \cancel{unit}}{\cancel{1,000} \; \cancel{mU}} \times \frac{\cancel{1,000} \; \cancel{mL}}{10 \; \cancel{units}} \times \frac{60 \; mcgtt}{\cancel{mL}} = 18 \frac{mcgtt}{min}$$

So, you will administer 18 *mcgtt/min.*

NOTE

1 *unit* = 1,000 *milliunits* (mU)

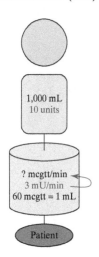

Converting IV Flow Rates to Dosage Rates

The next three examples illustrate how to convert IV flow rates (*volume of solution per time*) to dosage rates (*amount of medication per time*).

EXAMPLE 11.5

Calculate the number of units of Humulin R a patient is receiving per hour if the order is **500 *mL* NS with 300 *units of Humulin R infuse at the rate of 12.5 mL per hour via the pump.***

You want to convert the flow rate from *mL* per hour to the dosage rate in units per hour.

$$\frac{12.5 \; mL}{h} \longrightarrow ? \; \frac{units}{h}$$

Using the strength of the solution (300 *units*/500 *mL*), you do this in one line as follows:

$$\frac{12.5 \; \cancel{mL}}{h} \times \frac{300 \; units}{500 \; \cancel{mL}} = \frac{37.5 \; units}{5 \; h} \; \text{or} \; 7.5 \; \frac{units}{h}$$

So, the patient is receiving 7.5 units per hour.

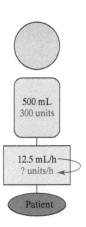

Safe Dose Range

The following examples, 11.6 and 11.7, involve the safe dose range.

EXAMPLE 11.6

An IV bag contains 1,000 *mL* of NS with 500 mg of a drug. It is infusing at 12 *gtt/min*. The drop factor is 10 *gtt/mL*.

(a) Find the dosage rate in *mg/min*.

(b) If the recommended dose is 0.5–2.5 *mg/min*, is this infusion in the safe dose range?

(a) The problem is to change the flow rate of 12 *gtt/min* to a dosage rate in *mg/min*.

$$\frac{12 \; gtt}{min} = ? \; \frac{mg}{min}$$

The strength of the solution (500 *mg* = 1,000 *mL*) and the drop factor (10 *gtt* = 1 *mL*) will both be used to construct the necessary unit fractions.

$$\frac{12 \; \cancel{gtt}}{min} \times \frac{\cancel{mL}}{10 \; \cancel{gtt}} \times \frac{500 \; mg}{1,000 \; \cancel{mL}} = \frac{0.6 \; mg}{min}$$

So, the dosage rate is 0.6 *mg/min*.

(b) Because 0.6 is between 0.5 and 2.5, this infusion is in the safe dose range.

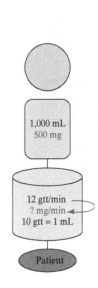

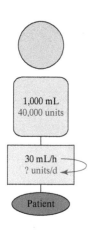

EXAMPLE 11.7

Order: *heparin* 40,000 *units continuous IV in* 1,000 *mL of D5W infuse at* 30 *mL/h.* Find the rate in *units/day*, and determine if it is in the safe dose range (the normal heparinizing range is between 20,000 to 40,000 *units per day*).

You want to convert the flow rate from milliliters per hour to units per day.

$$\frac{30 \; mL}{1 \; h} \longrightarrow \; ?\frac{units}{day}$$

Using the strength of the solution (40,000 *units*/1,000 *mL*) and the fact that there are 24 *hours* in a day, you do this on one line as follows:

$$\frac{30 \; \cancel{mL}}{\cancel{h}} \times \frac{40,000 \; units}{1,000 \; \cancel{mL}} \times \frac{24 \; \cancel{h}}{day} = 28,800 \; \frac{units}{day}$$

So, your patient is receiving 28,800 *units* of heparin per day. This rate is within the safe dosage range of 20,000 to 40,000 *units per day*.

Determining Infused Volume and Duration of Infusion

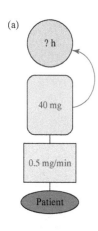

EXAMPLE 11.8

A patient is receiving an infusion at 0.5 *mg/min*. The concentration in the IVPB bag is 100 *mg* in 200 *mL*.

(a) How long will it take for the patient to receive 40 *mg*?

(b) How many milliliters will the patient receive in 30 *minutes*?

(a) Convert 40 *mg* to hours.

$$40 \; mg = ? \; h$$

Use the dosage rate (0.5 *mg/min*) as a unit fraction.

$$\frac{40 \; \cancel{mg}}{1} \times \frac{\cancel{min}}{0.5 \; \cancel{mg}} \times \frac{1 \; h}{60 \; \cancel{min}} = \frac{1.33 \; h}{1}$$

So, it will take 1 *hour and* 20 *minutes* for the patient to receive 40 *mg*.

(b) Convert 30 *minutes* to *milliliters*.

$$30 \; min = ? \; mL$$

Use the dosage rate (0.5 *mg/min*) and the concentration in the bag (100 *mg*/200 *mL*) as unit fractions.

$$\frac{30 \; \cancel{min}}{1} \times \frac{0.5 \; \cancel{mg}}{1 \; \cancel{min}} \times \frac{200 \; mL}{100 \; \cancel{mg}} = \frac{30 \; mL}{1}$$

So, the patient will receive 30 *milliliters* in 30 *minutes*.

EXAMPLE 11.9

A patient is receiving an infusion of a drug at the rate of 3 *units/min* IVPB. The bag contains 250 *units* of the drug in 100 *mL* of solution.

(a) How many units of the drug will the patient receive in 20 *minutes*?

(b) How many minutes will it take for 50 *mL* of the solution to infuse?

(a) Convert 20 *minutes* to *units*.

$$20 \ min = ? \ units$$

Use the dosage rate (3 *units/min*) as a unit fraction.

$$\frac{20 \ \overline{min}}{1} \times \frac{3 \ units}{1 \ \overline{min}} = \frac{60 \ units}{1}$$

So, the patient will receive 60 *units* in 20 *minutes*.

(b) Convert 50 *milliliters* to *minutes*.

$$50 \ mL = ? \ min$$

Use the dosage rate *(3 units/min) and the concentration in the bag (250 units per 100 mL) as the unit fractions.*

$$\frac{50 \ \overline{mL}}{1} \times \frac{250 \ \overline{units}}{100 \ \overline{mL}} \times \frac{1 \ min}{3 \ \overline{units}} = \frac{41.67 \ min}{1}$$

So, it will it take 42 *minutes* for 50 *mL* of the solution to infuse.

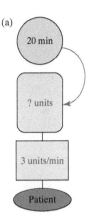

(a)

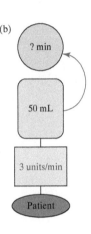

(b)

IV Push

To infuse a small amount of medication in a short period of time, a syringe can be inserted directly into a vein, or a saline lock or heparin lock can be attached to an IV catheter. For patients who have a primary IV line, the medication should be administered through the port closest to the patient. The medication can then be "pushed" directly into the vein. This route of medication administration is referred to as **IV push (IVP)**. See ● Figure 11.5.

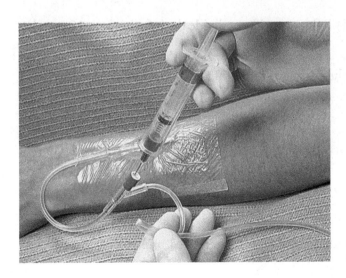

● **Figure 11.5**
IV push administration.

ALERT

An IV push generally involves medications administered over a short period of time. Be sure to verify the following: need for the drug, route, concentration, dose, expiration date, and clarity of the solution. It is also essential to verify the rate of injection with the package insert. Some medications (e.g., adenosine) require rapid administration, whereas others (e.g., verapamil) are administered more slowly.

Because the IVP flow rate is determined by the speed at which the plunger of the syringe is manually pushed, it is important to control that speed. It is difficult to maintain the desired flow rate over the entire infusion. Therefore, the infusion may be mentally divided into smaller segments or pieces to make the flow rate easier to control.

For example, suppose that 4 *mL* of solution must be infused IVP in 1 *minute* (60 *seconds*). Because the total infusion volume (4 *mL*) and duration (60 *sec*) are known, the flow rate is 4 *mL*/60 *sec*. You may choose to divide numerator and denominator of this fraction by any convenient number. By doing so, you will make the numbers in the numerator and denominator smaller and thereby obtain an equivalent infusion rate using the smaller quantities, as shown in the following:

- If you divide both the numerator and denominator of the flow rate of $\frac{4\ mL}{60\ sec}$ by 2, you obtain

$$\frac{4\ mL}{60\ sec} = \frac{4 \div 2\ mL}{60 \div 2\ sec} = \frac{2\ mL}{30\ sec}$$

and the flow rate of $\frac{4\ mL}{60\ sec}$ is equivalent to $\frac{2\ mL}{30\ sec}$. So, you would push 2 *mL* every 30 *seconds* until the 4 *mL* of medication in the syringe are infused.

- On the other hand, if you divide both the numerator and denominator of the flow rate of $\frac{4\ mL}{60\ sec}$ by 4, you obtain

$$\frac{4\ mL}{60\ sec} = \frac{4 \div 4\ mL}{60 \div 4\ sec} = \frac{1\ mL}{15\ sec}$$

and the flow rate of $\frac{4\ mL}{60\ sec}$ is equivalent to $\frac{1\ mL}{15\ sec}$. So, you would push 1 *mL* every 15 *seconds* until the 4 *mL* of medication in the syringe are infused.

EXAMPLE 11.10

750 *mg* of a drug is ordered IVP stat over 5 *minutes*, and the concentration of the drug is 75 *mg/mL*.

(a) Find the total number of milliliters you will administer.

(b) Determine the IVP flow rate if you divide the infusion into 5 equal segments.

(c) Determine the IVP flow rate if you divide the infusion into 10 equal segments.

(a) You must find the number of milliliters of solution that contain the 750 *mg* dose.

$$750\ mg = ?\ mL$$

The strength of 75 *mg* = 1 *mL* will be used to form the unit fraction.

$$\frac{750\ mg}{1} \times \frac{1\ mL}{75\ mg} = 10\ mL$$

So, you would administer 10 *mL* over the 5 *minutes*.

(b) From part (a), the rate of infusion is $\frac{10\,mL}{5\,min}$. Because you want to cut the infusion into 5 equal segments, divide both the numerator and denominator of the flow rate by 5.

$$\frac{10\,mL \div 5}{5\,min \div 5} = \frac{2\,mL}{1\,min}$$

So, 2 *mL* will be pushed during every 1-*minute* interval. If a 10 *mL* syringe is used, each tick represents 1 *mL*, and the plunger will move 2 ticks each *minute*.

(c) In part (a), the flow rate was determined to be 10 *milliliters* in 5 *minutes*. Because you want to cut the infusion into 10 equal segments, divide both the numerator and denominator of the flow rate by 10.

$$\frac{10\,mL \div 10}{5\,min \div 10} = \frac{1\,mL}{0.5\,min}$$

Substitute 30 seconds for 0.5 *minutes* to obtain

$$\frac{1\,mL}{0.5\,min} = \frac{1\,mL}{30\,sec}$$

So, each milliliter is administered in 30 *seconds*. If a 10 *mL* syringe is used, the plunger will move 1 tick on the syringe every 30 *seconds*.

EXAMPLE 11.11

Order: *Cefizox (ceftizoxime sodium) 1,500 mg IVP stat over 4 min.* The 2 *g* Cefizox vial has strength of 1 *g*/10 *mL*.

(a) Find the total number of milliliters you will administer.

(b) Determine the number of mL you will push during each 30-*second* interval.

(c) Determine the number of seconds needed to deliver each 1 *mL* of the solution.

(a) The problem is to change the dose of 1,500 *mg* to a dose measured in *mL*.

$$1,500\,mg = ?\,mL$$

The strength of 1 *g* = 10 *mL*, and the equivalence 1 *g* = 1,000 *mg* will be used to form the unit fractions.

$$\frac{1,500\,mg}{1} \times \frac{1\,g}{1,000\,mg} \times \frac{10\,mL}{1\,g} = 15\,mL$$

So, you would administer a total of 15 *mL* of Cefizox over 4 *minutes*.

(b) From part (a), the rate of infusion is $\frac{15 \ mL}{4 \ min}$. Because $4 \ min = 240 \ sec$, the flow rate is $\frac{15 \ mL}{240 \ sec}$. You want to divide the 240-*second* infusion time into 30-*second* segments and

$$\frac{240 \ sec}{30 \ sec} = 8$$

So, divide both the numerator and the denominator of the flow rate by 8.

$$\frac{15 \ mL \div 8}{240 \ sec \div 8} = \frac{1.875 \ mL}{30 \ sec} \approx \frac{1.9 \ mL}{30 \ sec}$$

So, 1.9 *mL* of Cefizox should be pushed during every 30-*second* interval. This amount cannot be measured accurately on a 20 *mL* syringe; it is only a guideline. Because each tick on a 20 *mL* syringe represents 1 *mL*, the plunger will move about 2 ticks on the syringe each 30 *seconds*.

(c) In part (a) the flow rate was determined to be $\frac{15 \ mL}{240 \ sec}$
You want to divide the 15 *mL* into 1 *mL* pieces and

$$\frac{15 \ mL}{1 \ mL} = 15$$

So, both numerator and denominator of the IVP rate must be divided by 15.

$$\frac{15 \ mL \div 15}{240 \ sec \div 15} = \frac{1 \ mL}{16 \ sec}$$

So, 1 *mL* is administered each 16 seconds. If a 20 *mL* syringe is used, the plunger will move 1 tick on the syringe every 16 seconds.

Compound Rates

In Chapter 6, you calculated dosages based on the *size of the patient*, measured in either kilograms or meters squared. For example, if a patient weighing 100 *kg* has an order to receive a drug at the rate of 2 *micrograms per kilogram (2 mcg/kg)*, the dose would be obtained by multiplying the size of the patient by the rate in the order, as follows:

$$\text{Size of Patient} \times \text{Order} = \text{Dose}$$

$$100 \ kg \times \frac{2 \ mcg}{kg} = 200 \ mcg$$

So, the dose is 200 *mcg*, and the single unit of measurement (100 *kg*) was converted to another single unit of measurement (200 *mcg*).

In this chapter, some IV medications are prescribed not only based on the patient's size; the amount of drug the patient receives also depends on *time*. For example, an order might indicate that a drug is to be administered at the rate of 2 *micrograms per kilogram per minute (2 mcg/kg/min)*. This means that the patient is to receive *each minute* 2 *mcg* of the drug for every *kg* of body weight. Therefore, the amount of medication the patient receives depends on two things: body weight and time.

This new type of rate, called a **compound rate**, for computational purposes is written as follows:

$$\frac{2\ mcg}{kg \cdot min}$$

where the dot in the denominator stands for multiplication.

Suppose a patient weighing 100 *kg* has an order to receive a drug at the compound rate of 2 *mcg/kg/min*. The dosage rate would be obtained by multiplying the size of the patient by the compound rate in the order as follows:

Size of Patient × Order = Dosage Rate

$$100\ kg \times \frac{2\ mcg}{kg \cdot min} = \frac{200\ mcg}{min}$$

So, the dosage rate is 200 *mcg/min*, and the single unit of measurement (100 *kg*) was converted to a dosage rate (200 *mcg/min*).

EXAMPLE 11.12

The prescriber ordered: **250 *mL* 5% D/W *with* 60 *mg* of a drug 0.006 *mg/kg/min* IVPB daily. The patient weighs 75 *kg*, and the drop factor is 20 *gtt/mL*. Calculate the flow rate for this drug in drops per minute.**

Given:	75 *kg* (weight of the patient)
Known equivalences:	0.006 *mg/kg/min* (order)
	60 *mg*/250 *mL* (strength)
	20 *gtt/mL* (drop factor)
Find:	? *gtt/min* (flow rate)

Because the order is based on the size of the patient, start with the size of the patient and use the formula:

Size of Patient × Order = Dosage Rate

$$\frac{75\ kg}{1} \times \frac{0.006\ mg}{kg \cdot min} = \frac{0.45\ mg}{min}$$

Now, change the dosage rate to the desired flow rate.

$$\frac{0.45\ mg}{min} = ?\ \frac{gtt}{min}$$

Use the concentration in the bag (60 *mg*/250 *mL*) and the drop factor (20 *gtt/mL*) as unit fractions.

$$\frac{0.45\ mg}{min} \times \frac{250\ mL}{60\ mg} \times \frac{20\ gtt}{1\ mL} = \frac{37.5\ gtt}{min}$$

So, the flow rate is 38 *gtt/min*.

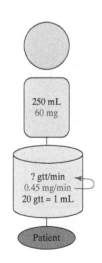

250 mL
60 mg

? gtt/min
0.45 mg/min
20 gtt = 1 mL

Patient

EXAMPLE 11.13

The prescriber ordered: *Ifex (ifosfamide)* **1.2 g/m²/d IVPB, infuse over 30 min. Repeat for 5 consecutive days.** The IV solution strength is **50 mg/mL**. The patient has BSA of **1.50 m²**. Find the flow rate in **mL/h**.

Notice that the order contains the compound rate of 1.2 *g/m²/d*. Multiply the size of the patient by this compound rate as follows:

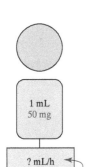

$$1.50 \; \cancel{m^2} \times \frac{1.2 \; g}{\cancel{m^2} \cdot d} = \frac{1.8 \; g}{d}$$

This means that the patient should receive 1.8 *g* of Ifex per day. Because the drug must be administered over 30 *minutes*, the dosage rate is $\frac{1.8 \; g}{30 \; min}$, and it must be changed to the flow rate in $\frac{mL}{h}$.

$$\frac{1.8 \; g}{30 \; min} = ? \; \frac{mL}{h}$$

Use the concentration in the bag of 50 *mg/mL* to form a unit fraction.

$$\frac{1.8 \; \cancel{g}}{30 \; \cancel{min}} \times \frac{60 \; \cancel{min}}{1 \; h} \times \frac{1,000 \; \cancel{mg}}{1 \; \cancel{g}} \times \frac{1 \; mL}{50 \; \cancel{mg}} = \frac{72 \; mL}{h}$$

So, the flow rate is 72 *mL/h*.

EXAMPLE 11.14

The patient weighs **80 kg** and must receive dopamine hydrochloride at the rate of **3 mcg/kg/min**.

(a) How many mg/min should the patient receive?

(b) How long will it take for the patient to receive 50 *mg* of the drug?

(a) Multiply the size of the patient by the order as follows:

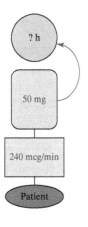

$$80 \; \cancel{kg} \times \frac{3 \; mcg}{\cancel{kg} \times min} = \frac{240 \; mcg}{min}$$

So, the patient should receive the drug at the rate of 240 *mcg/min*.

(b) You want to convert 50 *mg* to *hours*, using the dosage rate of 240 *mcg/min* as a unit fraction.

$$50 \; mg = ? \; h$$

$$\frac{50 \; \cancel{mg}}{1} \times \frac{1,000 \; \cancel{mcg}}{1 \; \cancel{mg}} \times \frac{1 \; \cancel{min}}{240 \; \cancel{mcg}} \times \frac{1 \; h}{60 \; \cancel{min}} = \frac{3.472 \; h}{1}$$

So, it will take about $3\frac{1}{2}$ *hours* for the patient to receive 50 *mg* of the drug.

Adding Medication to an IVPB Bag

Although premixed IVPB bags are generally supplied, sometimes the drug must be added to the bag at the time of administration. The next three examples illustrate this.

EXAMPLE 11.15

A patient must receive a drug at the recommended rate of 15 *mg/kg/d.*

(a) If the patient weighs 100 kg, how many mg/d must the patient receive?

(b) The drug is to be administered IVPB in 200 *mL* D/5/W over 60 *min.* The vial contains 1.5 *g* of the drug in powdered form. This vial is used with a reconstitution device similar to that shown in • Figure 11.6. Find the IV flow rate in *mL/h.*

(c) How many mg/min will the patient receive?

(a) Multiply the size of the patient by this compound rate as follows:

$$100 \ kg \times \frac{15 \ mg}{kg \cdot d} = \frac{1,500 \ mg}{d}$$

This means that the patient should receive the dosage rate of 1,500 *milligrams* per day.

(b) Because the drug is dissolved in 200 *mL* and the infusion time is 60 *minutes,* the IV flow rate is

$$\frac{200 \ mL}{60 \ min}$$

Replace 60 *minutes* with 1 *hour.*

$$\frac{200 \ mL}{60 \ min} = \frac{200 \ mL}{1 \ h}$$

So, the IV flow rate is 200 *mL/h.*

(c) The problem is to find the dosage rate in *mg/min.*

Because the patient is receiving 1,500 *mg* in 60 *min,* the dosage rate is

$$\frac{1,500 \ mg}{60 \ min} = \frac{1,500}{60} \ \frac{mg}{min} = 25 \ \frac{mg}{min}$$

So, the dosage rate is 25 *mg/min.*

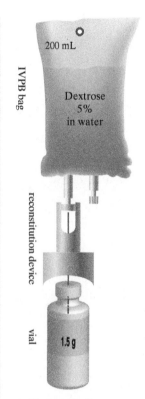

• **Figure 11.6**
Reconstitution system.

There are reconstitution systems that enable the healthcare provider to reconstitute a powdered drug and place it into an IVPB bag without using a syringe. One such device is shown in Figure 11.6. With this device, when the IVPB bag is squeezed, fluid is forced into the vial, dissolving the powder. The system is then placed in a vertical configuration, with the vial on top and the IVPB bag on the bottom. The IVPB bag is then squeezed and released, thereby creating a negative pressure, which allows the newly reconstituted drug to flow into the IVPB bag.

Another reconstitution device is the ADD-Vantage system, which employs an IV bag containing intravenous fluid. The bag is designed with a special port, which will accept a vial of medication. When the vial is placed into this port, the contents of the vial and the fluid mix to form the desired solution. See • **Figure 11.7**.

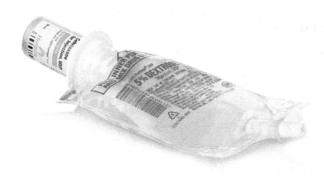

• Figure 11.7
ADD-Vantage System.

EXAMPLE 11.16

A patient is to receive 150 *mg* of a drug IVPB in 200 *mL* NS over 1 *hour*. The vial of medication indicates a strength of 75 *mg/mL*.

(a) How many milliliters must be withdrawn from the vial and added to the NS?

(b) At what rate in mL/h should the pump be set?

(a) The problem is to change the dose of 150 *mg* to *mL* of solution to be taken from the vial.

$$150 \ mg = ? \ mL$$

In the vial, the strength is 75 *mg/mL*. Use this to make the unit fraction.

$$\frac{150 \ \cancel{mg}}{1} \times \frac{1 \ mL}{75 \ \cancel{mg}} = \frac{2 \ mL}{1}$$

So, 2 *mL* of the drug must be withdrawn from the vial and added to the normal saline.

(b)

Method 1: *Include the volume of drug added to the IV bag.*	**Method 2:** *Do not include the volume of drug added to the IV bag.*

Method 1: *Include the volume of drug added to the IV bag.*

After 2 *mL* of drug are withdrawn from the vial and added to the 200 *mL* of NS, the IVPB bag will then contain (200 + 2) 202 *mL* of solution. Because the infusion will last 1 *hour*, the pump rate would be set at 202 *mL/h*.

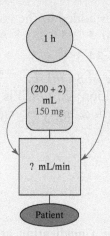

Method 2: *Do not include the volume of drug added to the IV bag.*

When the 2 *mL* of drug from the vial are added to the 200 *mL* of NS, the volume of the bag increases by $\left(\frac{Change}{Original} = \frac{2}{200}\right)$ 1%. Because this increase in volume is relatively small, some institutional guidelines permit it to be excluded in IV flow rate calculation. If the increase in volume is excluded, the pump rate would be set at 200 *mL/h*.

Consult facility protocols to determine which calculation method to use. In the worked-out solutions to the Practice Sets, Method 1 will be used.

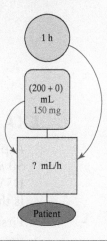

EXAMPLE 11.17

The order is: *a drug* 100 *mg/m² IVPB in* 250 *mL NS infuse over 3 h.* The patient's BSA is 1.65 *m²*, and the drug is available in a vial labeled 60 *mg/mL*.

(a) How many milligrams of the drug must the patient receive?

(b) How many milliliters must be withdrawn from the vial and added to the IV bag?

(c) The order indicates that the drug should be added to 250 *mL* of NS. At what rate in *mL/h* should the pump be set?

(a) Multiply the size of the patient by the order.

$$1.65 \; m^2 \times \frac{100 \; mg}{m^2} = 165 \; mg$$

So, the patient should receive 165 *mg* of the drug.

(b) The problem is to change the dose of 165 *mg* to *mL* of solution to be taken from the vial.

$$165 \; mg = ? \; mL$$

Use the strength in the vial, 60 *mg/mL*, to make the unit fraction.

$$\frac{165 \; \cancel{mg}}{1} \times \frac{1 \; mL}{60 \; \cancel{mg}} = 2.75 \; mL$$

So, 2.8 *mL* of the drug must be withdrawn from the vial and added to the IV bag.

(c) If the additional volume of the drug is added to the volume of the IVPB bag, the bag will contain (250 + 2.8) 252.8 *mL*, and the pump rate would be set at $\frac{252.8 \; mL}{3 \; h} = 84.3 \; \frac{mL}{h}$

So, the pump would be set at the rate of 84 *mL/h*.

If only the volume of the IV solution (250 *mL*) is considered, the pump rate would be set at $\frac{250 \; mL}{3 \; h} \approx 83.3 \; \frac{mL}{h}$. So, the pump would be set at the rate of 83 *mL/h*.

EXAMPLE 11.18

A patient who weighs 55 *kg* is receiving a medication at the rate of 30 *mL/h*. The concentration of the medication is 400 *mg* in 500 *mL* of D5W. The recommended dose range for the drug is 2–5 *mcg/kg/min*. Is the patient receiving a safe dose?

First use the *minimum* recommended dose of 2 *mcg/kg/h* to determine the minimum IV rate in *mL/h* that the patient may receive. Multiply the size of the patient by the order.

$$55 \; kg \times \frac{2 \; mcg}{kg \cdot min} = \frac{110 \; mcg}{min}$$

Change the dosage rate of 110 *mcg/min* to an IV rate in *mL/h*.

$$\frac{110 \; mcg}{1 \; min} = ? \; \frac{mL}{h}$$

Use the strength of the solution (400 *mg* = 500 *mL*) to form a unit fraction.

$$\frac{110 \; \cancel{mcg}}{1 \; \cancel{min}} \times \frac{1 \; \cancel{mg}}{1,000 \; \cancel{mcg}} \times \frac{500 \; mL}{400 \; \cancel{mg}} \times \frac{60 \; \cancel{min}}{1 \; h} = \frac{8.25 \; mL}{1 \; h}$$

So, the *minimum* IV flow rate is 8.25 *mL/h*.

Now use the *maximum* recommended dose of 5 *mcg/kg/h* to determine the *maximum* IV flow rate in *mL/h* that the patient should receive. It can be done in one line as follows:

$$\frac{55 \; kg}{1} \times \frac{5 \; \cancel{mcg}}{kg \cdot \cancel{min}} \times \frac{1 \; \cancel{mg}}{1,000 \; \cancel{mcg}} \times \frac{500 \; mL}{400 \; \cancel{mg}} \times \frac{60 \; \cancel{min}}{1 \; h} = \frac{20.625 \; mL}{1 \; h}$$

So, the *maximum flow rate* is 21 *mL/h*.

ALERT

Whenever your calculations indicate that the prescribed dose is not within the safe range, you must verify the order with the prescriber.

The safe dose range of 2–5 *mcg/kg/min* is equivalent to the flow rate range of 8–21 *mL/h* for this patient. The patient is receiving an IV rate of 30 *mL/h*. Because 30 *mL/h* is larger than the maximum allowable flow rate of 21 *mL/h*, the patient is not receiving a safe dose. The patient is receiving an overdose. Turn off the IV and contact the prescriber.

Titrated Medications

The process of adjusting the dosage of a medication based on patient response is called **titration**. Orders for titrated medications are often prescribed for critical care patients. Such orders require that therapeutic effects, such as pain reduction, be monitored. The dose of the medication must be adjusted accordingly until the desired effect is achieved.

An order for a titrated medication generally includes a purpose for titrating and a maximum dose. If either the initial dose or directions for subsequent adjustments of the initial dose are not included in the order, the medication cannot be given, and you must contact the prescriber.

Dosage errors with titrated medications can quickly result in catastrophic consequences. Therefore, a thorough knowledge of the particular medication and its proper dosage adjustments is crucial. Dosage increment choices are medication-specific, and depend on many factors that go beyond the scope of this book.

> **ALERT**
>
> Drugs that are titrated are administered according to protocol. Therefore, it is imperative to know the institution's protocols.

Suppose an order indicates that a certain drug must be administered with an initial dosage rate of 10 *mcg/min* and that the rate should be increased by 5 *mcg/min* every 3–5 *min* for chest pain until response, up to a maximum rate of 30 *mcg/min*. The IV bag has a strength of 50 *mg/250 mL*.

To administer the drug, first determine the IV rate in *mL/h* for the initial dose rate of 10 *mcg/min*.

That is

$$\frac{10\ mcg}{min} = ?\ \frac{mL}{h}$$

Use the strength of the solution ($50\ mg = 250\ mL$) to form a unit fraction.

$$\frac{10\ \cancel{mcg}}{1\ \cancel{min}} \times \frac{1\ \cancel{mg}}{1{,}000\ \cancel{mcg}} \times \frac{250\ mL}{50\ \cancel{mg}} \times \frac{60\ \cancel{min}}{1\ h} = \frac{3\ mL}{1\ h}$$

So, the initial IV rate is 3 *mL/h*.

After the initial dose is administered, the patient is monitored. If the desired response is not achieved, the order indicates to increase the dose rate by 5 *mcg/min*. This requires that you find the corresponding IV rate in *mL/h* for the new dosage rate. This titration may also require other dosage changes. Every time the dose rate is changed, recalculation of the corresponding IV rate is necessary. Rather than performing such calculations each time a dose is modified, it is useful to compile a *titration table* that will quickly provide the IV rate for any possible drug dosage rate choice.

Construction of the titration table for each incremental dose change of 5 *mcg/min*, up to the maximum rate of 30 *mcg/min*, could be accomplished by repeating a procedure similar to that which was used to determine the initial flow rate. Instead, however, the table can be quickly compiled by first finding the incremental IV flow rate for a dosage rate change of 5 *mcg/min*.

$$5 \frac{mcg}{min} = ? \frac{mL}{h}$$

Use the strength of the solution $(50 \ mg = 250 \ mL)$ to form a unit fraction.

$$\frac{5 \ \cancel{mcg}}{1 \ \cancel{min}} \times \frac{1 \ \cancel{mg}}{1,000 \ \cancel{mcg}} \times \frac{250 \ mL}{50 \ \cancel{mg}} \times \frac{60 \ \cancel{min}}{1 \ h} = \frac{1.5 \ mL}{1 \ h}$$

So, for each change of 5 *mcg/min*, the incremental IV flow rate is 1.5 *mL/h*.

Table 11.1 shows the titration table for the order. It contains the various dosage rates in *mcg/min* and their corresponding flow rates. As you move down the columns, the dosage rate increases in 5 *mcg/min* increments, while the corresponding flow rate increases in 1.5 *mL/h* increments.

Table 11.1 **Titration Table**

Dosage Rate (mcg/min)	Flow Rate (mL/h)
10 *mcg/min* (initial)	3 *mL/h*
15 *mcg/min*	4.5 *mL/h*
20 *mcg/min*	6 *mL/h*
25 *mcg/min*	7.5 *mL/h*
30 *mcg/min* (maximum)	9 *mL/h*

EXAMPLE 11.19

To induce labor, the order is: *Pitocin (oxytocin) start at 1 mU/min IV, may increase by 2 mU/min q15 min to a max of 11 mU/min.* The IV strength is 10 *mU/mL*.

(a) Calculate the initial pump setting in *mL/h*.

(b) Construct a titration table for this order.

(a) Determine the flow rate in mL/h for the initial dosage rate of $1\ mU/min$.

The problem is

$$\frac{1\ mU}{min} = ?\,\frac{mL}{h}$$

Use the strength of the solution ($10\ mU = 1\ mL$) to form a unit fraction.

$$\frac{1\ \cancel{mU}}{1\ \cancel{min}} \times \frac{1\ mL}{10\ \cancel{mU}} \times \frac{60\ \cancel{min}}{1\ h} = \frac{6\ mL}{1\ h}$$

Therefore,

$$1\frac{mU}{min} = 6\frac{mL}{h}$$

and the initial flow rate is $6\ mL/h$.

(b) The order indicates that the dosage rate may be changed in $2\,\dfrac{mu}{min}$.

increments. The problem now is to change these dosage rate increments to flow rate increments; that is,

$$2\frac{mU}{min} = ?\,\frac{mL}{h}$$

Again, use the strength of the solution ($10\ mU = 1\ mL$) to form a unit fraction.

$$\frac{2\ \cancel{mU}}{1\ \cancel{min}} \times \frac{1\ mL}{10\ \cancel{mU}} \times \frac{60\ \cancel{min}}{1\ h} = \frac{12\ mL}{h}$$

Therefore, the flow rate increments are $12\ mL/h$.

Table 11.2 shows the entire titration table. Notice that the dose rates increase in $2\ mU/min$ increments, whereas the flow rates increase in $12\ mL/h$ increments.

Table 11.2 Titration Table for Example 11.19	
Dosage Rate (mU/min)	**Flow Rate (mL/h)**
1 mU/min (initial)	6 mL/h
3 mU/min	18 mL/h
5 mU/min	30 mL/h
7 mU/min	42 mL/h
9 mU/min	54 mL/h
11 mU/min (maximum)	66 mL/h

Summary

In this chapter, the IV medication administration process was discussed. IVPB and IVP infusions were described, and orders based on body weight and body surface area were illustrated.

- A secondary line is referred to as an IV piggyback.
- IV push, or bolus, medications can be injected into a heplock/saline lock or directly into the vein.
- In a gravity system, the IV bag that is hung highest will infuse first.

- An order containing a compound rate of the form *mg/kg/min* directs that each minute the patient must receive the stated number of milligrams of medication for each kilogram of the patient's body weight.
- For calculation purposes, write *mg/kg/min* as $\frac{mg}{kg \cdot min}$.
- When the size of the patient is multiplied by a compound rate, the dosage rate is obtained.
- When titrating medications, the dose is adjusted until the desired therapeutic effect is achieved.

Case Study 11.1

Read the Case Study and answer the questions. Answers can be found in Appendix A.

A woman is admitted to the labor room with a diagnosis of preterm labor. She states that she has not seen a physician because this is her third baby and she "knows what to do while she is pregnant." Her initial workup indicates a gestational age of 32 weeks, and she tests positive for chlamydia and Strep-B. Her vital signs are T 100° F; P 98; R 18; B/P 140/88. The fetal heart rate is 140–150. The orders include the following:

- NPO
- IV fluids: D5/RL 1,000 *mL* q8h
- Continuous electronic fetal monitoring
- Vital signs q4h
- Dexamethasone 6 *mg* IM q12h for 2 doses
- Brethine (terbutaline sulfate) 0.25 *mg* subcutaneous q30 *minutes* for 2h
- Rocephin (ceftriaxone sodium) 250 *mg* IM stat

- Penicillin G 5 million units IVPB stat; then 2.5 *million units* q4h
- Zithromax (azithromycin) 500 *mg* IVPB stat and daily for 2 *days*

1. Calculate the rate of flow for the D5/RL in *mL/h*.
2. The label on the dexamethasone reads 8 *mg/mL*. How many milliliters will you administer?
3. The label on the terbutaline reads 1 *mg/mL*. How many milliliters will you administer?
4. The label on the ceftriaxone states to reconstitute the 1 *g* vial with 2.1 *mL* of sterile water for injection, which results in a strength of 350 *mg/mL*. How many milliliters will you administer?
5. The instructions state to reconstitute the penicillin G (use the minimum amount of diluent), add to 100 *mL* D5W, and infuse in 1 hour. The drop factor is 15. What is the rate of flow of the stat dose in *gtts/min*? See the label in • **Figure 11.8**.

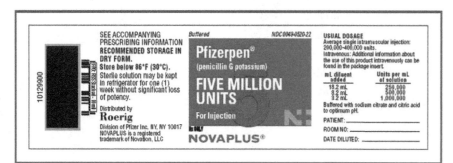

• **Figure 11.8**
Drug label for penicillin G.

(Reg. Trademark of Pfizer Inc. Reproduced with permission.)

6. The instructions for the azithromycin state to reconstitute the 500 *mg* vial with 4.8 *mL* until dissolved, to yield a strength of 100 *mg/mL*, and then to add it to 250 *mL* of D5W and administer over at least 60 *minutes*. At what rate will you set the infusion pump if you choose to administer the medication over 90 *minutes*?

7. The patient continues to have uterine contractions, and a new order has been written: *magnesium sulfate 4g IV bolus over 20 minutes, then 1 g/h.*

   The label on the IV bag states "magnesium sulfate 40 g in 1,000 *mL*."

   (a) What is the rate of flow in *mL/h* for the bolus dose?

   (b) What is the rate of flow in *mL/h* for the maintenance dose?

The patient continues to have contractions and her membranes rupture. The following orders are written:

- Discontinue the magnesium sulfate.
- Pitocin (oxytocin) 10 units/1,000 *mL* RL, start at 0.5 *mU/min* increase by 1 *mU/min* q20 minutes.
- Stadol (butorphanol tartrate) 1 *mg* IVP stat.

8. What is the rate of flow in *mL/h* for the initial dose of Pitocin?

9. The Pitocin is infusing at 9 *mL/h*. How many *mU/h* is the patient receiving?

10. The vial of butorphanol tartrate is labeled 2 *mg/mL*. How many milliliters will you administer?

Practice Sets

The answers to *Try These for Practice, Exercises,* and *Cumulative Review Exercises* are found in Appendix A. Ask your instructor for the answers to the *Additional Exercises.*

Try These for Practice

Test your comprehension after reading the chapter.

1. An IV bag contains 600 *mg* of a drug in 200 *mL* of NS, and it must infuse over 2 *hours*. Find the flow rate in *mL/h* and the dosage rate in *mg/min*.

2. Order: *Alimta 500 mg/m² IV on day 1 of a 21-day cycle infuse in 10 min.* Read the label in • **Figure 11.9**. The directions on the package insert of this antineoplastic drug state: "reconstitute the vial with 20 *mL* NS and further dilute with NS for a total volume of 100 *mL*." The patient has BSA of 1 *m²*. Find the

   (a) pump setting in *mL/h*.
   (b) dosage rate in *mg/min*.

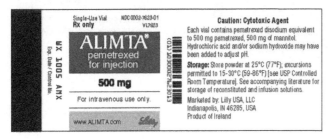

• **Figure 11.9**
Drug label for Alimta.

Workspace

Workspace

3. An IVPB bag containing 50 *mg* of drug in 100 *mL* of solution must infuse at the rate of 2 *mg/min*. If the infusion begins at 0800h, when will it finish?

4. A dosage of 4 *mcg/kg/min* has been ordered for an adult weighing 83 *kg*. The solution used has a strength of 100 *mg* in 250 *mL*. Calculate the dosage rate in *mcg/min* and the flow rate in *mL/h*.

5. To induce labor, the prescriber orders *LR 1,000 mL IVc̄ Pitocin 20 units continuous drip. Infuse at an initial rate of 2 milliunits/min, increase by 2 milliunits/min every hour to a maximum of 20 milliunits/min.* Make a titration table showing the dosage rate (*milliunits/min*) and flow rate in *mL/h* for this titration.

Exercises

Reinforce your understanding in class or at home.

1. An IV is infusing at 300 *milliunits per minute*. The solution available is 20 *units* in 250 *mL* D5W. The drop factor is 15 *gtt/mL*. What is the drip rate in *gtt/min*?

2. An IVPB is infusing at 20 *gtt/min*. The concentration of the solution is 40 *mg* of drug in 250 *mL* of D5W. The drop factor is 10 *gtt/mL*. What is the dosage rate in *mcg/min*?

3. An IVPB is infusing at 0.5 *mcg/min*. The solution concentration is 50 *mcg* in 100 *mL* NS. What is the pump setting in *mL/h*?

4. An IVPB is infusing at 120 *mL/h*. The concentration is 50 *mg* in 100 *mL* of NS. What is the dosage rate in *mg/min*?

5. Order: *Gemzar (gemcitabline HCl) 1,000 mg/m² IVPB add to 200 mL NS infuse in 30 min.* The BSA is 0.91 *m²*. Read the label of this antineoplastic drug in • **Figure 11.10** and determine the

   (a) number of *mL* of diluent you would add to the Gemzar vial.

   (b) number of *mL* you would take from the Gemzar vial.

   (c) pump setting in *mL/h*.

   (d) dosage rate in *mg/min*.

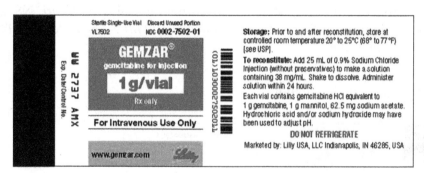

• **Figure 11.10**
Drug label for Gemzar.

6. Order: *ampicillin sodium 500 mg IVPB q6h infuse in 15 min.* Find the dosage rate of this antibiotic in *mg/min*.

7. A patient with a systemic infection must receive 500 *mg* of ampicillin sodium IV over 60 *minutes*. The concentration of the IV solution is 30 *mg/mL*. What is the flow rate of this antibiotic drug in *mcgtt/min*?

8. Order: *morphine sulfate 4 mg IVP over 5 minutes*. Directions: Further dilute with NS to *5 mL*. The concentration in the morphine sulfate vial is 10 *mg/mL*.

    (a) How many milliliters will be withdrawn from the vial?

    (b) Find the flow rate in *mL/min*.

    (c) How many *mL* will be administered every 30 *seconds*?

    (d) Using a 12 *mL* syringe, find the number of seconds for each calibration on the syringe. [Hint: Each milliliter on the 12 *mL* syringe is divided into 5 segments.]

9. Order: *Paraplatin (carboplatin) 360 mg/m^2 IVPB over 15 minutes once q4wk*. The BSA of the patient is 1.39 *m^2*. The Paraplatin vial has a concentration of 10 *mg/mL*.

    (a) How many *mg* must be administered?

    (b) How many milliliters must be withdrawn from the vial.

10. A drug is ordered at 0.3 *mg/kg/min*. If the patient weighs 148 *pounds*, find the dosage rate in *mg/min*.

11. A drug is ordered at 0.3 *mg/kg/min*. If the patient weighs 148 *kilograms*, find the dosage rate in mg/min.

12. An IVPB bag contains 200 *mg* of drug in 100 *mL* of solution. If the medication will infuse at the rate of 10 *mg/min*, how long will the infusion take?

13. An IVPB bag contains 400 *mg* of drug in 50 *mL* of solution. If the medication will infuse at the rate of 50 *mg/min*, how many *mL* will infuse in 2 *minutes*?

14. A drug is ordered to start at a rate of 3 *mcg/min IV*. This rate may, depending on the response of the patient, be increased by 2 *mcg/min q15 min* to a maximum of 11 *mcg/min*. The IV has a concentration of 5 mcg/mL.

    (a) Calculate the initial pump setting in *mL/h*.

    (b) Construct the titration table.

15. The physician orders *morphine sulfate 200 mg IVPB in NS 1,000 mL to be infused at a rate of 20 mcg/kg/h stat*. The patient weighs 134 *kg*.

    (a) How many *mg/h* of this narcotic analgesic will the patient receive?

    (b) How many *mL/h* of the solution will the patient receive?

16. Order: *Elspar (asparaginase) 200 units/kg/day IV over 60 min for 28 days*. Add 10,000 *units* to 100 *mL* of D5W. The patient weighs 196 *lb*. Calculate the dosage rate for this antineoplastic enzyme in units/day.

17. Order: *Humulin R 100 units IVPB in 500 mL NS infuse at 0.1 unit/kg/h stat*. The patient weighs 46 *kg*. How long will it take for the infusion of this U-100 insulin to complete?

18. Order: *amikacin sulfate 7.5 mg/kg IVPB q8h in 200 mL D5W to infuse in 30 min*. The vial reads 500 *mg/2 mL*. Calculate the flow rate of this aminoglycoxide antibiotic drug in *mL/h* for a patient whose weight is 144 *lb*.

19. A drug must be administered IVPB at the initial rate of 2 *mg/min*, and the rate may be increased as needed every hour thereafter by 3 *mg/min*, up to a maximum of 20 *mg/min*. The strength of the IV solution is 300 *mg* in 100 *mL D5W*. Make a titration table showing the dosage rate (*mg/min*) and flow rate (*mL/h*).

20. The physician ordered *Platinol (cisplatin)* 100 *mg/m²* IV *to infuse over 6 hours once every 4 weeks* for a patient who has a BSA of 1.66 *m²*.

    (a) How many *mg* of this antineoplastic drug should the patient receive?

    (b) If the dose of cisplatin were administered in 1,000 *mL* D5 1/2 NS, at how many *mL/h* would the IV run?

Additional Exercises

Now, test yourself!

1. An IV is infusing at 80 *mL/h*. The concentration in the IV bag is 40 *mg* in 200 *mL* NS. What is the dosage rate in *mg/min*?

2. An IV is infusing at 0.5 *mg/min*. The concentration in the IV bag is 25 *mg* in 200 *mL* 0.9% NaCl. What is the pump setting in *mL/h*?

3. An IV is infusing at 15 *gtt/min*. The concentration in the IV bag is 40 *mg* in 250 *mL* NS. The drop factor is 10 *gtt/mL*. What is the dosage rate in *mg/min*?

4. An IV is infusing at 40 *milliunits/min*. The concentration in the IV bag is 10 units in 250 *mL* D5W. The drop factor is 10 *gtt/mL*. What is the drip rate in *gtt/min*?

5. The concentration in the IV bag is 150 *mg* in 200 *mL*. If the IV begins on Monday at 0800 *hours* and it must infuse with a dosage rate of 1.5 *mg/min*, then

    (a) what should be the pump setting in *mL/h*?

    (b) when will the IV finish?

6. Order: *lidocaine drip 0.75 mg/kg IV in 500 mL D5W stat*. The patient weighs 169 *pounds*.

    (a) How many milliliters of lidocaine 2% will be added to prepare the IV solution?

    (b) Calculate the flow rate in *mL/h* in order for the patient to receive the dosage rate of 5 *mg/h*.

7. An IVPB infusion begins at 8:00 P.M. The bag contains 150 *mg* of drug in 200 *mL* of NS. The patient is receiving 3 *mg/min*. In military time, when will the infusion finish?

8. Order: *digoxin 0.75 mg IVP stat over 5 min*. The digoxin vial has a concentration of 0.1 *mg/mL*. Find the

    (a) total number of milliliters you will administer.

    (b) number of *mL* you will push during each 30-*second* interval.

    (c) number of seconds needed to deliver each *mL* of the solution.

9. Order: *adenosine 140 mcg/kg/min IVP stat*. Read the label for this antiarrhythmic drug in • **Figure 11.11**. The patient weighs 43 *kg*.

    (a) Find the dosage rate in *mg/min*.

    (b) How many *mL* will you push every 15 *seconds*?

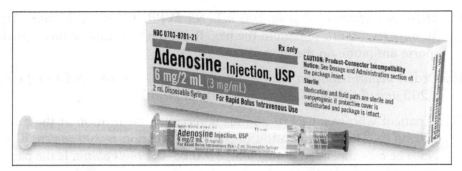

● **Figure 11.11**
Adenosine prefilled syringe.

10. The prescriber orders the cardiac stimulant dopamine hydrochloride at a rate of 3 *mcg/kg/min*. The patient weighs 155 *lb*. The pharmacist sends a solution of dopamine hydrochloride 200 *mg* in 250 *mL* of D5W.

   (a) How many *mcg/min* will the patient receive?
   (b) How many *mL/h* will the patient receive?

11. Order: *heparin 1,500 units/h via infusion pump stat.* The premixed IV bag is labeled heparin 25,000 *units* in 500 *mL* 0.45% Sodium Chloride. At what rate will you set the infusion pump in *mL/h*?

12. The prescriber ordered an insulin drip to run at 10 *units* per hour. The IV bag is labeled 100 *units* regular insulin in 250 *mL* NS.

   (a) At what rate will you set the infusion pump in *mL/h*?
   (b) How many hours will the IV run?

13. The prescriber ordered Covert (*ibutilide fumarate*) 0.01 *mg/kg* IVPB in 50 *mL* of 0.9% *NaCl* to infuse in 10 *min stat*. The vial label reads 1 *mg*/10 *mL*. The patient weighs 125 *pounds*.

   (a) How many milliliters of this antiarrhythmic drug will you need?
   (b) Calculate the flow rate in milliliters per minute.

14. Order: *desmopressin acetate* 0.3 *mcg/kg* IVPB 30 *minutes before surgery*. The vial label reads 4 *mcg/mL* and the patient weighs 80 *kg*.

   (a) Calculate the dose of this antidiuretic in mcg.
   (b) Add the dose to 50 *mL* 0.9% *NaCl*; and calculate the flow rate in milliliters/hour.

15. Nipride 3 *mcg/kg/min* has been ordered for a patient who weighs 82 *kg*. The solution has a strength of 50 *mg* in 250 *mL* of D5W. Calculate the flow rate of this antihypertensive in *mL/h*. _____

16. A medication is ordered at 75 mg/m^2 IVP. The patient has a BSA of 2.33 m^2. How many milliliters of the medication will be administered if the vial is labeled 50 *mg/mL*? _____

17. A liter of D5/NS with 10 *units* of Regular insulin is started at 9:55 A.M. at a rate of 22 *gtt/min*. If the drop factor is 20 *gtt/mL*, when will the infusion finish? _____

Workspace

18. *Mefoxin (cefoxitin) 2 g in 100 mL NS IVPB. Infuse in 1 hour.* After 30 *minutes*, 70 *mL* remain in the bag. Reset the flow rate of this cephalosporin antibiotic on the pump in *mL/h*. _____

19. Order: *heparin sodium 40,000 units IV in 500 mL of $\frac{1}{2}$ NS to infuse at 1,200 units/hour.* What is the flow rate in *mL/h*? _____

20. A patient who weighs 150 pounds is receiving medication at the rate of 100 *mL/h.* The concentration of the IVPB solution is 200 *mg* in 50 *mL* NS. The recommended dosage range is 0.05–0.1 *mg/kg/min.* Is the patient receiving a safe dose? _____

Cumulative Review Exercises

Review your mastery of previous chapters.

1. What is the reading at the arrow on this scale in *mL*? _____

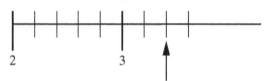

2. What is the weight in pounds and ounces of a neonate who weighs 4,773 *g*? _____

3. Read the label in • **Figure 11.12** and determine the total number of micrograms contained in two tablets of this antiplatelet drug. _____

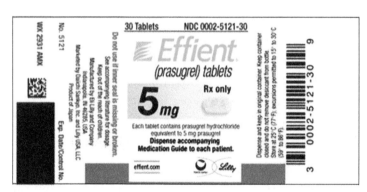

• **Figure 11.12**
Drug label for Effient.

4. Estimate the BSA of a person who is 161 *cm* tall and who weighs 89 *kg*.

5. A patient who has hypertension and weighs 154 *pounds* is to receive an infusion of Nitropress (nitroprusside sodium) at a rate of 1 *mL/h,* to be followed by upward titration. The solution contains 50 *mg* of Nitropress in 500 *mL* of D5W. The safe dose range for this drug is 0.3–10 *mcg/kg/min.* Is this initial dose safe?

6. Order: *quinidine gluconate 7.5 mg/kg administer IVPB over 4 hours for 7 days.* The patient weighs 165 *lb.* See • **Figure 11.13**.

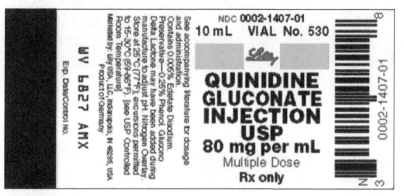

• **Figure 11.13**
Drug label for quinidine gluconate.

Workspace

(a) How many *mg* of this antimalarial drug would be prescribed for the patient? _____

(b) How many *mL* would be needed from the vial? _____

(c) Add the quinidine to 100 *mL*. What would be the pump setting in *mL/h*? _____

(d) What would be the dosage rate in *mg/min*? _____

7. A wound has a diameter of 42 *mm*. What is the diameter in centimeters? _____

8. Three teaspoons equal how many milliliters? _____

9. Your calculations lead to a result of 3.88 *mL*.

   (a) Round off this calculation to one decimal place. _____
   (b) Round down this calculation to one decimal place. _____

10. Order: *Uniphyl (theophylline) 5 mg/kg po loading dose stat*. The strength of the Uniphyl is 400 *mg* per tablet. How many tablets of this bronchodilator would you administer to a patient who weighs 76 *kg*? _____

11. How many grams of NaCl are contained in 500 *mL* of a 0.9% NaClsolution? _____

12. What is the strength as a percent of a lidocaine solution that has 20 *mg* of lidocaine in each *mL* of the solution? _____

13. An IV is infusing at 70 *mL/h*. What is this flow rate in *mcgtt/min*? _____

14. An IV is infusing at 25 *mL/h*. The concentration in the IV bag is 50 *mg* in 200 *mL* NS. What is the dosage rate in *mg/min*? _____

15. An IV is infusing at 125 *milliunits/min*. The concentration in the IV bag is 15 *units* in 300 *mL* D5W. The drop factor is 15 *gtt/mL*. What is the drip rate in *gtt/min*? _____

Chapter

12 Pediatric Dosages

Learning Outcomes

After completing this chapter, you will be able to

1. Determine if a pediatric dose is within the safe dose range.
2. Calculate pediatric oral and parenteral dosages based on body weight.
3. Calculate pediatric oral and parenteral dosages based on body surface area (BSA).
4. Perform calculations necessary for administering medications using a volume-control chamber.
5. Calculate daily fluid maintenance.

Because the metabolism and body mass of children are different from those of adults, children are at greater risk of experiencing adverse effects of medications. Refer to your pharmacology and pediatric texts for a complete discussion of the physiological and developmental considerations of administering medications to children. Therefore, with pediatric and high-risk medications, it is essential to *carefully calculate* the dose, determine if the dose is in the *safe dose range* for the patient, and *validate your calculations* with another healthcare professional. As always, before administering any medication it is imperative to know its *indications*, *uses*, *side effects*, and possible *adverse reactions*.

In this chapter, you will be applying many of the techniques you have already learned in the previous chapters to the calculation of pediatric dosages.

Pediatric dosages are generally based on the weight of the child. It is important to *verify* that the dose ordered is safe for the particular child. Pediatric dosages are sometimes rounded down, instead of rounded off, because of the danger that overdose poses to infants and children. Consult your facility's policy on rounding pediatric dosages. In this chapter, dosages will be rounded down (rather than rounded off) to provide practice in rounding down.

Pediatric Drug Dosages

Most pediatric doses are based on body weight. Body surface area (BSA) is also used, especially in pediatric oncology and critical care. You must be able to determine whether the amount of a prescribed pediatric dosage is within the recommended range. To do this, you must compare the child's ordered dosage to the recommended safe dosage as found in a reputable drug resource. The recommended dose or dosage range can be found in the package insert, hospital formulary, *Physician's Desk Reference (PDR)*, *United States Pharmacopeia*, manufacturer's Web site prescribing information, or drug guide books. In order to reduce the chance of errors, the trend is for the pharmacy to supply medication in unit doses. However, the nurse is still responsible for verifying the accuracy of the prepared drug dose, form, and route of administration.

Oral Medications

When prescribing medications for the pediatric population, the oral route is preferred. However, if a child cannot swallow or the medication is ineffective when given orally, the parenteral route is used.

The developmental age of the child must be taken into consideration when determining the device needed to administer oral medication. For example, an older child may be able to swallow a pill or drink a liquid medication from a cup. Children younger than five years of age, however, generally are not able to swallow tablets and capsules. Therefore, most medications for these children are in the form of elixirs, syrups, or suspensions. An *oral syringe, calibrated dropper, or measuring spoon* can be selected when giving medication to an infant or younger child. Do NOT mix medications in essential foods or fluids (milk, juice, or formula). If the child does not like the taste, he or she may refuse to accept the food or fluid again. Medications should be placed in the smallest amount of nonessential food or fluid to ensure that the child will take the entire amount. An oral syringe is different from a parenteral syringe in two ways. Generally, an oral syringe does not have a Luer-Lok™ hub and has a cap on the tip that must be removed before administering a medication. Because a needle does not fit on an oral syringe, the chance of administering a medication via a wrong route is decreased. See • **Figures 12.1** and **12.2**.

> **NOTE**
>
> Many oral pediatric medications are suspensions. Remember to shake them well immediately before administering.

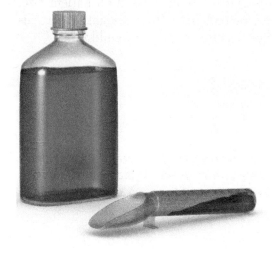

• **Figure 12.1**
A bottle of oral medication and a measuring spoon.

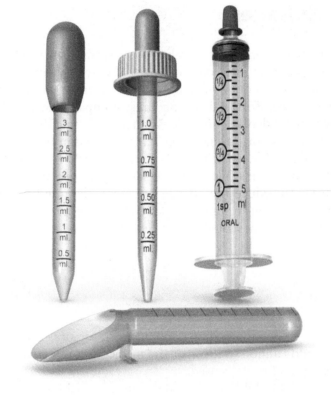

● **Figure 12.2**
Liquid medication administration devices: Two droppers, an oral syringe, and a measuring spoon.

Parenteral Medications

Subcutaneous or intramuscular routes may be necessary, depending on the type of medication to be administered. For example, many childhood immunizations are administered subcutaneously or intramuscularly. Intramuscular injections are rarely ordered on a routine basis for children because of limited sites, developmental considerations, and the possibility of trauma. Because of the small muscle mass of children, the amount injected is usually not more than 2 *mL*. You should consult a current pediatric text for the equipment, injection sites, and procedure.

Dosages Based on Body Size

Drug manufacturers can recommend pediatric dosages based on patient size, as measured by either body weight (*kg*) or BSA (m^2). Body weight in particular is frequently used when prescribing drugs for infants and children.

Dosages Based on Body Weight

EXAMPLE 12.1

The prescriber ordered *Biaxin (clarithromycin) oral suspension 15 mg/kg/day po divided in two equal doses*. Read the label in ● Figure 12.3 and calculate how many milliliters of this macrolide antibiotic a child who weighs 30 *kg* will receive.

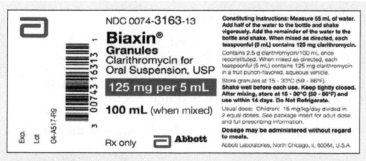

● **Figure 12.3**
Drug label for Biaxin.

The child's weight is 30 *kg*, and the order is for 15 *mg/kg/d* in two equally divided doses. Multiply the *size of the patient by the order* to determine the dose of Biaxin.

$$30 \; kg \times \frac{15 \; mg}{kg \cdot day} = \frac{450 \; mg}{day}$$

Now, change the *mg* to *mL*.

Because the strength is 125 *mg per 5 mL*, use the unit fraction $\dfrac{5 \; mL}{125 \; mg}$

$$\frac{450 \; \overline{mg}}{d} \times \frac{5 \; mL}{125 \; \overline{mg}} = \frac{18 \; mL}{d}$$

The medication is to be administered in two equally divided doses, so the child will receive 9 *mL* of Biaxin twice a day.

EXAMPLE 12.2

The prescriber ordered cephalexin 19 *mg/kg* PO oral suspension q8h for a child who weighs 50 *kg* and has otitis media. Read the label in ● Figure 12.4 and calculate the number of milliliters of this cephalosporin antibiotic the child will receive.

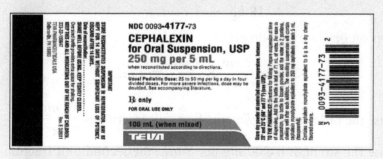

● **Figure 12.4**
Drug label for cephalexin.

You want to convert the body weight to the dose in milliliters.

$$50 \; kg \longrightarrow ? \; mL$$

Do this problem on one line as follows:

$$50 \ kg \times \frac{? \ mg}{? \ kg} \times \frac{? \ mL}{? \ mg} = ? \ mL$$

Because the order is 19 mg/kg, the first unit fraction is $\dfrac{19 \ mg}{1 \ kg}$

Because the strength is 250 mg/5 mL, the second unit fraction is $\dfrac{5 \ mL}{200 \ mg}$

You cancel the kilograms and milligrams and obtain the dose in milliliters.

$$50 \ kg \times \frac{19 \ \widetilde{mg}}{1 \ \widetilde{kg}} \times \frac{5 \ mL}{250 \ \widetilde{mg}} = 19 \ mL$$

So, you would administer 19 mL of cephalexin to the child.

EXAMPLE 12.3

The prescriber ordered: *Zithromax (azithromycin) 10 mg/kg PO stat, then give 5 mg/kg/day for 4 days.* The child weighs 18 kg. Read the information on the label in • Figure 12.5 and determine the number of milliliters that would contain the stat dose.

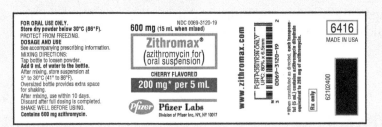

• **Figure 12.5**
Drug label for Zithromax.
(*Reg. Trademark of Pfizer Inc. Reproduced with permission.*)

You want to convert the body weight to a dose in milliliters.

$$18 \ kg \longrightarrow ? \ mL$$

Do this on one line as follows:

$$18 \ kg \times \frac{? \ mg}{? \ kg} \times \frac{? \ mL}{? \ mg} = ? \ mL$$

Because the order is 10 mg/kg, the first unit fraction is $\dfrac{10 \ mg}{kg}$

Because the strength is 200 mg per 5 mL, the second unit fraction is $\dfrac{5 \ mL}{200 \ mg}$.

$$18 \ kg \times \frac{10 \ \widetilde{mg}}{\widetilde{kg}} \times \frac{5 \ mL}{200 \ \widetilde{mg}} = 4.5 \ mL$$

So, you would prepare 4.5 mL of zithromax.

EXAMPLE 12.4

The recommended dose for neonates receiving amikacin sulfate is 7.5 *mg/kg* IM q12h. If an infant weighs 2,600 *grams,* how many milligrams of amikacin would the neonate receive in one day?

You want to convert the body weight to the dose in milligrams.

$$2,600 \text{ } g \text{ (body weight)} \rightarrow ? \text{ } mg \text{ (drug)}$$

Do this problem on one line as follows:

$$2,600 \text{ } g \times \frac{? \text{ } kg}{? \text{ } g} \times \frac{? \text{ } mg}{? \text{ } kg} = ? \text{ } mg$$

Because 1 *kg* = 1,000 *g*, the first unit fraction is $\dfrac{1 \text{ } kg}{1,000 \text{ } g}$

Because the recommended dose is 7.5 *mg/kg*, the second unit fraction is $\dfrac{7.5 \text{ } mg}{1 \text{ } kg}$

$$2,600 \text{ } \cancel{g} \times \frac{1 \text{ } \cancel{kg}}{1,000 \text{ } \cancel{g}} \times \frac{7.5 \text{ } mg}{\cancel{kg}} = 19.5 \text{ } mg \text{ per dose}$$

Because the neonate receives two doses per day, the total daily dose is 39 *mg*.

Dosages Based on BSA

Pediatric dosages may also be based on body surface area (BSA). For example, antineoplastic agents used in the treatment of cancer are often ordered using the BSA. To calculate the BSA accurately, it is important that the *actual* height and weight be assessed, not just estimated. In most instances, the prescriber will calculate the BSA. However, it is the responsibility of the person who administers the drug to verify that the BSA is correct and that the dose is within the safe dosage range.

ALERT

When calculating BSA, be sure to check your calculations with another professional.

EXAMPLE 12.5

The prescriber ordered *Cytarabine* 200 *mg/m²* IV over 24h. Read the label in • Figure 12.6 and determine how many milliliters of this bone marrow suppressant you will need for a child who has a BSA of 0.49 *m²*.

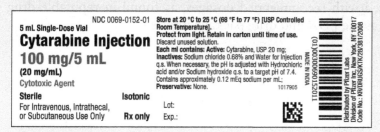

• **Figure 12.6**
Drug label for Cytarabine injection.

The child's BSA is 0.49 m^2. *Multiply the BSA of the child by the order to determine how many milligrams of Cytarabine are needed.*

$$0.49 \ m^2 \times \frac{200 \ mg}{m^2} = 98 \ mg$$

Now, convert 98 *milligrams* to *mL*. Because the strength on the label is 100 *mg per 5 mL*, use the unit fraction $\frac{5 \ mL}{100 \ mg}$

$$98 \ mg \times \frac{5 \ mL}{100 \ mg} = 4.9 \ mL$$

So, 4.9 *mL* of Cytarabine are required.

EXAMPLE 12.6

Order: *Leucovorin Calcium* 10 *mg/m^2 PO q6h until serum methotrexate level is less than* 10^{-8} *M.* **The strength of the leucovorin tablets are 5** *mg.* **Calculate the number of tablets that contain the dose for a child who is 85** *cm* **tall and weighs 12** *kg.*

You want to find the body surface area and convert it to a dose in milligrams. Calculate the BSA using the formula

$$\text{BSA} = \sqrt{\frac{85 \times 12}{3600}} \approx 0.532 \ m^2$$

So, the child has a BSA of approximately 0.53 m^2.
Multiply the size of the patient by the order to obtain the dose.

$$0.53 \ m^2 \times \frac{10 \ mg}{m^2} \times \frac{1 \ tab}{5 \ mg} = 1.06 \ tab$$

So, one 5 *mg* tablet of Leucovorin contains the dose.

ALERT

Both overdoses and underdoses are dangerous. Too much medication results in the risk of possible life-threatening effects, whereas too little medication risks suboptimal therapeutic effects.

Determining Safe Dosage Range

The following example illustrates that pediatric dosage orders should always be compared with recommended dosages, as found in reputable drug references such as the *PDR* and drug package inserts.

EXAMPLE 12.7

The prescriber ordered *Dilantin (phenytoin)* 100 *mg oral suspension PO daily.* The recommended daily maintenance dosage is 4–8 *mg/kg/d.* Is the ordered dose safe for a child who weighs 30 *kg?*

Use the *minimum* recommended dosage of 4 *mg/kg* to determine the minimum number of milligrams the child should receive daily.

Multiply the size of the patient by the minimum daily recommendation.

$$30 \: kg \times \frac{4 \: mg}{kg} = 120 \: mg$$

So, the *minimum daily safe dose* is 120 *mg.*

Now use the *maximum* recommended dosage of 8 *mg/kg* to determine the maximum number of milligrams the child should receive daily.

Multiply the size of the patient by the maximum daily recommendation.

$$30 \: kg \times \frac{8 \: mg}{kg} = 240 \: mg$$

So, the *maximum daily safe dose* is 240 *mg.*

The recommended dosage of 4–8 *mg/kg/d* is equivalent to a dose range of 120–240 *mg* daily for this child. The ordered dose of 100 *mg* is smaller than the minimum recommended dose of 120 *mg.* Therefore, the ordered dose is not in the safe dose range, and it should not be administered. The healthcare provider must contact the prescriber.

EXAMPLE 12.8

The prescriber ordered *gentamicin* 60 *mg IM q8h* for a child who weighs 60 *lb.* The recommended dosage is 6–7.5 *mg/kg/d* in 3 divided doses.

(a) What is the recommended dosage in mg/day, and is the order safe?

(b) The strength on the vial is 80 *mg/2 mL.* Determine the number of milliliters you would administer.

(a) You want to convert the body weight in pounds to kilograms and then convert the body weight in kilograms to the recommended dose in milligrams of gentamicin per day.

$$60 \: lb \: (\text{body weight}) \longrightarrow kg \: (\text{body weight}) \longrightarrow mg \: (\text{drug})$$

Do this on one line as follows:

$$\frac{60 \: lb}{1} \times \frac{? \: kg}{? \: lb} \times \frac{? \: mg}{? \: kg \times d} = \frac{? \: mg}{d}$$

Because 1 kg = 2.2 lb, the first unit fraction is $\dfrac{1\ kg}{2.2\ lb}$

Because the *minimum recommended* dose is 6 mg/kg per day, the second unit fraction is $\dfrac{6\ mg}{kg \times d}$

$$\frac{60\ \cancel{lb}}{1} \times \frac{1\ \cancel{kg}}{2.2\ \cancel{lb}} \times \frac{6\ mg}{\cancel{kg} \cdot d} = \frac{163.6\ mg}{d}$$

So, the *minimum* safe dose is 163.6 *mg/d*.

Now, use the *maximum recommended* dose of 7.5 *mg/kg* to determine the maximum number of milligrams the child may receive. Because the *maximum recommended* dose is 7.5 *mg/kg per day*,

the second unit fraction is $\dfrac{7.5\ mg}{kg \times d}$

$$\frac{60\ \cancel{lb}}{1} \times \frac{1\ \cancel{kg}}{2.2\ \cancel{lb}} \times \frac{7.5\ mg}{\cancel{kg} \cdot d} = \frac{204.5\ mg}{d}$$

So, the *maximum* safe dose is 204.5 *mg/d*.

The safe dose range of 6–7.5 *mg/kg/d* is equivalent to a dose range of 163.6–204.5 *mg/d* for this child.

The ordered dose of 60 *mg q8h* is a total of 180 *mg/d* and is within the recommended safe dose range.

(b) You want to convert the ordered dose in *milligrams* to *milliliters*.

$$mg\ (\text{drug}) \longrightarrow mL\ (\text{drug})$$

Do this on one line as follows:

$$60\ mg \times \frac{?\ mL}{?\ mg} = ?\ mL$$

Because the strength of the gentamicin is 80 *mg/2 mL*, the unit fraction is $\dfrac{2\ mL}{80\ mg}$

$$\frac{60\ \cancel{mg}}{1} \times \frac{2\ mL}{80\ \cancel{mg}} = 1.5\ mL$$

So, you would administer 1.5 *mL* of gentamicin IM q8h.

EXAMPLE 12.9

Valium (diazepam) 3.75 *mg* IVP stat was ordered for a child with status epilepticus. The package insert says that the recommended dose is 0.2–0.5 *mg/kg/d* IVP slowly. The child weighs 33 *lb*, and the label on the vial reads 5 *mg/mL*.

(a) Is the ordered dose within the safe range?

(b) How many milliliters would you administer?

(a) You want to convert the body weight in *pounds* to *kilograms* and then convert the body weight in *kilograms* to a recommended dose in *milligrams*.

33 *lb* (body weight) $\longrightarrow$? *kg* (body weight) $\longrightarrow$? *mg* (drug)

Do this on one line as follows:

$$33\ lb \times \frac{?\ kg}{?\ lb} \times \frac{?\ mg}{?\ kg} = ?\ mg$$

Because 1 *kg* = 2.2 *lb*, the first unit fraction is $\frac{1\ kg}{2.2\ lb}$.

Because the recommended dosage is 0.2 *mg* to 0.5 *mg/kg* per day, you need to find the minimum and the maximum recommended doses in milligrams for this patient. Use the unit fractions $\frac{0.2\ mg}{kg}$ and $\frac{0.5\ mg}{kg}$

$$\frac{33\ lb}{1} \times \frac{1\ kg}{2.2\ lb} \times \frac{0.2\ mg}{kg} = 3\ mg\ (minimum\ dose)$$

$$\frac{33\ lb}{1} \times \frac{1\ kg}{2.2\ lb} \times \frac{0.5\ mg}{kg} = 7.5\ mg\ (maximum\ dose)$$

The safe dose range for this patient is 3–7.5 *mg*.
Because the ordered dose of 3.75 *mg* is between 3 *mg* and 7.5 *mg*, it is a safe dose.

(b) You want to convert the ordered dosage in milligrams to the liquid daily dose in milliliters.

$$3.75\ mg\ (drug) \longrightarrow ?\ mL\ (drug)$$

Do this on one line as follows:

$$3.75\ mg \times \frac{?\ mL}{?\ mg} = ?\ mL$$

Because the vial label says 5 *mg/mL*, the unit fraction is $\frac{1\ mL}{5\ mg}$.

$$\frac{3.75\ mg}{1} \times \frac{1\ mL}{5\ mg} = 0.75\ mL$$

So, you would administer 0.75 *mL* of the Valium IVP slowly.

Intravenous Medications

When a child is to have nothing by mouth (NPO), needs pain relief, or needs a high concentration of a medication, the intravenous (IV) route is the most effective route to use. In addition, when the duration of the therapy is long term, or when gastrointestinal absorption is poor, the IV route is indicated.

Methods of intravenous infusions include peripheral intravenous catheters, peripherally inserted central catheters (PICC lines), central lines, and long-term central venous access devices (VAD) or ports. The method chosen is based on the age and size of the child and the duration of therapy.

Most IV medications must be further diluted once the correct dose is calculated. Follow the directions precisely for the reconstitution process. An electronic infusion device and a volume-control chamber should always be used to administer IV fluids and intravenous piggyback (IVPB) medications, especially high-alert drugs, to infants and children.

Using a Volume-Control Chamber

To avoid fluid overload, pediatric IV medications are frequently administered using a volume-control chamber (VCC) (burette, Volutrol, Buretrol, Soluset).

A VCC is calibrated in 1 *mL* increments and has a capacity of 100–150 *mL*. It can be used as a primary or secondary line. When administering IVPB medications, the medication is added to the top injection port of the VCC. Fluid is then added from the IV bag to further dilute the medication. After the infusion is complete, additional IV fluid is added to the VCC to flush any remaining medication left in the tubing. See • **Figure 12.8.**

Volume-Control Chamber

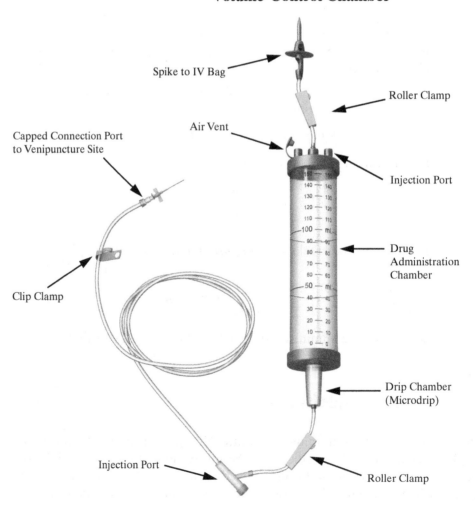

• **Figure 12.8**
Volume-control chamber.

The following example illustrates the use of a VCC.

EXAMPLE 12.10

Order: *sulfamethoxazole and trimethoprim (SMZ-TMP) 75 mg in 100 mL D₅ W IVPB q6h.* The recommended dose is 6–10 *mg/kg/day every 6 hours.* The child weighs 40 *kg.*

(a) **Is the prescribed dose in the safe range?**

(b) **Read the label in • Figure 12.9. The manufacturer directions state that "weight-based doses are calculated on the TMP component." How many milliliters will you withdraw from the vial?**

(c) **Using a volume-control chamber, how many milliliters of IV solution will you add?**

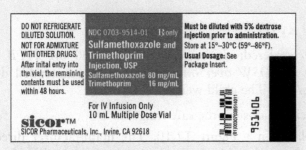

• **Figure 12.9**
Drug label for Sulfamethoxazole and Trimethoprim.

(a) Convert both the *safe dose range* and the *prescribed dose* to *mg/day.* First, use the *minimum safe dose (6 mg/kg/day)* to determine how many *mg/day* the child should minimally receive, as follows:

$$40 \ kg \times \frac{6 \ mg}{kg \cdot day} = 240 \ \frac{mg}{day} \quad \textit{Minimum}$$

Now, use the *maximum safe dose (10 mg/kg/day)* to determine how many *mg/day* the child should maximally receive, as follows:

$$40 \ kg \times \frac{10 \ mg}{kg \cdot day} = 400 \ \frac{mg}{day} \quad \textit{Maximum}$$

So, the safe dose range for this child is 240–400 *mg/day.*

The ordered dose is 75 *mg* every 6 *hours* (4 *times* per day). Therefore, the ordered dose is (75 × 4) 300 *mg daily.* Because 300 *mg/d* is in the range of 240–300 *mg/d*, the child is receiving a safe dose.

(b) You want to convert the order of 75 *mg* to *mL.*

$$75 \ mg \longrightarrow ? \ mL$$

$$75 \ mg \times \frac{? \ mL}{? \ mg} = ? \ mL$$

The directions state to use the TMP (trimethoprim) component. The strength of the TMP on the label is 16 *mg/mL*. So, the unit fraction is $\dfrac{1\ mL}{16\ mg}$

$$\frac{75\ mg}{1} \times \frac{1\ mL}{16\ mg} = 4.6875\ mL$$

So, you would withdraw 4.6 *mL* of sulfamethoxazole and trimethoprim from the vial. Note that rounding *down* was used here.

(c) You would add 4.6 *mL* of sulfamethoxazole and trimethoprim to the VCC, then add D5W to the 100 *mL* mark. This means that 95.4 *mL* of D5W are added to the VCC.

EXAMPLE 12.11

The prescriber ordered: *doxycycline hyclate* 100 *mg IVPB daily. Infuse in* 100 *mL D5W over one hour.* The recommended dose is 2.2–4.4 *mg/kg/day.* The child weighs 45 *kg.*

(a) Is the prescribed dose in the safe range?

(b) Read the label in • Figure 12.10. The manufacturer directions state that the medication "must be reconstituted with 10 *mL* of sterile water for injection." How many milliliters must be withdrawn from the doxycycline vial and added to the VCC?

(c) How many milliliters of IV solution will you add to the volume-control chamber?

(d) At what rate will you set the IV pump?

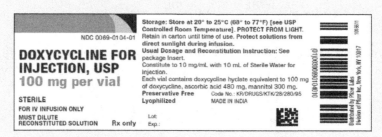

NDC 0069-0104-01

DOXYCYCLINE FOR INJECTION, USP
100 mg per vial

STERILE
FOR IV INFUSION ONLY
MUST DILUTE
RECONSTITUTED SOLUTION   Rx only

Storage: Store at 20° to 25°C (68° to 77°F) [see USP Controlled Room Temperature]. PROTECT FROM LIGHT. Retain in carton until time of use. Protect solutions from direct sunlight during infusion.
Usual Dosage and Reconstitution Instruction: See package insert.
Constitute to 10 mg/mL with 10 mL of Sterile Water for injection.
Each vial contains doxycycline hyclate equivalent to 100 mg of doxycycline, ascorbic acid 480 mg, mannitol 300 mg.
Preservative Free   Code No.: KR/DRUGS/KTK/28/280/95
Lyophilized   MADE IN INDIA

Lot:
Exp.:

Distributed by Pfizer Labs
Division of Pfizer Inc., New York, NY 10017

• **Figure 12.10**
Drug label for doxycycline.

(a) Convert both the *recommended dose range* and the *prescribed dose* to *mg/day.*

First, use the *minimum recommended dose* (2.2 *mg/kg/day*) to determine how many *mg/day* the child should minimally receive as follows:

$$45\ kg \times \frac{2.2\ mg}{kg \cdot day} = 99\ \frac{mg}{day}\ Minimum$$

Now, use the *maximum recommended dose* (4.4 *mg/kg/d*) to determine how many *mg/day* the child should maximally receive as follows:

$$45 \ kg \times \frac{4.4 \ mg}{kg \cdot day} = 198 \ \frac{mg}{day} \ Maximum$$

So, the safe dose range for this child is 99–198 *mg/day*. The ordered dose of 100 *mg/day* is within the safe dose range. So, the child is receiving a safe dose.

(b) The directions state to reconstitute the 100 *mg* vial of doxycycline with 10 *mL* of sterile water for injection. The strength of the reconstituted solution will then be 100 *mg* per 10 *mL*. Because the ordered dose is 100 *mg*, the entire 10 *mL* of solution must be withdrawn from the vial and added to the VCC.

(c) Because the directions say to infuse in 100 *mL* of D5W, add 100 *mL* of D5W to the VCC.

(d) The VCC contains 10 *mL* of doxycycline and 100 *mL* of D5W, for a total of 110 *ml*. The infusion must last 1 *hour*. So, you would set the pump rate to 110 *mL/h*.

Calculating Daily Fluid Maintenance

The administration of pediatric IV medication requires careful and exact calculations and procedures. Infants and severely ill children are not able to tolerate extreme levels of hydration and are quite susceptible to dehydration and fluid overload. Therefore, you must closely monitor the amount of fluid a child receives. The fluid a child requires over a 24-*hour* period is referred to as *daily fluid maintenance needs*. Daily fluid maintenance includes both oral and parenteral fluids. The amount of maintenance fluid required depends on the weight of the patient (see the formula in Table 12.1). The daily maintenance fluid does not include body fluid losses through vomiting, diarrhea, or fever. Additional fluids referred to as *replacement fluids* (usually Lactated Ringer's or 0.9% NaCl) are used to replace fluid losses and are based on each child's condition (e.g., if 20 *mL* are lost, then 20 *mL* of replacement fluids are usually added to the daily maintenance).

Table 12.1 Daily Fluid Maintenance Formula

Pediatric Daily Fluid Maintenance Formula		
For the *first*	10 *kg* of body weight:	100 *mL/kg*
For the *next*	10 *kg* of body weight:	50 *mL/kg*
For *each kg above*	20 *kg* of body weight:	20 *mL/kg*

EXAMPLE 12.12

Determine the normal 24 *hr* fluid requirement for a child who weighs 33 *lb*.

First, convert the child's weight to kilograms.

$$\frac{33 \ lb}{1} \times \frac{1 \ kg}{2.2 \ lb} = 15 \ kg$$

Divide the weight (in kilograms) into three portions, following the formula in Table 12.1.

$$15 \ kg = 10 \ kg + 5 \ kg + 0 \ kg$$

For each of these portions, the number of milliliters must be calculated. A table will be useful for organizing the calculations (see Table 12.2).

Table 12.2 Daily Fluid Maintenance Computations for Example 12.12					
1st Portion	10 kg	$\times$	$\frac{100 \ mL}{kg}$	=	1,000 mL
2nd Portion	5 kg	$\times$	$\frac{50 \ mL}{kg}$	=	250 mL
3rd Portion	0 kg	$\times$	$\frac{20 \ mL}{kg}$	=	0 mL
Total	15 kg				1,250 mL

So, the child who weighs 33 *lb* has a daily fluid requirement of 1,250 *mL*.

EXAMPLE 12.13

If the order is *half-maintenance* for a child who weighs 35 *kg*, at what rate should the pump be set in *mL/h*?

Because the child weighs 35 *kg*, this weight would be divided into three portions following the formula in Table 12.1, as follows:

$$35 \ kg = 10 \ kg + 10 \ kg + 15 \ kg$$

For each of these three portions, the number of milliliters must be calculated. A table will be useful for organizing the calculations (Table 12.3). The daily "maintenance" was determined to be 1,800 *mL*. "half-maintenance" ($\frac{1}{2}$ of maintenance) is, therefore, $\frac{1}{2}$ of 1,800 *mL*, or 900 *mL*.

Table 12.3   Daily Fluid Maintenance Computations for Example 12.13

1st Portion	10 kg	×	$\dfrac{100\ mL}{kg}$	=	1,000 mL
2nd Portion	10 kg	×	$\dfrac{50\ mL}{kg}$	=	500 mL
3rd Portion	15 kg	×	$\dfrac{20\ mL}{kg}$	=	300 mL
Total	35 kg				1,800 mL

Now, you must change $\dfrac{900\ mL}{1\ day}$ to $\dfrac{mL}{h}$.

Replace 1 day with 24 *hours* to obtain

$$\frac{900\ mL}{1\ day} = \frac{900\ mL}{24\ h} = 37.5\ \frac{mL}{h}$$

So, the pump would be set at the rate of 37 *mL*/h.

Summary

In this chapter, you learned to calculate oral and parenteral dosages for pediatric patients. Some dosages were based on the size of the patient: body weight (*kg*) or BSA (*m*²). The calculations needed for the use of the volume-control chamber, as well as the method for determining daily fluid maintenance, were explained.

- Taking shortcuts in pediatric medication administration can be fatal to a child.
- Always verify that the order is in the safe dose range.
- Consult a reliable source when in doubt about a pediatric medication order.
- Question the order or check your calculations if the ordered dose differs from the recommended dose.
- Pediatric dosages are sometimes rounded down (truncated) to avoid the danger of an overdose.
- Know your institution's policy on rounding.
- IV bags of no more than 500 *mL* should be hung for pediatric patients.
- No more than 2 *mL* should be given intramuscularly to a pediatric patient.

- Because accuracy is crucial in pediatric infusions, electronic control devices or volume-control chambers should always be used.
- Minimal and maximal dilution volumes for some IV drugs are recommended to prevent fluid overload, minimize irritation to veins, and reduce toxic effects.
- When preparing IV drug solutions, the smallest added volume (minimal dilution) results in the strongest concentration; the largest added volume (maximal dilution) results in the weakest concentration.
- For a volume-control chamber, a flush is always used to clear the tubing after the medication is infused.
- Know the facility policy regarding the inclusion of medication volume as part of the total infusion volume.
- Daily fluid maintenance depends on the weight of the child and includes both oral and parenteral fluids.

Case Study 12.1

Read the Case Study and answer the questions. Answers can be found in Appendix A.

An 8-year-old boy is admitted to the hospital with a diagnosis of sickle cell crisis and pneumonia. He complains of pain in his legs and abdomen, wheezing, and pain in his chest. He has a history of asthma and epilepsy and is allergic to peanuts, tomatoes, and aspirin. He is 40 *inches* tall and weighs 55 *pounds*. Vital signs are T 102°F; B/P 90/66; P 112; R 30. Chest X-ray confirms right upper-lobe pneumonia, and the throat culture is positive for Group A streptococcus. His orders include the following:

- Bed Rest
- Diet as tolerated, encourage PO fluids
- IV D5 $\frac{1}{3}$ NS @ 110 *mL/h*
- morphine sulfate 0.025 *mg/kg/h* IV
- penicillin G 100,000 *units/kg/day* divided q6h, infuse via pump in 100 *mL* D5W, over 1 *hour*

- methylprednisolone 1 *mg/kg* IM now, then 1 *mg/kg* PO daily in the A.M.
- Flovent HFA (fluticasone propionate) inhalation aerosol 2 puffs B.I.D.
- Folic Acid 1 *mg* PO daily
- Depakene (valproic acid) 30 *mg/kg* PO b.i.d.
- Tylenol (acetaminophen) 12 *mg/kg* PO q4h prn temp over 101°F
- montelukast 5 *mg* PO qhs
- albuterol 2 *mg* PO T.I.D.

Use the labels in • **Figure 12.11** to answer the following questions:

1. Calculate the child's 24-*hour* fluid requirement.
2. How many milliliters of diluent will you add to the Pfizerpen vial to obtain a strength of

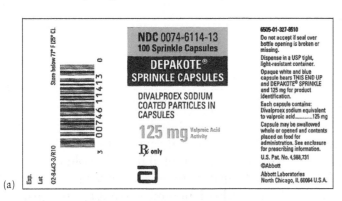
(a)

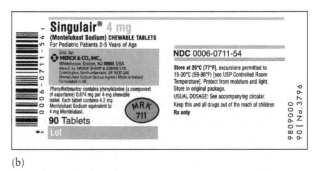
(b)

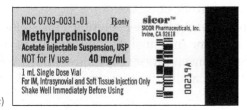
(c)

(d)

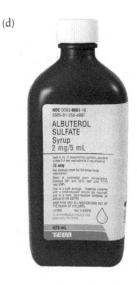

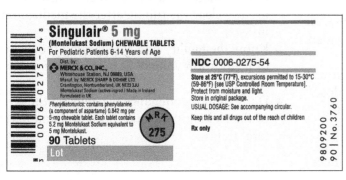
(e)

• **Figure 12.11**
Drug labels for Case Study.

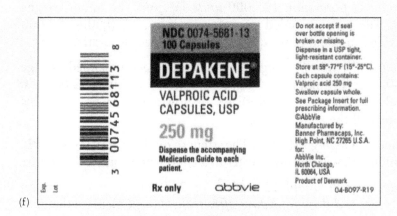

(f)

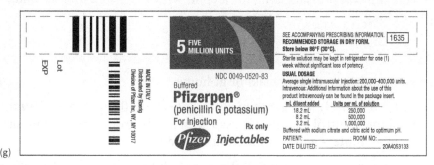

(g)

● **Figure 12.11**
(Continued)

250,000 *units/mL*, and how many milliliters will you withdraw to obtain the prescribed dose?

3. At what rate will you set the pump to infuse the Penicillin G?

4. The recommended dose for morphine is 0.05–0.1 *mg/kg IV q4h*. Is the prescribed dose safe?

5. How many milliliters of methylprednisolone will you administer for the IM dose?

6. Select the correct label for valproic acid, and determine how many capsules you will administer.

7. The folic acid is available in 1 *mg* tablets. How many micrograms is the child receiving per day?

8. Select the correct label for montelukast, and determine how many tablets you will administer.

9. The Tylenol available is labeled 160 *mg/5 mL*. How many milliliters will the child receive for a temperature of 102°F?

10. Select the correct label for albuterol, and determine how many milliliters you will administer.

11. The strength of the Flovent is 44 *mcg/inhalation*. How many mcg is the patient receiving/day?

Practice Sets

The answers to *Try These for Practice*, *Exercises*, and *Cumulative Review Exercises* are found in Appendix A. Ask your instructor for the answers to the *Additional Exercises*.

Workspace

Try These for Practice

Test your comprehension after reading the chapter.

1. Order: *Dycill (dicloxacillin sodium) 50 mg po q6h*. The recommended dosage for a 35-*pound* child is 12.5–25 *mg/kg/d in 4 equally divided doses*. Is the prescribed order safe for this child, and if so, how many milligrams will you administer?

2. Order: *penicillin G potassium* 125,000 *units IV q6h*. The infant weighs 2,500 *grams*. The recommended dose for infants is 150,000–300,000 *units/kg/d* divided in equal doses q4–6h. Is the ordered dose safe?

3. Order: *Proventil (albuterol)* 2 *mg PO T.I.D.* The recommended dosage range is 0.1–0.2 *mg/kg* t.i.d. max 4 *mg/dose*. The child weighs 32 *pounds*. The label reads 2 *mg/5 mL*. If the dose is safe, how many teaspoons of this bronchodilator will the child receive?

4. Order: *amikacin* 7.5 *mg/kg IM q12h*. The strength on the vial is 250 *mg/mL*. How many milliliters will you administer to a child who weighs 54 *pounds*?

5. Order: *Simulect (basiliximab)* 12 *mg/m²* for 2 *doses. Give 1st dose 2h before surgery, second dose four days after transplant*. Calculate the dose of this immunosuppressant drug for a child who weighs 22 *pounds* and is 28 *inches* long.

Exercises

Reinforce your understanding in class or at home.

1. Order: *D₅NS with* 40 *mg gentamicin IV infuse at 30 mL/h over 30 min q8h*. A volume-control chamber is used with an electronic infusion pump. How many milliliters will be infused in one day?

2. Order: *cefaclor oral suspension* 200 *mg po q8h* for a child who has otitis media and weighs 33 *pounds*. The recommended dose is 40 *mg/kg/d* in 3 divided doses. Is the ordered dose safe?

3. Order: *Rocephin (ceftriaxone)* 1 *g IV q12h*. The patient is a child who has an infection and weighs 30 *pounds*. The recommended dose is 50–75 *mg/kg/d* given once a day, or daily in 2 equally divided doses, not to exceed 2 *g/day*. Is the prescribed order safe?

4. Order: *Narcan (naloxone hydrochloride)* 0.01 *mg/kg subcut stat* for a neonate who weighs 3,300 *g*. The strength available is 0.4 *mg/mL*. How many milliliters will you administer?

5. A seven-year-old patient weighs 66 *pounds*. The recommended dose of Kantrex (kanamycin) is 15 *mg/kg/d* IM in equally divided doses q8–12h. How many milligrams will the prescriber order per day?

6. Order: *Omnicef (cefdinir) oral suspension* 7 *mg/kg q12h for* 10 *days*. Read the information on the label in • **Figure 12.12.** Calculate the number of milliliters of this cephalosporin antibiotic you would administer to a child who weighs 77 *pounds*.

7. Calculate the daily fluid maintenance and the hourly flow rate for a child who weighs 17 *kg*.

8. Order: *aminophylline* 27 *mg/kg/day po divided in* 6 *doses*. The strength on the label is 105 *mg/5 mL*. Calculate how many milliliters of this bronchodilator you will administer to a child who weighs 45 *pounds*.

9. Order: *Pediapred (prednisolone sodium phosphate)* 60 *mg/m²/day PO in three divided doses for* 4 *weeks*. Calculate how many milliliters of this anti-inflammatory agent you will administer to a child who has nephrotic

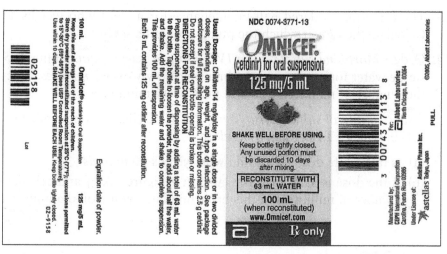

• **Figure 12.12**
Drug label for Omnicef.

syndrome and weighs 30 *pounds* and is 36 *inches* tall. The strength on the vial is *5 mg* per *5 mL*.

10. Order: *aminophylline 5 mg/kg IV loading dose to infuse in 250 mL D5W over 30 min.*

   (a) Calculate how many *mg* of aminophylline a child who weighs 30 *pounds* will receive.

   (b) At what rate will you set the pump in *mL/h*?

11. Order: *ampicillin 50 mg/kg/day in 4 equally divided doses IVPB in 50 mL NS infuse over 30 minutes.* The directions state to "reconstitute the 1 g vial with 10 *mL* of NS." The child weighs 40 *kilograms*. How many milliliters of this antibiotic will you withdraw from the vial?

12. Order: *ProQuad 1 dose subcut now.* The label reads Single-Dose 0.5 *mL* vial. Draw a line on the most appropriate syringe indicating the number of milliliters you will administer to a 12-month-old infant in • Figure 12.13.

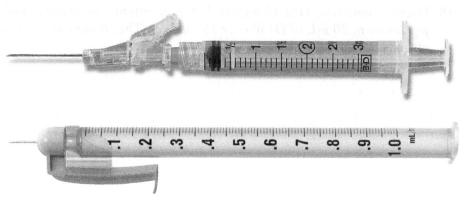

• **Figure 12.13**
Box label for Syringes for question 12.

13. The prescriber ordered half-maintenance for a child who weighs 15 *kg*. Calculate the rate at which the pump should be set in *mL/h*.

14. Order: *Morphine sulfate 3 mg IVP q3h prn severe pain*. Dilute in *5 mL* sterile water for injection and administer slowly over *5 minutes*. Calculate the number of milliliters you will push every minute.

15. Order: *albuterol sulfate syrup 3 mg PO T.I.D*. The recommended dose is 0.1–0.2 *mg/kg* T.I.D (max 4 *mg/dose*).

    (a) Is this a safe dose for a child who weighs 60 *pounds*?
    (b) If the dose is safe, read the label in • **Figure 12.14** and calculate the number of milliliters of this bronchodilator you would administer.

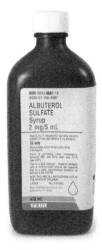

• **Figure 12.14**
Bottle of albuterol sulfate.

16. Order: *Children's Motrin (ibuprofen) 400 mg PO q4h prn temp over 101°F*. The recommended dose range is 5–10 *mg/kg* q4–6h up to 40 *mg/kg/day*. Is the ordered dose of this NSAID safe for a child who weighs 45 *kg*?

17. Order: *Cleocin (clindamycin phosphate) 600 mg IVPB q8h, infuse in 50 mL of D5W over 20 minutes*. At what rate in *mL/h* will you set the pump to infuse this cephalosporin antibiotic?

18. Order: *granisetron HCl 10 mcg/kg IVPB, 30 minutes before chemotherapy. Infuse in 20 mL of D5W over 15 minutes*. The strength of the granisetron is 0.1 *mg/mL*.

(a) Calculate how many milliliters of this antiemetic a child who weighs 10 *kg* will need.

(b) At what rate will you set the infusion to run in *mL/h*?

19. The prescriber ordered 2,000 *units/m²/h* IVPB of a drug. The solution is labeled 10,000 *units* in 100 *ml* D5W. Calculate the flow rate in *mL/h* for a child who has a BSA of 1.2 *m²*.

20. Order: 150 *units of regular insulin in 250 mL NS, infuse at 6 mL/h*. Calculate the number of units of insulin the child is receiving per hour.

Additional Exercises

Now, test yourself!

1. The prescriber ordered *dicloaxacillin 75 mg oral suspension PO q6h* for a child who weighs 38 *kg*. The recommended dose for a child is 12.5–25 *mg/kg/day* in divided doses q6h. Is the prescribed dose of this penicillin antibiotic safe?

2. Order: *Biaxin (clarithromycin) oral suspension 7.5 mg/kg PO q12h*. Read the label in • **Figure 12.16,** and calculate the number of milliliters of this macrolide antibiotic you would administer to a child who weighs 18 *pounds*.

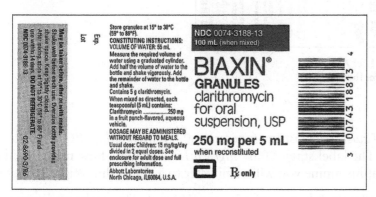

• **Figure 12.16**
Drug label for Biaxin.

Workspace

3. Order: *theophylline* 300 *mg PO q6h.* The strength available is 150 *mg/15 mL.* How many milliliters of this bronchodilator will you administer to the child?

4. The prescriber ordered *cephradine* 275 *mg IVPB q6h* for a child who weighs 31 *pounds.* The recommended dose is 50–100 *mg/kg/day* divided in four doses (maximum 8 *g/day*). Is the prescribed dose of this cephalosporin antibiotic safe?

5. Order: *acyclovir* 250 *mg/m²* *IV q8h.* The child has a BSA of 0.8 *m²*, and the vial is labeled "50 *mg/mL.*" How many milliliters of this antiviral will you prepare?

6. What is the daily fluid maintenance for a child who weighs 82 *pounds*?

7. Order: *Humatrope (somatropin)* 0.18 *mg/kg/week subcut divided into equal doses give on Mon/Wed/Fri.* Read the label in • **Figure 12.17** and calculate how many milliliters of this growth hormone you will administer to a child who weighs 40 *pounds*. The package insert states to "reconstitute the 5 *mg* vial with 5 *mL* of diluent."

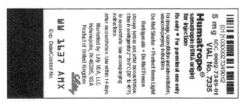

• **Figure 12.17**
Drug label for Humatrope.

8. Order: *Tavist (clemastine fumarate)* 0.05 *mg/kg/day PO divided into 2 doses.* The label states "0.67 *mg/5 mL.*" Calculate how many milliliters of this antihistamine you will administer to a child who weighs 35 *pounds*.

9. Order: *Dilantin (phenytoin)* 150 *mg IVP stat.* The packages insert states give 1 *mg/kg/min*, and the label reads 250 *mg/5 mL.* Over how many minutes should you administer this anticonvulsant to a child who weighs 10 *kg*?

10. Order: *Cefadyl (cephapirin sodium)* 40 *mg/kg/day IVPB divided into 4 doses. Infuse in 50 mL D5W over 30 min.* The child weighs 20 *kg*, and the directions state to reconstitute the 500 *mg* vial with 1 *ml* of diluent, yielding 500 *mg/1.2 mL.* How many *mL/h*, of this cephalosporin antibiotic, will you infuse?

11. Order: *Zostavax (zoster vaccine live)* 1 *dose subcut now*, has been prescribed for a child. Read the information on the labels in • **Figure 12.18**, and use the diluent supplied to reconstitute the vaccine. Draw a line on the appropriate syringe in • **Figure 12.19** indicating the number of milliliters of this reconstituted vaccine you will administer.

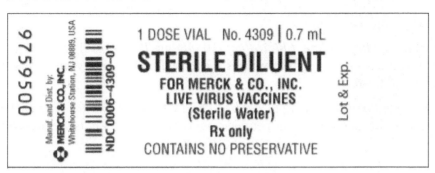

● Figure 12.18
Drug labels for Zostavax and Diluent.

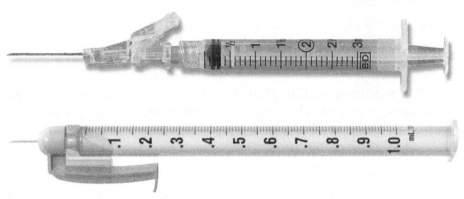

● Figure 12.19
Syringes for Question 11.

12. Order: *IV D5 $\frac{1}{3}$ NS, infuse at* 40 *mL/h.* What is the rate in microdrops per minute?

13. The prescriber ordered 1/3 maintenance for a child who weighs 10 *kg.* Calculate the rate at which the pump should be set in *mL/h.*

14. A child who weighs 33 *pounds* has diarrhea. To prevent dehydration, his fluid requirements are 100 *mL/kg/day.* The pediatrician tells the mom to give the child Pedialyte solution or "freezer pops." The label on the box states "62.5 *mL* per pop." What is the maximum number of Pedialyte freezer pops that the child may have in 1 *hour?*

15. Order: *erythromycin estolate* 125 *mg* PO q4h. The child weighs 14.5 *kg.* The recommended dosage is 30–50 *mg/kg/day* in equally divided doses. The label reads 125 *mg/mL.*

    (a) Is the ordered dose safe? _____

    (b) How many milliliters would you administer? _____

16. Order: *Vancocin (vancomycin)* 40 *mg/kg/d IVPB q6h to infuse over* 90 *minutes in* 200 *mL NS*. The child weighs 41 *kg*. The Vancocin vial has a concentration of 50 *mg/mL*. At what rate in *mL/h* will you set the pump?

17. A medication of 100 *mg* in 1 *mL* is diluted to 15 *mL* and administered IVP over 20 *minutes*. How many *mg/min* is the patient receiving?

18. 40 *mL* of IV fluid is to infuse over 60 *minutes*. What is the rate of flow in microdrops per minute?

19. Order: *Pediaprophen (ibuprofen)* 10 *mg/kg PO q4h*. The label reads 100 *mg/2.5 mL*. The child weighs 35 *pounds*. How many milliliters will you administer?

20. Order: *ampicillin* 125 *mg PO q6h.* A child weighs 22 *pounds.* The package insert states that the recommended dose is 50 *mg/kg/24* h. Is the prescribed dose safe?

Cumulative Review Exercises

Review your mastery of previous chapters.

1. 42 *mm* = ? *cm*

2. How many grams of sodium chloride are contained in 1 *liter* of 0.9% NaCl?

3. An IV is infusing at 120 *mL/h* via a pump. If this infusion were switched to a gravity system, what would be the flow rate in drops per minute? The drop factor of the tubing is 15 *gtt/mL*.

4. An IVPB bag with a concentration of 300 *milligrams* of a drug in 200 *mL* of D_5W is infusing at the rate of 90 *mL/h*. What is the dosage rate in *mg/min*?

5. Order: *Cefizox (ceftizoxime)* 1,500 *mg IV push q8h infuse over* 7.5 *minutes*. The concentration available is 1 *gram* in 10 *mL* of sterile water. How many *mL* will you infuse every 15 *seconds*?

6. Order: *Nipride (nitroprusside sodium)* 2 *mcg/kg/min IV stat for hypertensive crisis*. The pharmacy has sent an IV labeled Nipride 50 *mg/* 250 *mL* NS. The patient weighs 250 *pounds*. Calculate the rate at which you will set the IV pump in milliliters per hour.

7. Order: *D5W/0.45% NaCl* 1,000 *mL infuse at* 25 *gtt/min*. Calculate the number of hours it will take for this solution to infuse. The drop factor is 15 *gtt/mL*.

8. The physician ordered *Mirapex (pramipexole dihydrochloride)* 0.125 *mg PO T.I.D.* for a patient who has Parkinson's disease. How many milligrams per day is the patient receiving?

9. The prescriber ordered *Hemabate (carboprost tromethamine)* 250 *mcg deep IM stat. Repeat q15 min not to exceed* 8 *doses*. What is the maximum number of milligrams that may be administered in total?

10. What is the BSA of a person who is 75 *inches* tall and weighs 210 *pounds*?

11. Order: *Ticar (ticarcillin disodium)* 1 g *IVPB q6h, infuse in 50 mL D5W over 45 minutes*. The instructions for the 1 g vial state to reconstitute with 2 *mL* of sterile water for injection yielding 1g/2.6 *mL*. At what rate in *mL/h* will you set the pump? _____

12. Order: *morphine sulfate 3 mg IV stat*. The label reads 10 *mg/ml*. How many milliliters of this narcotic analgesic will you administer? _____

13. Order: *Videx (didanosine) 250 mg PO B.I.D.* The directions state to reconstitute the 4-g bottle, add 200 *mL* of water. How many milliliters of this antiretroviral will you administer? _____

14. Order: *Nalfon (fenoprofen calcium) 900 mg/m² PO daily in two divided doses*. How many milligrams of this analgesic would a child who weighs 23 *kg* and is 128 *cm* tall receive per day? _____

15. Which is the strongest solution? 1:1,000; 1:10,000; 1:15,000 _____

Workspace

Comprehensive Self-Tests

Comprehensive Self-Test 1

Answers to *Comprehensive Self-Tests* 1–4 can be found in Appendix A at the back of the book.

1. Order: *Omnicef (cefdinir) for oral suspension 300 mg PO q12h for 10 days.* Read the label in • **Figure S.1** and calculate how many grams of this antibiotic the patient will receive.

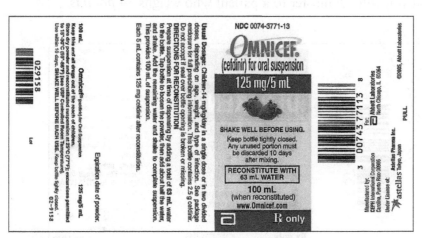

• **Figure S.1**
Drug label for Omnicef.

2. Order: *Kaletra (lopinavir/ritonavir) 400 mg lopinavir/100 mg ritonavir PO b.i.d* Read the label in • **Figure S.2** and calculate how many milliliters of this antiviral drug you will administer.

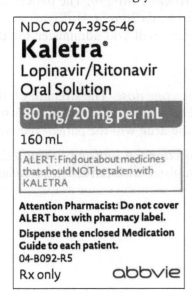

• **Figure S.2**
Drug label for Kaletra.

3. Order: *Ativan (lorazepam) 2 mg IVP stat inject slowly over 1 minute.* The label on the 10 *mL* multiple-dose vial reads 2 *mg/mL*.
   (a) How many milliliters of this anxiolytic will you prepare?
   (b) How many milliliters will you administer every 15 *seconds*?

4. Order: *morphine sulfate 10 mg IM stat.* The label reads 15 *mg* per *mL*.
   (a) How many milliliters of this analgesic will you administer?
   (b) What size syringe will you use?

5. *Dopamine hydrochloride 5 mcg/kg/min via continuous IV infusion* is ordered for a patient who weighs 176 *pounds*. The premixed IV solution reads dopamine 200 *mg* in D_5W 250 *mL* and is infusing via pump at 30 *mL/h*. How many milligrams per hour of this sympathomimetic agent is the patient receiving?

6. Order: *Depakene (valproic acid) 15 mg/kg/day PO*. Read the label in
   • **Figure S.3** and calculate how many capsules of this antiseizure medication you will administer to a patient who weighs 34 *pounds*.

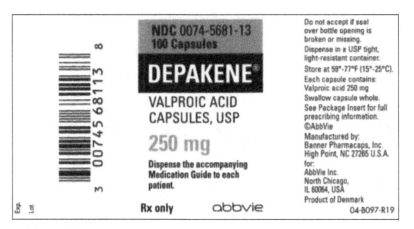

• **Figure S.3**
Drug label for Depakene.

7. Order: *vasopressin 5 units IM stat, then 10 units IM q4h*. The patient has abdominal distention. The label on the vial reads 20 *units/mL*.
   (a) How many milliliters of this antidiuretic will you administer for the stat dose?
   (b) What size syringe will you use?

8. Order: *vinblastine sulfate 5.5 mg/m^2 IV for one dose*. The strength on the 10 *mL* multiple-dose vial is 1 *mg/mL*. The patient has BSA of 1.66 *m^2*. How many milligrams of this antineoplastic drug will the patient receive?

9. Order: *insulin glargine (rDNA origin) injection 0.4 units/kg subcut daily*. Calculate how many units you will administer to a patient who weighs 150 *pounds*.

10. Order: *Pipracil (piperacillin sodium) 1.5 g IVPB q6h, infuse in 50 mL 0.9% NS over 20 minutes.* The reconstitution directions on the 3 g vial of this antibiotic indicate to add 5 mL of sterile water. At what rate will you set the IV pump in *mL/h*?

11. Order: *Gemzar (gemcitabine HCl) 1,390 mg IV once a week for 7 weeks, infuse in 100 mL of NS over 30 minutes.* The patient has pancreatic cancer. The patient is 155 *cm* tall and weighs 45 *kg*. The recommended dose is 1,000 *mg/m²* once weekly for up to 7 *weeks*, followed by 1 *week* of rest from treatment.
    (a) Is the prescribed dose safe?
    (b) At what rate will you set the infusion pump in *mL/h*?

12. Order: *gentamycin sulfate 3mg/kg IV daily in three equally divided doses. Infuse in 50 mL NS over 60 min.* The patient weighs 154 *pounds*. How many *mcgtt/min* of this aminoglycoside will the patient receive?

13. Order: *Flumadine (rimantadine hydrochloride) syrup 5 mg/kg PO twice a day.* The strength on the label is 50 *mg* per 5 *mL*. How many milliliters will a child who weighs 54 *pounds* receive?

14. Calculate the daily fluid maintenance for a child who weighs 58 *pounds*.

15. Order: *DDAVP (desmopressin acetate) 0.2 mL nasal spray daily in two equally divided doses.* The label on the 5 *mL* bottle states the strength is 10 *mcg/0.1 mL*. How many doses are contained in the bottle?

16. A patient has an IV of 250 *mL* with 1 *g* of lidocaine infusing via pump at a rate of 10 *mL/h*.
    (a) What is the concentration of lidocaine measured in *mg/mL*?
    (b) How many milligrams of lidocaine is the patient receiving per hour?
    (c) How many milliliters per minute of the lidocaine solution is the patient receiving?

17. Order: *Motrin (ibuprofen) 10 mg/kg PO q8h.* The strength on the label is 100 *mg/5 mL*. How many milliliters will you prepare for a child who weighs 70 *pounds*?

18. Order: *hyoscyamine sulfate oral solution 0.025 mg PO 1h before meals and at bedtime.* The recommended dose for this anticholinergic drug is 0.0625–0.125 *mg* q4h prn (max: 0.75 *mg/d*).
    (a) Is the prescribed dose safe?
    (b) If the dose is safe, how many milliliters will you administer? The label reads 0.125 *mg/mL* (0.2 *mL*).

19. The prescriber ordered *Vitamin B₁₂ alpha (hydroxocobalamin) 34 mcg IM/month* for a child who weighs 20 *kg*. The label reads 1,000 *mcg/mL*.
    (a) How many milliliters will the child receive?
    (b) What size syringe will you use?

20. The prescriber ordered *Zanosar (streptozocin) 500 mg/m²/d IV for 5 days.* Read the label in • **Figure S.5**.
    (a) How many grams will a patient who has a BSA of 1.8 *m²* receive in 5 *days*? The medication is to be infused in 250 *mL* of D5W over 50 *minutes* via pump.
    (b) At what rate will you set the pump in *mL/h*?

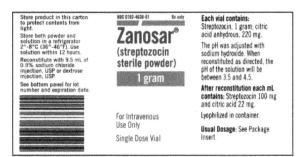

● **Figure S.5**
Drug label for Zanosar.

21. Order: *Tegopen (cloxacillin) oral suspension 400 mg PO q6h.* The label reads 125 *mg/5 mL*, and the recommended dose is 12.5 *mg–25 mg/kg/q6h* (max: 4 *g/d*).

    (a) Is the prescribed dose safe for a child who weighs 66 *pounds*?

    (b) If the dose is safe, how many milliliters will the child receive?

22. Order: *M-M-R II vaccine 1 dose subcut now.* Read the label in ● **Figure S.6.** The vaccine must be reconstituted with 0.5 *mL* of diluent. Indicate the dose on the most appropriate syringe.

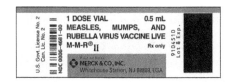

● **Figure S.6**
Drug label for M-M-R II.

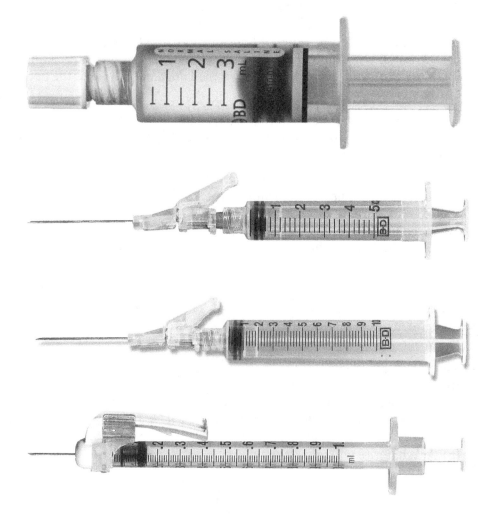

23. Order: *Prinvil (lisinopril) 0.07 mg/kg PO daily*. The label reads 1 *mg/mL*. Calculate the number of milliliters of this angiotensin-converting enzyme (ACE) inhibitor you will administer to a child who weighs 70 *pounds*.

24. Order: *Ativan (lorazepam) 3 mg IV push stat*. The strength on the vial is 4 *mg/mL*. The package insert recommends diluting the medication with an equal volume of compatible solution and to infuse slowly at a maximum rate of 2 *mg/min*.
    (a) How many milliliters of Ativan (lorazepam) will you prepare?
    (b) Over how many minutes will you administer the Ativan (lorazepam)?

25. Order: *heparin 1,000 units in 500 mL 0.9% NaCl, infuse at 100 mL/h*. How many units per hour is the patient receiving?

Comprehensive Self-Test 2

Answers to *Comprehensive Self-Tests* 1–4 can be found in Appendix A at the back of the book.

1. Order: *Biaxin (clarithromycin) 500 mg PO q12h*. Read the label in
   • **Figure S.7(a)** and determine how many milliliters of this antibiotic you will administer. Draw a line at the appropriate measurement on the medication cup in • **Figure S.7(b).**

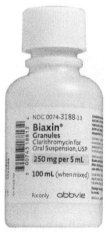

• **Figure S.7(a)**
Drug label for Biaxin.

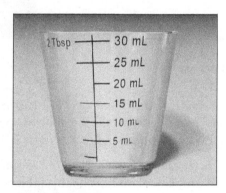

• **Figure S.7(b)**
Medication cup.

2. The prescriber ordered *acetazolamide 500 mg IVP over 1 minute* preoperatively for a patient who has secondary glaucoma. The directions on the 500 *mg* vial state to reconstitute with 5 *mL* of sterile water for injection.
   (a) How many milliliters of this diuretic will you prepare?
   (b) How many milliliters will you administer every 30 *seconds*?

3. Order: *Zovirax (acyclovir) 200 mg PO q4h while awake (max 1,000 mg/ day) for 10 days*. How many grams of this antiviral drug will the patient have received in total after 7 *days*?

4. Order: *ampicillin 250 mg IM q6h*. The directions on the 1 g vial state to add 3.5 *mL* of diluent yielding 250 *mg/mL* and use the solution within 1 *hour*. How many milliliters of this antibiotic will you administer?

5. The prescriber ordered *Tegretol (carbamazepine) suspension 150 mg PO b.i.d.* for a 5-year-old child who weighs 50 *pounds*. The recommended

dosage for this anticonvulsant is 10–20 *mg/kg/day* in three to four divided doses. The label on the Tegretol bottle reads 100 *mg/5 mL*.

(a) Is the ordered dose safe?

(b) If it is safe, how many milliliters will you administer?

6. The prescriber ordered *Myleran (busulfan) 2.1 mg/m² PO daily* for a child who is 42 *inches* tall and weighs 70 *pounds*. How many milligrams of this antineoplastic drug will you administer?

7. The prescriber ordered *Enbrel (etanercept) 0.4 mg/kg subcut two times a week* for a child who has rheumatoid arthritis and weighs 40 *pounds*. The label on the vial reads 25 *mg/mL*. How many milliliters will you administer?

8. Order: *amoxicillin oral suspension 120 mg PO q8h*. The recommended dosage is 20–40 *mg/kg/day*.

(a) Is this a safe dose for a child who weighs 37 *pounds*?

(b) If the dose is safe, refer to the information on the label in ● **Figure S.8** and calculate how many milliliters of this antibiotic the child would receive.

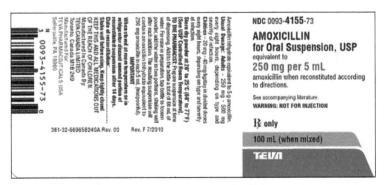

● **Figure S.8**
Drug label for amoxicillin.

9. Order: *Doxycin (doxycycline hyclate) 100 mg IVPB q12h. Infuse in 100 mL D5W over 1 hour*. At what rate in drops per minute will you set the infusion for this antibiotic if the drop factor is 10 *gtt/mL*?

10. Order: *Zocor (simvastatin) 10 mg PO daily*. Read the information in ● **Figure S.9** and calculate how many tablets the patient will receive in one week.

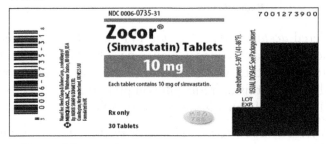

● **Figure S.9**
Drug label for Zocor (simvastatin).

11. Order: *heparin 30,000 units IV in 500 mL of D5W, infuse at 1,500 units/h*. Calculate the flow rate in *mL/h*.

12. Order: *heparin 50,000 units in 500 mL of NS, infuse at 25 mL/h*. Calculate the number of units per hour of this anticoagulant the patient is receiving.

13. The prescriber ordered an *insulin drip of Humulin R Regular insulin 50 units IV in 100 mL 0.9% NaCl, infuse at 6 mL/h.* How many units of insulin per hour is the patient receiving?

14. The prescriber ordered *morphine sulfate 4 mg IVP stat, give slowly over 5 minutes.* The strength on the label is 10 *mg/mL*, and the directions state to dilute to *5 mL* of sterile water.
    (a) How many milliliters of this narcotic analgesic will be withdrawn from the vial?
    (b) How many milliliters will be administered every 30 *seconds*?

15. Order: *Primaxin (imipenem-cilastatin sodium) 500 mg IVPB q6h.* The recommended dosage is 15–25 *mg/kg* q6h. Is the prescribed dose of this antibiotic safe for a child who weighs 55 *pounds*?

16. Calculate the daily fluid maintenance requirements for a child who weighs 33 *kg*.

17. The prescriber ordered *Azactam (aztreonam) 1 g IV q6h* for a child who has cystic fibrosis. The recommended dosage range is 50–200 *mg/kg* q6h (maximum 8 *g/day*). Is the prescribed dose safe for a child who weighs 70 *pounds*?

18. The prescriber ordered *dopamine 2 mcg/kg/min IV* for a patient who weighs 110 *pounds*. The label on the IV bag reads dopamine 200 *mg/250 mL* D5W. At what rate will you set the infusion pump in *mL/h*?

19. Order: *Solu-Cortef (hydrocortisone sodium succinate) 150 mg IM stat.* The strength on the label is 250 *mg/2 mL*. How many milliliters will the patient receive?

20. Order: *Dynapen (dicloxacillin sodium) mg 500 mg PO q6h.* The recommended dosage range for a child with a severe infection is 50–100 *mg/kg/day* divided into doses given q6h. Is the prescribed dose of this antibiotic safe for a child who weighs 77 *pounds*?

21. The prescriber ordered *Mannitol 12.5 g IVP stat.* The label on the 50 *mL* vial reads 25%. How many milliliters of this osmotic diuretic will you prepare?

22. Order: *Norvir (ritonavir) 250 mg/m² PO B.I.D.* How many milligrams are required for a child who weighs 15 *kg* and is 77 *cm* tall?

23. Order: *D5W 500 mL IV, infuse over 5 hours.* Calculate the flow rate in drops per minute. The drop factor is 15 *gtt/mL*.

24. The prescriber ordered *Synthroid (levothyroxine sodium) 0.05 mg PO daily.* The strength on the label is 25 *mcg* (0.025 *mg*)/*tab*. Calculate how many tablets you will administer.

25. Order: *heparin 8,000 units subcut q12h.* The strength on the vial is 10,000 *units/mL*. How many milliliters will you administer?

Comprehensive Self-Test 3

Answers to *Comprehensive Self-Tests* 1–4 can be found in Appendix A at the back of the book.

1. The prescriber ordered *dobutamine 10 mcg/kg/min via continuous IV infusion* for a patient who weighs 143 *pounds*. The IV is labeled D5/W 500 *mL*

with dobutamine 250 *mg*. How many micrograms of this beta-adrenergic agent is the patient receiving per minute?

2. Order: *Vistaril (hydroxyzine pamoate) 75 mg PO Q.I.D.* Read the label in • **Figure S.10** and calculate how many milliliters of this anxiolytic medication you will administer.

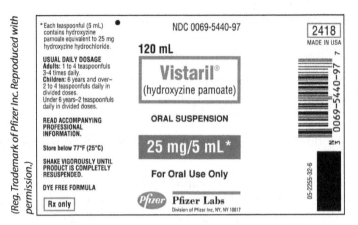

• **Figure S.10**
Drug label for Vistaril.

3. You need to prepare 15 *mg* of lidocaine HCl injection. The label reads lidocaine 2%. How many milliliters of this antiarrhythmic will you prepare?

4. Order: *heparin 4,000 units subcut q12h.* The label on the 10 *mL* multidose vial reads 10,000 *units* per *mL*. How many milliliters of this anticoagulant will you administer?

5. Order: *D₅NS 150 mL IV infuse in 1 hour.* The drop factor is 15 *gtt/mL*. Calculate the flow rate in drops per minute.

6. Calculate the number of grams of dextrose in 500 *mL* of D10W.

7. Order: *Humulin Regular insulin U-100 8 units and Humulin NPH insulin 12 units subcutaneous ac breakfast.* Read the labels in • **Figure S.11** and place an arrow on the syringe, indicating the total amount of insulin you will give.

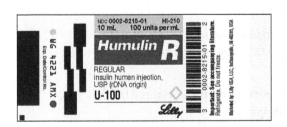 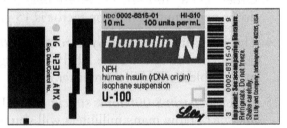

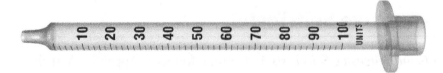

• **Figure S.11**
Drug labels for Humulin R and Humulin N and syringe.

(Copyright Eli Lilly and Company. Used with permission)

8. The prescriber ordered *Dilaudid (hydromorphone HCl) oral solution 4 mg PO q6h*. The label on the bottle states that each teaspoon contains 5 *mg* of the drug. How many milliliters of this narcotic analgesic will you administer?

9. The prescriber ordered *ampicillin sodium 500 mg IVPB q6h to infuse in 100 mL of D5W over 30 minutes.*
   (a) Calculate the flow rate in milliliters per hour.
   (b) How many grams of this antibiotic will the patient receive per day?

10. Order: *Dilaudid HP (HYDROmorphone HCl) 1 mg subcut q2h prn moderate pain*. The strength on the vial is 4 *mg* per *mL*. Calculate the dose in milliliters of this narcotic analgesic and place an arrow on the syringe below, indicating the dose.

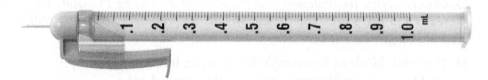

11. Order: *Adrenalin (epinephrine) 0.3 mg subcut stat*. The strength on the label is 1:1000. How many milliliters of this sympathomimetic catecholamine will you administer?

12. Order: *dopamine hydrochloride 200 mg in 500 mL NS, infuse at 2 mcg/kg/min for systolic B/P less than 90. Increase rate up to 10 mcg/kg/min as needed*. The patient weighs 165 *pounds*. At what flow rate in milliliters per hour will you begin the infusion of this cardiac stimulant?

13. Order: *Humulin R insulin 100 units in 100 mL NS, infuse at 0.2 unit/kg/h*. The patient weighs 200 *pounds*. How many units per hour is the patient receiving?

14. Order: *ZyPREXA (olanzapine) 10 mg IM stat*. Reconstitution instructions on the 10 *mg* vial state to "add 2.1 *mL* of sterile water for injection and dissolve contents completely. Each milliliter will contain 5 *mg*. Solution must be used within 1 *hour*." How many milliliters of this antipsychotic drug will you administer to the patient?

15. Order: *Sandostatin (octreotide acetate) 0.25 mg subcut daily*. The label states that the strength is 500 *mcg* per *mL*. How many milliliters will the patient receive?

16. Order: *EryPED200 (erythromycin ethylsuccinate) oral suspension 120 mg PO q4h*. The child weighs 32 *pounds* and the recommended dose is 30–50 *mg/kg/day*.
   (a) What is the minimum daily dose in *mg/day*?
   (b) What is the maximum daily dose in *mg/day*?
   (c) Is the ordered dose of this antibiotic safe?

17. *Vibramycin (doxycycline hyclate) 4.4 mg/kg IVPB daily* is ordered for a child who weighs 80 *pounds*. The premixed IV solution bag is labeled Vibramycin 200 *mg/250 mL* D5W to infuse in 4 *hours*.
   (a) How many milligrams of Vibramycin will the patient receive?
   (b) Calculate the flow rate in *mL/h*.

18. Order: *Levaquin (levofloxacin) 500 mg in 100 mL D5W IVPB daily for 14 days to infuse in 1 h.* Calculate the flow rate in drops per minute if the drop factor is 15 *gtt/mL.*

19. Calculate the BSA of a child who is 44 *inches* and *weighs* 72 *pounds.*

20. Order: *heparin 5,000 units subcutaneous q12h.* The multidose vial label reads 10,000 *units/mL.* How many milliliters will you give the patient?

21. Order: *D10W 1,000 mL to infuse at 75 mL/h.* The drop factor is 20 *gtt/mL.*
    (a) What is the rate of flow in $\frac{mL}{min}$?
    (b) How many drops per minute will you set the IV to infuse?
    (c) How long will it take for the infusion to be complete?

22. Calculate the total daily fluid maintenance for a child who weighs 45 *kg.*

23. Order: *Keflex (cephalexin) oral suspension 50 mg/kg PO q6h.* The label reads 125 *mg/5 mL.* The patient weighs 33 *pounds.* How many milliliters will you give?

24. The 5 mL bottle of furosemide has a strength of 40 *mg/5 mL.*
    (a) How many milligrams of furosemide are in 1 *mL?*
    (b) How many milliliters of furosemide are in the bottle?

25. The prescriber ordered *ReoPro (abciximab) 0.125 mcg/kg/min IV* for a patient who weighs 75 *kg.* Calculate the dosage rate in micrograms per minute.

Comprehensive Self-Test 4

Answers to *Comprehensive Self-Tests* 1–4 can be found in Appendix A at the back of the book.

1. A patient has an IV of 250 *mL* 0.9% NaCl with 25,000 *units* of heparin infusing at 15 *mL/h.* How many units of heparin is the patient receiving per hour?

2. The prescriber ordered *Phenergan (promethazine HCl) 20 mg IM q6h prn nausea* for a child who weighs 45 *kg.* The recommended dosage of this antiemetic drug is 0.25–0.5 *mg/kg* q4–6h prn (max: 25 *mg*/dose). The label reads 25 *mg/mL.*
   (a) Is the dose safe?
   (b) If the dose is safe, how many milliliters will you administer?

3. Order: *vinblastine sulfate 3.7 mg/ m² IVP infuse over one minute once a week*. The patient's BSA is 1.66 *m²*. The package insert states to reconstitute the 10 *mg* vial with 10 *mL* NS, yielding a concentration of 1 *mg/mL*.
   (a) How many milligrams of this antineoplastic drug will the patient receive?
   (b) How many milliliters contain the dose?
   (c) How many milliliters will you push every 15 *seconds*?

4. Order: *midazolam HCl 20 mcg/kg IM one hour before surgery*. The label on the vial reads 1 *mg/mL*. How many milliliters of this central nervous system agent will you prepare for a patient who weighs 150 *pounds*?

5. Order: *verapamil ER 120 mg PO daily each morning*. Calculate the dose of this calcium channel blocker in grams.

6. An IV of D₅RL (1,000 *mL*) is infusing at 50 *mL/h*. The infusion started at 1500h. What time will it finish?

7. A patient is to receive *Zofran (ondansteron HCl) 8 mg PO 30 minutes before chemotherapy, then 8 mg 8 hr later, followed by 8 mg q12h for 24 hours*. The label reads 4 *mg* per tab. How many tablets of this antiemetic drug will the patient receive in total?

8. The physician ordered *methotrexate 15 mg PO daily* for a child who has leukemia. The child has a BSA of 1.10 *m²*. The recommended daily dosage is 7.5–30 *mg/m²*. Is the prescribed dose safe?

9. Order: *Haldol LA (haloperidol decanoate) 60 mg IM stat*. The strength on the label is 50 *mg/mL*.
   (a) How many milliliters will you administer?
   (b) Place an arrow on the syringe, indicating the dose.

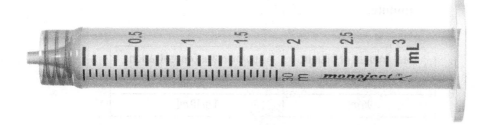

10. The prescriber ordered *Tagamet (cimetidine) 165 mg PO q6h* or a child who weighs 48 *pounds*. The recommended dose is 20–40 *mg/kg/day* divided into 4 *doses*. The strength on the label is 300 *mg* per 5 *mL*.
    (a) Calculate the minimum safe daily dose in *mg/day*.
    (b) Calculate the maximum safe daily dose in *mg/day*.
    (c) Calculate how many milliliters of this histamine H2-antagonist you will administer.

11. Calculate how many grams of lidocaine are contained in 100 *ml* of 2% lidocaine solution.

12. A patient has an IV infusing at 25 *gtt/min*. How many *mL/h* is the patient receiving? The drop factor is 20 *gtt/mL*.

13. Calculate the total volume and hourly IV flow rate for a child who weighs 70 *kg* and is receiving maintenance fluids.

14. Order: *nicardipine 25 mg in 250 ml NS infuse at 80 mL/h. The recommended dosage range is 3–15mg/min.* Is the prescribed dose of this calcium channel blocker safe?

15. Order: *dobutamine 250 mg in 50 mL NS, infuse at 5 mcg/kg/min.* Calculate the flow rate in milliliters per hour of this beta-adrenergic agonist. The patient weighs 165 *pounds.*

16. Order: *Humulin R insulin 100 units in 100 mL NS, infuse at 6 units per hour.* Calculate the milliliters per hour at which you will set the IV pump.

17. Order: *Ticar (ticarcillin disodium) 1 g IM q6h.* The package insert states to reconstitute each 1 *g* vial with 2 *mL* of sterile water for injection. Each 2.5 *mL* = 1g. How many milliliters will you administer?

18. Order: *Indocin SR (indomethacin) 150 mg PO t.i.d. for 7 days.* The label reads Indocin SR 75-*mg* capsules.
    (a) How many capsules will you give the patient for each dose?
    (b) Calculate the entire 7-*day* dosage in grams.

19. Order: *Colace (docusate sodium) syrup 100 mg via PEG t.i.d.* The label reads 50 *mg*/15 *mL.* How many *mL* will you give?

20. Order: *theophylline 0.8 mg/kg/h IV via pump.* The premixed IV bag is labeled theophylline 800 *mg* in 250 *mL* D5W. The patient weighs 185 *pounds.* At how many *mL/h* will you set the pump?

21. Order: *cefazolin 1 g IVPB q6h, add to 50 mL D5W and infuse over 20 minutes.* Read the reconstitution information from the cefazolin label in • **Figure S.13.**
    (a) How many milliliters of diluent will you add to the vial, so that 1 *gram* of cefazolin is contained in 5 *mL* of the solution?
    (b) Based on the answer in part (a), calculate the flow rate in milliliters per minute.

Total Amount of Diluent	Approximate Concentration
45 mL	1 g/5 mL
96 mL	1 g/10 mL

• **Figure S.13**
Reconstitution information from the cefazolin label.

22. The nurse has prepared 7 *mg* of dexamethasone for IV administration. The label on the vial reads 10 *mg/mL.* How many milliliters did the nurse prepare?

23. Order: *Cogentin (benztropine mesylate) 2 mg IM stat and then 1 mg IM daily.* The label reads 2 *mg*/2 *mL.*
    (a) How many milliliters will you administer daily?
    (b) What size syringe will you use?

24. Order: ⅔ *strength Sustacal 900 mL via PEG give over 8h.* How will you prepare this solution?

25. An IV of 250 *mL* NS is infusing at 25 *mL/h.* The infusion began at 1800*h.* What time will it be completed?

Appendices

Appendix A

Diagnostic Test of Arithmetic

1. $\frac{3}{8}$
2. 0.285
3. 6.5
4. 0.83
5. 3.2
6. 3.8
7. 0.0639
8. 500
9. 2
10. $\frac{1}{4}$ and 0.25
11. $2\frac{1}{3}$
12. $\frac{1}{25}$
13. $\frac{9}{20}$
14. 0.025
15. $\frac{18}{7}$
16. 12
17. 7.6
18. 6
19. 0.4
20. $\frac{3}{4}$

Chapter 1

Try These for Practice

1. 0.44
2. 13.5
3. $\frac{3}{5}$ 0.6 60%
   $\frac{9}{20}$ 0.45 45%
   $\frac{3}{100}$ 0.03 3%
4. 22
5. $\frac{3}{10}$

Exercises

1. $\frac{11}{20}$
2. 8
3. $1\frac{1}{3}$
4. $\frac{11}{28}$
5. 40
6. $1\frac{3}{5}$
7. $\frac{1}{6}$
8. 0.37
9. 0.64
10. 6.7
11. 0.015
12. 0.21
13. 0.457
14. 0.0131
15. 0.84
16. 0.6
17. 0.9
18. 0.17
19. 0.009
20. 0.27
21. 65.7
22. 0.047
23. 52.94
24. 0.02
25. 7.3
26. 1.8
27. $\frac{10}{49}$ 0.2
28. $6\frac{3}{7}$ 6.4
29. $0.1\frac{1}{8}$
30. $0.4\frac{3}{8}$
31. $\frac{1}{2}$
32. $\frac{2}{3}$
33. 60
34. 6
35. 9.95
36. 0.838
37. 0.7
38. 16
39. 25% increase
40. 30% decrease

Chapter 2

Try These for Practice

1. Xanax
2. intravenous
3. indinavir sulfate
4. Hyzaar 100/25
5. 2 *mcg* per capsule

Exercises

1. Xanax
2. 4 *mL* Cleocin
3. 200 *mg/cap*
4. 25 *mg*
5. indinavir sulfate

6. (a) Levemir and Tylenol with codeine #3
   (b) 1000h, 1400h, 1800h
   (c) Four
   (d) Subcutaneous
   (e) Neurontin, digoxin, Norvasc

7. (a) metoclopramide HCl
   (b) digoxin, Mevacor, Cozaar,
   (c) two times a day
   (d) Intravenous push
   (e) Up to a maximum of 8 *times per day*

8. (a) olanzapine tablet
   (b) acute agitation associated with schizophrenia and bipolar I mania
   (c) orthostatic hypotension
   (d) 5-10 *mg* once daily
   (e) no

9.

Standard	Military
9:30 AM	0930 *h*
2:43 PM	1443 *h*
12 midnight	2400 *h*
11:20 PM	2320 *h*
9:48 AM	0948 *h*
11:40 PM	2340 *h*
8:42 PM	2042 *h*
2:15 AM	0215 *h*
12:02 AM	0002 *h*
7:15 AM	0715 *h*

10. (a) Administer five hundred milligrams of Glucophage by mouth twice a day
    (b) Administer ten thousand units of heparin subcutaneously every eight hours
    (c) Apply one-half inch of 2 *percent* NITRO-BID ointment to the chest wall every six hours
    (d) Administer 5 *milligrams* of Accupril by mouth once every day
    (e) Administer six hundred fifty milligrams of Tylenol by mouth every four hours whenever temperature is more than one hundred one degrees Fahrenheit

11. (a) dose and frequency or time
    (b) dosage strength and route
    (c) route and frequency or time
    (d) dose, and route
    (e) dosage strength, route

12. (a) 10 *mg*   (b) 10 *mg*   (c) 10 *mg*   (d) 5 *mg*

Chapter 3

Try These for Practice

1. 390 *sec*
2. 70 *oz*
3. $1\frac{1}{2}$ *hours*
4. 1.6 *oz/d*
5. 24 *in/min*

Exercises

1. 12 *min*
2. 18 *mon*
3. 66 *h*
4. 84 *oz*
5. 900 *sec*
6. 12 *in/min*
7. 60 *ft/hr*
8. 12 *hours*
9. 30 *pt/h*
10. 70 *oz*
11. $\frac{1}{4}h$
12. $480
13. 604,800 *sec*
14. 5 *ft* 10 *in*
15. $2\frac{qt}{min}$
16. $120\frac{pt}{hr}$
17. $6\frac{qt}{h}$
18. 10 *ft/h*
19. $\frac{7\ lb}{8\ wk}$
20. $6\frac{ft}{h}$

Chapter 4

Try These for Practice

1. (a) 1,000 *mL*
   (b) 1 *cc*
   (c) 1,000 *cm*^{3}
   (d) 1,000 *g*
   (e) 1,000 *mg*
   (f) 1,000 *mcg*
   (g) 10 *mm*
   (h) 2 *pt*
   (i) 2 *cups*
   (j) 8 *oz*
   (k) 2 *T*
   (l) 3 *t*
   (m) 12 *in*
   (n) 16 *oz*
2. 15,000 *mcg*
3. 0.03 *mg*
4. 0.9 *g*
5. 6 *T*

Exercises

1. 56,000 *mcg*
2. 0.6 *g*
3. 4 *qt*
4. 56 *mm*
5. 72 *oz*
6. 10,000 *mcg*
7. 0.84 *g/wk*
8. 0.65 *g*
9. 1.4 *L*
10. 42 *mg*
11. 2.65 *kg*
12. 9 *pt*
13. 50,000 *mcg*
14. 0.175 *g*
15. 0.028 *g*
16. 3 *T*
17. 0.08 *g*
18. 0.4 *g*
19. 3,100 *g*
20. 1.7 *mg* is in the range of 1–2 *mg*. The order is safe.

Cumulative Review Exercises

1. 8.8 *cm*
2. 2.5 *lb*
3. 3,700 *mL*
4. 15 *t*
5. 60 *in*
6. 140 *oz/wk*
7. 0.9 *g*
8. 2 *cups*
9. 10 *mg*
10. Route of administration
11. 80 *mg*
12. 80 *mg*
13. 40 *mg*
14. 2130 *hours*
15. 0100 *h* the next day

Chapter 5

Try These for Practice

1. (a) 1,000 *mL*   (i) 2 *T*   (q) 30 *mL*
   (b) 1,000 *g*   (j) 3 *t*   (r) 240 *mL*
   (c) 1,000 *mg*   (k) 16 *oz*   (s) 500 *mL*
   (d) 1,000 *mcg*   (l) 12 *in*   (t) 1,000 *mL*
   (e) 10 *mm*   (m) 2.5 *cm*   (u) 2, 6, 30
   (f) 2 pt   (n) 2.2 *lb*   (v) 2, 4, 32, 1,000
   (g) 2 cups   (o) 5 *mL*
   (h) 8 *oz*   (p) 15 *mL*

2. 158 *cm*   3. 1 *t*

4. 480 *mL or* 500 *mL* – depending on the equivalents used   5. 9 *t*

Exercises

1. 20 *mL*	2. 240 *mL*	3. 3 *T*
4. $\frac{1}{2}$ *cup*	5. 68.2 *kg*	6. 1 *t*
7. 2 *in*	8. 8 *T*	9. 4 *oz*
10. 24 *t*	11. 6 *ft* 2 *in*	12. 0.2 *g*
13. 6 *lb* 13 *oz*	14. 1.44 *g*	

15. Take 2 *tablespoons*, three times a day, for a total of 6 *tablespoons* per day

16. 0.36 *g*	17. 1,365 *mL*	18. 1 *oz*
19. 10 *g*	20. 24 *doses*	

Cumulative Review Exercises

1. 80 *kg*	2. 0.08 *g*	3. 2,000 *mL*
4. 0.12 *L*	5. 2,273 *g*	6. 1$\frac{1}{2}$ *pt/d*
7. 105 *mL/wk*	8. 0.84 *g*	9. 1330 *h*
10. No, Harold is too light	11. 42.5 *mm*	12. 10 *mL*
13. 198 *lb*	14. 180 *cm*	15. 1 *cup* per hour

Chapter 6

Case Study

1. 1 *tab* [label c]	2. 2 *cap*	3. 4 *tab*
4. 8 $\frac{tab}{day}$	5. 4 *tab*	6. 0.075 *g*

7. 28 *tab*   8. 2 *tab*   9. 1 *cap*

10. 4 $\dfrac{cap}{day}$ 11. 2.73 *m²*

Practice Reading Labels

1. 10 *mg/tab*, 1 *tab*   2. 50 *mg/5 mL*, 5 *mL*
3. 500 *mg/tab*, 2 *tab*   4. 5 *mg/5 mL*, 15 *mL*
5. 20 *mg/cap*, 2 *cap*   6. 30 *mg/cap*, 2 *cap*
7. 10 *mEq/tab*, 2 *tab*   8. 2.5 *mg/20 mg* per *tab*, 2 *tab*
9. 2 *mg/mL*, 2 *mL*   10. 7.5 *mg/300 mg* per *tab*, 2 *tab*
11. 125 *mg/5 mL*, 20 *mL*   12. 100 *mg/tab*, 3 *tab*
13. 0.5 *mg/tab*, 2 *tab*   14. 10 *mg/tab*, 3 *tab*
15. 100 *mg/25 mg* per *tab*, 3 *tab*   16. 20 *mg/tab*, 2 *tab*
17. 60 *mg/tab*, 1 *tab*   18. 10 *mg/tab*, 6 *tab*
19. 2.5 *mg/tab*, 2 *tab*   20. 40 *mg/cap*, 2 *cap*
21. 2 *mcg/cap*, 3 *cap*   22. 120 *mg/tab*, 4 *tab*
23. 10 *mg/tab*, 2 *tab*   24. 250 *mg/5 mL*, 15 *mL*
25. 125 *mg/5 mL*, 20 *mL*   26. 30 *mg/cap*, 2 *cap*
27. 40 *mg/tab*, 2 *tab*   28. 5 *mg/12.5 mg* per *tab*, 2 *tab*
29. 20 *mg/mL*, 6 *mL*   30. 100 *mg/5 mL*, 4 t
31. 10 *mg/tab*, 2 *tab*   32. 80 *mg/20 mg* per *mL*, 1 t
33. 250 *mg/5 mL*, 2 t   34. 100 *mg/cap*, 3 *cap*
35. 2.5 *mg/tab*, 2 *tab*   36. 200 *mg/5 mL*, 10 *mL*
37. 0.4 *mg/tab*, 1 *tab*   38. 50 *mg/1,000 mg* per *tab*, 2 *tab*
39. 250 *mg/5 mL*, 10 *mL*   40. 25 *mg/cap*, 3 *cap*
41. 100 *mg/tab*, 6 *tab*   42. 80 *mg/mL*, 7.5 *mL*
43. 60 *mg/tab*, 1 *tab*   44. 40 *mg/tab*, 2 *tab*
45. 20 *mg/tab*, 2 *tab*   46. 400 *mg/tab*, 1 *tab*
47. 125 *mg/5 mL*, 20 *mL*   48. 250 *mg/5 mL*, 10 *mL*
49. 600 *mg/42.9 mg* per 5 *mL*, 10 *mL*   50. 10 *mg/mL*, 10 *mL*

Try These for Practice

1. 1.75 *m²*   2. 2 t   3. 0.5 *mL*   4. 4.2 g   5. 4 *mg*

Exercises

1. 3 *tab*   2. 4 t   3. 2.2–2.6 *mg/d*
4. No. It's an overdose.   5. 2 t   6. 1.92 *m²*

7. Yes, the order of 200 *mg/d* is in the recommended range.

8. 2.4 *g*   9. 3 *cap/day*   10. 9 *mL*

11. 2 *tab*   12. 0.25 *mL*   13. 1 *tab*

14. (a) prescribed dose is not safe   (b) Contact the prescriber

15. 1 *g*   16. 1.58 *m²* (using metric formula), 1.59 *m²* (using household formula)

17. 36 *mL*   18.   19. 3 *tab*   20. 2 *tab*

Cumulative Review Exercises

1. 60 *mL*   2. 20 *kg*   3. 30 *pt*
4. 4.7 *cm*   5. 4 *mL*   6. 2 *tab*

7. 20 *mL*

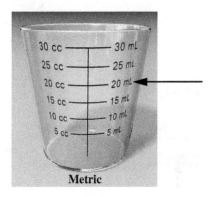

8. 2 *tab*   9. 2.19 *m²*   10. Tristan

11. 511 *mg*   12. 3.3 *mL*   13. 30 *mL/h*

14. 2 *tab*   15. 2230 *h*

Chapter 7

Case Study 7.1

1. (a) 0.4 *mL*
   (b) the 1-*mL* syringe

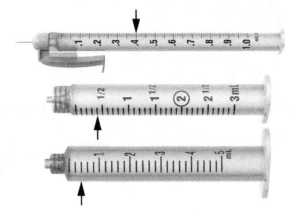

2. (a) 1 *mL* of Phenergan

(b) 75 *mg/mL* because no calculation would be necessary

(c)

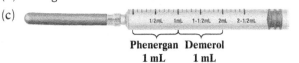

Phenergan Demerol
1 mL   1 mL

3.

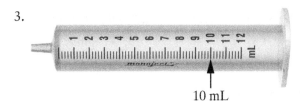

10 mL

4. 0.1 *mL*

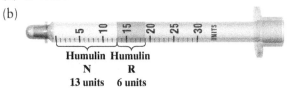

5. 0.2 *mL*

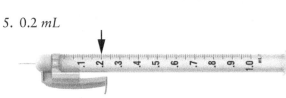

6. (a) 19 *units*

(b)

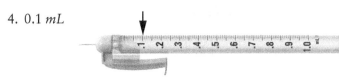

Humulin Humulin
   N   R
13 units   6 units

Try These for Practice

1. 1 *mL* tuberculin syringe; 0.68 *mL*

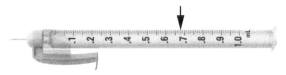

2. 12-*mL* syringe; 5.6 *mL*

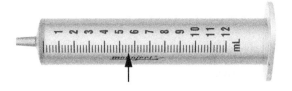

3. 3-*mL* syringe; 1.8 *mL*

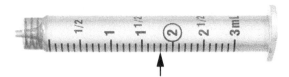

4. 5-*mL* syringe; 4.4 *mL*

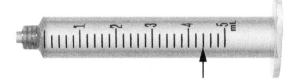

5. 1.5 *mL* using a 3-*mL* syringe

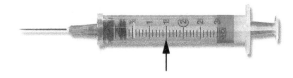

Exercises

1. 1-*mL* tuberculin syringe; 0.45 *mL*

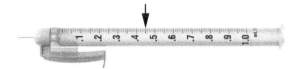

2. 30 *unit* Lo-Dose insulin syringe; 17 *units*

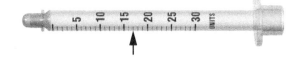

3. *5-mL* syringe; 1.8 *mL*

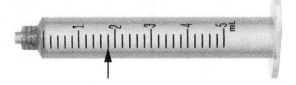

4. *3-mL* syringe; 1.8 *mL*

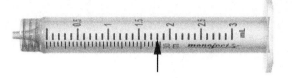

5. *35-mL* syringe; 18 *mL*

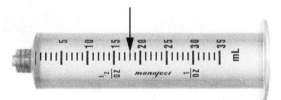

6. *12-mL* syringe; 9.2 *mL*

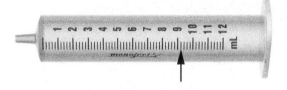

7. *50-unit* Lo-Dose insulin syringe; 33 *units*

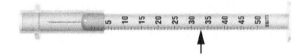

8. 100-unit insulin syringe; 66 *units*

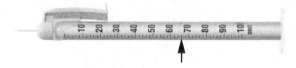

9. 0.5-*mL* syringe; 0.09 *mL*

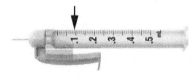

10. 100-unit insulin syringe; 67 *units*

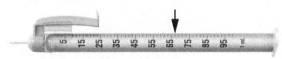

11. *12-mL* syringe; 10.4 *mL*

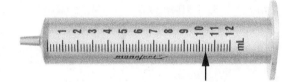

12. 1-*mL* tuberculin syringe; 0.75 *mL*

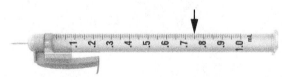

13. *12-mL* syringe; 11.2 *mL*

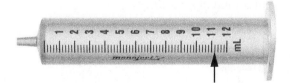

14. *35-mL* syringe; 24 *mL*

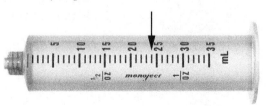

15. 1.5 *mL*

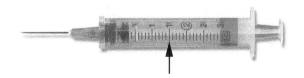

16. 50 *units*

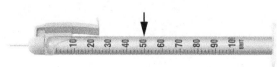

17. 2 *mL*

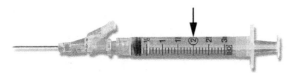

18. 0.4 *mL*

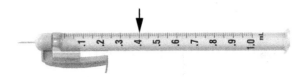

19. No, it is an overdose

20. 1.5 *mL*

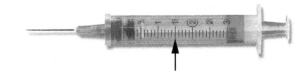

Cumulative Review Exercises

1. (a) no insulin   (b) 2 *units*   (c) notify MD stat

2. 4 *mL*   3. 4 *mL*   4. 2 *mL*   5. 4 *mL*

6. 2 *t*   7. 0.68 *g*   8. 90.9 *kg*   9. 3 *tab*

10. 1 *g*   11. 7 *g*   12. 1.64 *m²*   13. 75 *mg*

14. 100-*unit* insulin syringe   15. 0.67 *mL* in a 1-*mL* tuberculin syringe

Chapter 8

Case Study 8.1

1. label (d) 1 *tab*   2. label (f) 1 *tab*   3. 1 40-*mg tab*   4. 2 *tab*
5. 240 *mL/d*   6. 0.5 *mL*

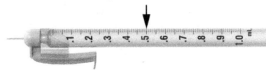

7. Withdraw 10 *units* of Humulin R insulin, then into the same syringe withdraw
34 *units* of Humulin N insulin for a total of 44 *units*.

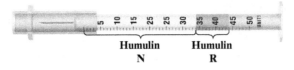

8. 4.5 *g*

Try These for Practice

1. $\frac{1}{5}$, 1:5, 20%   2. $\frac{2}{5}$, 2:5, 40%   3. 8 *g*

4. 500 *mL*   5. 4 *mL*

Exercises

1. $\frac{1}{4}$, 1:4, 25%

2. $\frac{3}{8}$, 3:8, 37.5%

3. $\frac{3}{50}$, 3:50, 6%

4. $\frac{1}{3}$, 1:3, 33.3%

5. 40 *mg/mL*

6. 6 *mL*

7.

Ratio	Fraction	Percent
1:5	$\frac{1}{5}$	20%
1:4	$\frac{1}{4}$	25%
1:10	$\frac{1}{10}$	10%
1:200	$\frac{1}{200}$	0.5%
9:1,000	$\frac{9}{1,000}$	0.9%

8. 25 *g*

9. 2 L

10. $\frac{1}{4}$ strength

11. 9,000 *mg*

12. 40 *oz*

13. 800 *mL*

14. 80 *g*

15. Take 8 *tablets*, dissolve, and dilute to 400 *mL*

16. 1,125 *mg*

17. 87 *mg*

18. Yes, they are equivalent.

19. (a) 8 *mL*   (b) 25 *mg*

20. 0.07 *mL*

Cumulative Review Exercises

1. 600 *mg*

2. $1\frac{1}{2}$ *oz*

3. 50 *kg*

4. 4.5 *cm*

5. 16 *oz*

6. 3.5 *lb/wk*

7. 0830*h* Wednesday

8. 3.5 *mL*

9. 40 *mg*

10. 15 *mcg*

11. 100 *kg*

12. 1/2 *tab*

13. 25 *mL*

14. 1,800 *mg*

15. 2,727 *g*

Chapter 9

Case Study 9.1

1. (a) 0.63 *mL*
   (b) Use a 1-*mL* syringe

2. (a) 1.5 *mL*
   (b) Use a 3-*mL* syringe

3. (a) 15.9 *mL*
   (b) Use a 20-*mL* syringe

4. 2.5 *mL*

5. (a) Label j
   (b) 1 *tablet*

6. (a) Label *h*
   (b) 1 *tablet*

7. (a) Label g
   (b) 15 *mL*

8. (a) Label i
   (b) 4 *tab*

9. *tab*

10. 60 *mg/day*

Try These for Practice

1. 1.4 *mL*   2. 1.6 *mL*   3. 4 *mL*   4. 0.68*mL*

5. (a) Use the 2-g vial   (b) 5 *mL*   (c) 6 *mL*

   (d) 330 *mg/mL*   (e) 4.5 *mL*   (f) one

Exercises

1. 0.5 *mL*   2. 0.92 *mL*   3. 0.65 *mL*   4. 2.6 *mL*   5. 0.8 *mL*

6. (a) 0.5 *mL*
   (b) use a 1 *mL* syringe

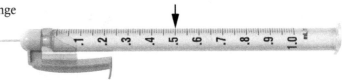

7. (a) 2.6 *mL*
   (b) use a 3-*mL* syringe

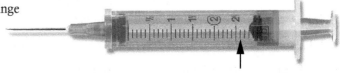

8. (a) 0.18 *mL*
   (b) 0.5 *mL*

9. (a) 0.38 *mL*
   (b) 0.5 *mL*

10. (a) 2.1 *mL*
    (b) sterile water
    (c) 1.5 *mL*
    (d) 3 *mL*

11. (a) 2 *mL*
    (b) 3 *mL*

12. (a) 0.91 *mL*
    (b) 1 *mL*

13. (a) 2 *mL*
    (b) 16 *mL*

14. (a) 480 *mcg* per 0.8 *mL* vial because 1.5 *mL* is too large a volume for a subcut
    (b) 0.76 *mL*

15. 2.6 *mL*

16. (a) 250 *mg*/1.5 *mL*
    (b) 3 *mL*

17. (a) 15 *units*
    (b) 300 *units*

18. 4 *units*

19. 1.5 *mg/d*
    (b) 2 *mg/d*

20. (a) 0.25 *mL*
    (b) 0.5-*mL* syringe
    (c) 0.5 *mL*/30 *min*

Cumulative Review Exercises

1. 150 *kg*

2. 4.5 *g*

3. No, it is an overdose.

4. 2.14 *m²*

5. 0.5 *mL*

6. dexamethasone sodium phosphate

7. 4 *mg/mL*

8. IV, IM, intra-articular, soft tissue, or intralesional

9. 0.75 *mL*

10. 30 *mL*

11. 200 *g*

12. 20 *mL*

13. 4 *cap*

14. Take 160 *mL* of Sustacal and add 80 *mL* of water.

15. (a) 0.75 *mL*

    (b) 1 *mL* syringe

Chapter 10

Case Study 10.1

1. 0.8 *mL*

2. 90 *mcgtt/min*

3. 0.21 *mL*

4.

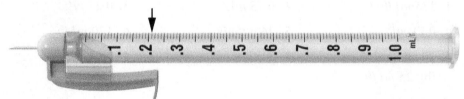

5. 126 *mg/day*

6. 80 *mL/h*

7. 2,160 *mL*

8. 24 *mL*

9. 6.7 *mL*

10. 785.5 *mL*

Try These for Practice

1. 42 *mL/h*

2. 10 *gtt/min*

3. 300 *mL*

4. 1705*h*

5. 75 *mL* (in)

Exercises

1. 63 $\frac{mL}{h}$

2. 125 *mcgtt/min*

3. 28 *gtt/min*

4. 30 *mL/h*

5. 80 *mL*

6. 42 *mL/h*

7. 28 *gtt/min*

8. (a) 133 *mL/h*

    (b) 250 *mL/h*

    (c) no 88% increase

9. 11:32 P.M. the same day

10. 8 h

11. 240 *mL*

12. 480 *mL*

13. (a) 28 *gtt/min*   14. 20 *mL*
    (b) 33 *gtt*/min
    (c) yes 18% increase

15. 10*h* 9 A.M. Thursday   16. 23 *gtt/min*

17. *6 h* 1300*h* the same day   18. 83 $\dfrac{mL}{h}$

19. 50 *mcgtt/min*   20. 140 *mL* (in)

Cumulative Review Exercises

1. 165 *cm*	2. 4 *oz*	3. 85 *kg*	4. 56 *mm*
5. 1655 *h*	6. 4,500 *mg*	7. 2.5%	8. 1.91 *m*^{2}
9. 40 *mg/mL*	10. 27.3 *mg*	11. 1 *mL*	12. 2 *tab*
13. 5 g	14. 150 *mL*	15. 1200h on Thursday	

Chapter 11

Case Study 11.1

1. 125 *mL/h*	2. 0.75 *mL*	3. 0.25 *mL*
4. 0.71 *mL*	5. 26 *gtt/min*	6. 170 *mL/h*
7. (a) 300 *mL/h*	8. 3 *mL/h*	9. 90 *mU/h*
(b) 25 *mL/h*		

10. 0.5 *mL*

Try These for Practice

1. 100 *mL/h*, 5 *mg/min*   2. (a) 600 *mL/h*   3. 0825 *h* the same day
                                      (b) 50 *mg/min*

4. 332 *mcg/min*, 50 *mL/h*

5.

Dosage Rate	Flow Rate
2 *mU/min*	6 *mL/h*
4 *mU/min*	12 *mL/h*
6 *mU/min*	18 *mL/h*
8 *mU/min*	24 *mL/h*
10 *mU/min*	30 *mL/h*
12 *mU/min*	36 *mL/h*
14 *mU/min*	42 *mL/h*
16 *mU/min*	48 *mL/h*
18 *mU/min*	54 *mL/h*
20 *mU/min*	60 *mL/h*

Exercises

1. 56 *gtt/min*
2. 320 *mcg/min*
3. 60 *mL/h*
4. 1 *mg/min*
5. (a) 25 *mL*
   (b) 23.9 *mL*
   (c) 448 *mL/h*
   (d) 30.3 *mg/min*
6. 33 *mg/min*
7. 17 *mcgtt/min*
8. (a) 0.4 *mL*
   (b) 1 *mL/min*
   (c) 0.5 *mL*
   (d) 12 sec
9. (a) 500 *mg*
   (b) 50 *mL*
10. 20 *mg/min*
11. 44 *mg/min*
12. 20 *min*
13. 12.5 *mL*
14. (a) 36 *mL/h*   (b)

Dosage Rate	Flow Rate
3 *mcg/min* (initial)	36 *mL/h*
5 *mcg/min*	60 *mL/h*
7 *mcg/min*	84 *mL/h*
9 *mcg/min*	108 *mL/h*
11 *mcg/min* (maximum)	132 *mL/h*

15. (a) 2.68 *mg/h*
    (b) 13.4 *mL/h*
16. 17,818 *units*
17. 21 *h* 44 *min*
18. 404 *mL/h*
19.

Dosage Rate	Flow Rate
2 *mg/min*	40 *mL/h*
5 *mg/min*	100 *mL/h*
8 *mg/min*	160 *mL/h*
11 *mg/min*	220 *mL/h*
14 *mg/min*	280 *mL/h*
17 *mg/min*	340 *mL/h*
20 *mg/min*	400 *mL/h*

20. (a) 166 *mg*
    (b) 167 *mL/h*

Cumulative Review Exercises

1. 3.4 *mL*
2. 10 *lb* 8 *oz*
3. 10,000 *mcg*
4. 2 *m²*
5. No, it is not safe.
6. (a) 563 *mg*
   (b) 7 *mL*
   (c) 27 *mL/h*
   (d) 2.3 *mg/min*
7. 4.2 *cm*
8. 15 *mL*
9. (a) 3.9 *mL*
   (b) 3.8 *mL*
10. 1 *tab*
11. 4.5 *g*
12. 2%
13. 70 *mcgtt/min*
14. 0.1 *mg/min*
15. 38 *gtt/min*

Chapter 12

Case Study 12.1

1. 1,600 *mL* DFM
2. add 18.2 *mL*, give 2.5 *mL*
3. 103 *mL/h*
4. Yes, the dose is safe.
5. 0.62 *mL* (rounding down)
6. 3 *cap* label (f)
7. 1,000 *mcg*
8. 1 *tab* label (e)
9. 9.3 *mL* (rounded down)
10. 5 *mL* label (d)
11. 176 *mcg/day*

Try These for Practice

1. Yes, it is safe; administer 50 *mg*.
2. Yes, it is safe.
3. 1 *t*
4. 0.73 *mL*
5. 5.28 *mg*

Exercises

1. 15 *mL*
2. Yes, it is safe.
3. No, it is an overdose
4. 0.08 *mL*
5. 450 *mg/d*
6. 9.8 *mL*
7. 56 *mL/h*
8. 4.3 *mL*
9. 11.7 *mL*
10. (a) 68 *mg*
    (b) 500 *mL/h*
11. 2 vials, withdraw 5 *mL*
12. 0.5 *mL*

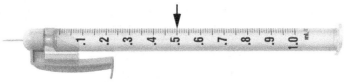

13. 26 *mL*
14. 1 *mL/min*
15. (a) Yes, the dose is safe
    (b) 7.5 *mL*
16. Yes, the dose is safe
17. 150 *mL/h*
18. (a) 1 *mL*
    (b) 84 *mL/h*
19. 24 *mL/h*
20. 3.6 *units/h*

Cumulative Review Exercises

1. 4.2 *cm*
2. 9 *g*
3. 30 *gtt/min*
4. 2.25 *mg/min*
5. 0.5 *mL*
6. 68 *mL/h*
7. 10 *h*
8. 0.375 *mg*
9. 2 *mg*
10. 2.24 *m*²
11. 70 *mL/h*
12. 0.3 *mL*
13. 12.5 *mL*
14. 813 *mg*
15. 1:1,000

Answers to the Comprehensive Self-Tests

Comprehensive Self-Test 1

1. 0.3 *g* of Omnicef
2. 5 *mL* of Kaletra
3. (a) 1 *mL*
   (b) 0.25 *mL*
4. (a) 0.67 *mL*
   (b) 1-*mL* syringe
5. 24 *mg/h*
6. 1 capsule of Depakene
7. (a) 25 *mL*
   (b) 0.5- or 1-*mL* syringe
8. 9.1 *mg*
9. 27.3 *units*
10. 158 *mL/h*
11. (a) yes
    (b) 200 *mL/h*
12. 50 *mcgtt/min*
13. 12.2 *mL*
14. 1,626 *mL/d*
15. 50 *doses*
16. (a) 4 *mg/mL*
    (b) 40 *mg/h*
    (c) 0.17 *mg/min*
17. 15.9 *mL*
18. (a) No the dose is not safe, it is not enough
    (b) Do not give the medication, contact the prescriber
19. (a) 0.03 *mL*
    (b) 1 *mL*
20. (a) 4.5 *g*
    (b) 311 *mL/h*
21. (a) Yes, the dose is safe, it is between the minimum dose of 375 *mg* and the maximum dose of 750 *mg*.
    (b) 16 *mL*

22.

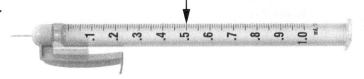

23. 2.2 *mL*   24. (a) 0.75 *mL*   (b) at least 1½ *minutes*   25. 200 *units/h*

Comprehensive Self-Test 2

1. 10 *mL*

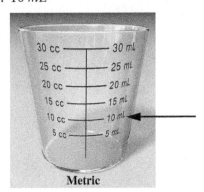

Metric

2. (a) 5 *mL*
   (b) 2.5 *mL* q30sec

3. 7 g of Zovirax

4. 1 *mL* of ampicillin

5. (a) Yes, it is safe
   (b) 7.5 *mL*

6. 2 *mg*

7. 0.29 *mL*

8. (a) yes
   (b) 2.4 *mL*

9. 17 *gtt/min*

10. 14 *tab*

11. 25 *mL/h*

12. 2,500 *units/h*

13. 3 *units/h*

14. (a) 0.4 *mL*
    (b) 0.5 *mL*

15. yes

16. 1,760 *mL/d*

17. No, the dose is too low, contact the prescriber

18. 7.5 *mL/h* of dopamine

19. 1.2 *mL* of Solu-Cortef (hydrocortisone sodium succinate)

20. Yes, the prescribed dose is safe

21. 50 *mL* of Mannitol

22. 141.6 *mg* of Norvir (ritonavir)

23. 25 *gtt/min* of D5W

24. 2 *tab* of Synthroid (levothyroxine)

25. 0.8 *mL* of heparin

Comprehensive Self-Test 3

1. 650 *mcg/min*

2. 15 *mL*

3. 0.75 *mL*

4. 0.4 *mL*

5. 38 *gtt/min*

6. 50 g

7.
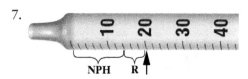

8. 4 *mL*

9. (a) 200 *mL/h*
   (b) 2 *g/d*

10. 0.25 *mL*

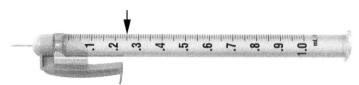

11. 0.3 *mL*

12. 22.5 *mL/h*

13. 18 *units/h*

14. 2 *mL*

15. 0.5 *mL*

16. (a) 436 *mg/d*
    (b) 727 *mg/d*
    (c) yes

17. 160 *mg*, 50 *mL/h*   18. 25 *gtt/min*   19. 1 m^2

20. 0.5 *mL*   21. 1.25 *mL/min*, 25 *gtt/min*, 13 *hours* 20 *minutes*

22. 2,000 *mL*   23. 30 *mL*   24. 10 *mg*, 60 *mL*   25. 21 *mL/h*

Comprehensive Self-Test 4

1. 1,500 *units/h*

2. (a) Yes the dose is safe
   (b) 0.8 *mL*

3. (a) 6 *mg*
   (b) 6 *mL*
   (c) 1.5 *mL* every 15 sec

4. 1.4 *mL*

5. 0.12 g

6. 1100*h* the next day

7. 8 *tab*

8. yes

9. (a) 1.2 *mL*
   (b)

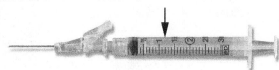

10. (a) 436 *mg/d*
    (b) 872 *mg/d*
    (c) 2.75 *mL*

11. 2g

12. 75 *mL/h*

13. 2,500 *mL/d*, 104 *mL/h*   14. no   15. 4.5 *mL/h*

16. 6 *mL/h*   17. 2.5 *mL*   18. 2 *cap*, 3.15 g

19. 30 *mL*   20. 21 *mL/h*   21. 45 *mL*, 2.75 *mL/h*

22. 0.7 *mL*   23. 3-*mL* syringe

24. Take 600 *mL* of Sustacal and dilute to 900 *mL*   25. 0400 h the next day

ISMP Institute for Safe Medication Practices

FDA and ISMP Lists of
Look-Alike Drug Names with Recommended *Tall Man Letters*

The look-alike drug names in the Tables that follow have been modified using tall man (mixed case) letters to help draw attention to the dissimilarities in their names. Several studies have shown that highlighting sections of drug names using tall man letters can help distinguish similar drug names,[1] making them less prone to mix-ups.[2-3] ISMP, FDA, The Joint Commission, and other safety-conscious organizations have promoted the use of tall man letters as one means of reducing confusion between similar drug names.

Table 1 provides an alphabetized list of FDA-approved established drug names with recommended tall man letters, which were first identified during the FDA Name Differentiation Project (www.fda.gov/Drugs/DrugSafety/MedicationErrors/ucm164587.htm).

Table 2 provides an alphabetized list of additional drug names with recommendations from ISMP regarding the use and placement of tall man letters. This is not an official list approved by FDA. It is intended for voluntary use by healthcare practitioners and drug information vendors. Any product label changes by manufacturers require FDA approval.

One of the difficulties with the use of tall man letters includes inconsistent application in health settings and lack of standardization regarding which letters to present in uppercase. A new study by Gerrett[4] describes several ways to determine which of the dissimilar letters in each drug name should be highlighted. To promote standardi-

zation, ISMP followed one of these tested methodologies whenever possible. Called the CD3 rule, the methodology suggests working from the left of the word first by capitalizing all the characters to the right once two or more dissimilar letters are encountered, and then, working from the right of the word back, returning two or more letters common to both words to lowercase letters. When the rule cannot be applied because there are no common letters on the right side of the word, the methodology suggests capitalizing the central part of the word only. ISMP suggests that the tall man lettering scheme provided in Tables 1 and 2 be followed when presenting these drug names to healthcare providers to promote consistency. At this time, scientific studies do not support the use of tall man letters when presenting drug names to patients.

References: 1) Filik R, Purdy K, Gale A, Gerrett D. Drug name confusion: evaluating the effectiveness of capital ("Tall Man") letters using eye movement data. *Social Science & Medicine* 2004;59(12):2597-2601. **2)** Filik R, Purdy K, Gale A, Gerrett D. Labeling of medicines and patient safety: evaluating methods of reducing drug name confusion. *Human Factors* 2006;48(1):39-47. **3)** Grasha A. Cognitive systems perspective on human performance in the pharmacy: implications for accuracy, effectiveness, and job satisfaction. Alexandria (VA): NACDS; 2000 Report No. 062100. **4)** Gerrett D, Gale AG, Darker IT, Filik R, Purdy KJ. Tall man lettering. Final report of the use of tall man lettering to minimize selection errors of medicine names in computer prescribing and dispensing systems. Loughborough University Enterprises Ltd.; 2009 (www.connectingforhealth.nhs.uk/systemsandservices/eprescribing/refdocs/tallman.pdf).

Table 1. FDA-Approved List of Generic Drug Names with Tall Man Letters	
Drug Name with Tall Man Letters	**Confused with**
aceta**ZOLAMIDE**	aceto**HEXAMIDE**
aceto**HEXAMIDE**	aceta**ZOLAMIDE**
bu**PROP**ion	bus**PIR**one
bus**PIR**one	bu**PROP**ion
chlorpro**MAZINE**	chlorpro**PAMIDE**
chlorpro**PAMIDE**	chlorpro**MAZINE**
clomi**PHENE**	clomi**PRAMINE**
clomi**PRAMINE**	clomi**PHENE**
cyclo**SERINE**	cyclo**SPORINE**
cyclo**SPORINE**	cyclo**SERINE**
DAUNOrubicin	**DOXO**rubicin
dimenhy**DRINATE**	diphenhydr**AMINE**
diphenhydr**AMINE**	dimenhy**DRINATE**
DOBUTamine	**DOP**amine
DOPamine	**DOBUT**amine

continued on next page

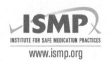

www.ismp.org

Institute for Safe Medication Practices

FDA and ISMP Lists of
Look-Alike Drug Names with Recommended Tall Man Letters (continued)

Table 1. FDA–Approved List of Generic Drug Names with Tall Man Letters (continued)

Drug Name with Tall Man Letters	Confused with
DOXOrubicin	**DAUNO**rubicin
glipi**ZIDE**	gly**BURIDE**
gly**BURIDE**	glipi**ZIDE**
hydr**ALAZINE**	hydr**OXY**zine
hydr**OXY**zine	hydr**ALAZINE**
medroxy**PROGESTER**one	methyl**PREDNIS**olone - methyl**TESTOSTER**one
methyl**PREDNIS**olone	medroxy**PROGESTER**one - methyl**TESTOSTER**one
methyl**TESTOSTER**one	medroxy**PROGESTER**one - methyl**PREDNIS**olone
ni**CAR**dipine	**NIFE**dipine
NIFEdipine	ni**CAR**dipine
predniso**LONE**	predni**SONE**
predni**SONE**	predniso**LONE**
sulf**ADIAZINE**	sulfi**SOXAZOLE**
sulfi**SOXAZOLE**	sulf**ADIAZINE**
TOLAZamide	**TOLBUT**amide
TOLBUTamide	**TOLAZ**amide
vin**BLAS**tine	vin**CRIS**tine
vin**CRIS**tine	vin**BLAS**tine

Table 2. ISMP List of Additional Drug Names with Tall Man Letters

Drug Name with Tall Man Letters	Confused with
ALPRAZolam	**LOR**azepam
a**MIL**oride	am**LODIP**ine
am**LODIP**ine	a**MIL**oride
ARIPiprazole	**RABE**prazole
AVINza*	**INV**anz*
aza**CITID**ine	aza**THIO**prine
aza**THIO**prine	aza**CITID**ine
car**BAM**azepine	**OX**carbazepine
CARBOplatin	**CIS**platin
ce**FAZ**olin	cefo**TE**tan – cef**OX**itin – cef**TAZ**idime – cef**TRIAX**one
cefo**TE**tan	ce**FAZ**olin – cef**OX**itin – cef**TAZ**idime – cef**TRIAX**one
cef**OX**itin	ce**FAZ**olin – cefo**TE**tan – cef**TAZ**idime – cef**TRIAX**one
cef**TAZ**idime	ce**FAZ**olin – cefo**TE**tan – cef**OX**itin – cef**TRIAX**one
cef**TRIAX**one	ce**FAZ**olin - cefo**TE**tan – cef**OX**itin – cef**TAZ**idime
Cele**BREX***	Cele**XA***
Cele**XA***	Cele**BREX***
chlordiaze**POXIDE**	chlorpro**MAZINE**
chlorpro**MAZINE**	chlordiaze**POXIDE**
CISplatin	**CARBO**platin
clonaze**PAM**	clo**NID**ine – clo**ZAP**ine – **LOR**azepam

* Brand names always start with an uppercase letter. Some brand names incorporate tall man letters in initial characters and may not be readily recognized as brand names. An asterisk follows all brand names in Table 2.

continued on next page

© **ISMP** 2011. Permission is granted to reproduce material for internal newsletters or communications with proper attribution. Other reproduction is prohibited without written permission from ISMP. Report actual and potential medication errors to the Medication Errors Reporting Program (MERP) via the Web at www.ismp.org or by calling 1-800-FAIL-SAF(E).

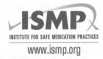
www.ismp.org

Table 2. ISMP List of Additional Drug Names with Tall Man Letters (continued)	
Drug Name with Tall Man Letters	**Confused with**
cloNIDine	clonazePAM – cloZAPine – KlonoPIN*
cloZAPine	clonazePAM – cloNIDine
DACTINomycin	DAPTOmycin
DAPTOmycin	DACTINomycin
DOCEtaxel	PACLitaxel
DOXOrubicin	IDArubicin
DULoxetine	FLUoxetine – PARoxetine
ePHEDrine	EPINEPHrine
EPINEPHrine	ePHEDrine
fentaNYL	SUFentanil
flavoxATE	fluvoxaMINE
FLUoxetine	DULoxetine – PARoxetine
fluPHENAZine	fluvoxaMINE
fluvoxaMINE	fluPHENAZine – flavoxATE
guaiFENesin	guanFACINE
guanFACINE	guaiFENesin
HumaLOG*	HumuLIN*
HumuLIN*	HumaLOG*
HYDROcodone	oxyCODONE
HYDROmorphone	morphine
IDArubicin	DOXOrubicin
inFLIXimab	riTUXimab
INVanz*	AVINza*
ISOtretinoin	tretinoin
KlonoPIN*	cloNIDine
LaMICtal*	LamISIL*
LamISIL*	LaMICtal*
lamiVUDine	lamoTRIgine
lamoTRIgine	lamiVUDine
levETIRAcetam	levOCARNitine
levOCARNitine	levETIRAcetam
LORazepam	ALPRAZolam – clonazePAM
metFORMIN	metroNIDAZOLE
metroNIDAZOLE	metFORMIN
mitoMYcin	mitoXANtrone
mitoXANtrone	mitoMYcin
NexAVAR*	NexIUM*
NexIUM*	NexAVAR*
niCARdipine	niMODipine – NIFEdipine
NIFEdipine	niMODipine – niCARdipine
niMODipine	NIFEdipine – niCARdipine
NovoLIN*	NovoLOG*

* Brand names always start with an uppercase letter. Some brand names incorporate tall man letters in initial characters and may not be readily recognized as brand names. An asterisk follows all brand names in Table 2.

continued on next page

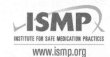

ISMP
INSTITUTE FOR SAFE MEDICATION PRACTICES
www.ismp.org

Table 2. ISMP List of Additional Drug Names with Tall Man Letters (continued)	
Drug Name with Tall Man Letters	**Confused with**
NovoLOG*	NovoLIN*
OLANZapine	QUEtiapine
OXcarbazepine	carBAMazepine
oxyCODONE	HYDROcodone – OxyCONTIN*
OxyCONTIN*	oxyCODONE
PACLitaxel	DOCEtaxel
PARoxetine	FLUoxetine – DULoxetine
PEMEtrexed	PRALAtrexate
PENTobarbital	PHENobarbital
PHENobarbital	PENTobarbital
PRALAtrexate	PEMEtrexed
PriLOSEC*	PROzac*
PROzac*	PriLOSEC*
QUEtiapine	OLANZapine
quiNIDine	quiNINE
quiNINE	quiNIDine
RABEprazole	ARIPiprazole
RisperDAL*	rOPINIRole
risperiDONE	rOPINIRole
riTUXimab	inFLIXimab
romiDEPsin	romiPLOStim
romiPLOStim	romiDEPsin
rOPINIRole	RisperDAL* – risperiDONE
SandIMMUNE*	SandoSTATIN*
SandoSTATIN*	SandIMMUNE*
SEROquel*	SINEquan*
SINEquan*	SEROquel*
sitaGLIPtin	SUMAtriptan
Solu-CORTEF*	Solu-MEDROL*
Solu-MEDROL*	Solu-CORTEF*
SORAfenib	SUNItinib
SUFentanil	fentaNYL
sulfADIAZINE	sulfaSALAzine
sulfaSALAzine	sulfADIAZINE
SUMAtriptan	sitaGLIPtin – ZOLMitriptan
SUNItinib	SORAfenib
TEGretol*	TRENtal*
tiaGABine	tiZANidine
tiZANidine	tiaGABine
traMADol	traZODone
traZODone	traMADol

* Brand names always start with an uppercase letter. Some brand names incorporate tall man letters in initial characters and may not be readily recognized as brand names. An asterisk follows all brand names in Table 2.

continued on next page

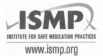

ISMP
INSTITUTE FOR SAFE MEDICATION PRACTICES
www.ismp.org

Table 2. ISMP List of Additional Drug Names with Tall Man Letters (continued)

Drug Name with Tall Man Letters	Confused with
TRENtal*	TEGretol*
valACYclovir	valGANciclovir
valGANciclovir	valACYclovir
ZOLMitriptan	SUMAtriptan
ZyPREXA*	ZyrTEC*
ZyrTEC*	ZyPREXA*

** Brand names always start with an uppercase letter. Some brand names incorporate tall man letters in initial characters
and may not be readily recognized as brand names. An asterisk follows all brand names in Table 2.*

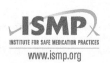

Appendix C

Commonly Used Abbreviations

To someone unfamiliar with prescription abbreviations, medication orders may look like a foreign language. To interpret prescriptive orders accurately and to administer drugs safely, a qualified person must have a thorough knowledge of common abbreviations. For instance, when the prescriber writes, **"hydromorphone 1.5 mg IM q4h prn,"** the healthcare professional knows how to interpret it as "hydromorphone, 1.5 milligrams, intramuscular, every four hours, whenever necessary." For measurement abbreviations, refer to Appendix D.

Abbreviation	Meaning	Abbreviation	Meaning
$\bar{a}$	before (*abante*)	IC	intracardiac
ac	before meals (*ante cibum*)	ID	intradermal
ad lib	as desired (*ad libitum*)	IM	intramuscular; intramuscularly
A.M., am	morning	IV	intravenous; intravenously
amp	ampule	IVP	intravenous push
aq	aqueous water	IVPB	intravenous piggyback
b.i.d.	two times a day	IVSS	IV Soluset
BP	blood pressure	kg	kilogram
$\bar{c}$	with	KVO	keep vein open
C	Celsius; centigrade	L	liter
cap	capsule	LA	long acting
CBC	complete blood count	lb	pound
cc	cubic centimeter	LIB	left in bag, left in bottle
CVP	central venous pressure	LOS	length of stay
d	day	MAR	medication administration record
D/W	dextrose in water	mcg	microgram
D5W or D5/W or D_5W	5% dextrose in water	mcgtt	microdrop
daw	dispense as written	mEq	milliequivalent
dr	dram	mg	milligram
Dx	diagnosis	min	minute
elix	elixir	mL	milliliter
ER	extended release	mU	milliunit
F	Fahrenheit	n, noct	night
g	gram	NDC	national drug code
gr	grain	NGT	nasogastric tube
GT	gastrostomy tube	NKA	no known allergies
gtt	drop	NKDA	no known drug allergies
h, hr	hour	NKFA	no known food allergies
hs	hour of sleep; bedtime (*hora somni*)	NPO	nothing by mouth (*per ora*)

Abbreviation	Meaning	Abbreviation	Meaning
NS	normal saline	q8h	every eight hours
NSAID	nonsteroidal anti-inflammatory drug	q12h	every 12 hours
OTC	over the counter	q.i.d.	four times a day *(quarter in die)*
oz	ounce	qn	every night *(quaque noct)*
p̄	after	qs	quantity sufficient or sufficient amount
PEG	percutaneous endoscopic		*(quantitas sufficiens)*
	gastrostomy tube	R	respiration
P	pulse	R/O	rule out
pc	after meals *(post cibum)*	Rx	prescription, treatment
PEJ	percutaneous endoscopic	s̄	without *(sine)*
	jejunostomy	SIG	directions to the patient
PICC	peripherally inserted central catheter	SL	sublingual
P.M., pm	afternoon, evening	SR	sustained release
PO	by mouth *(per os)*	stat	immediately *(statum)*
POST-OP	after surgery	subcut	subcutaneous
PR	by way of the rectum	supp	suppository
PRE-OP	before surgery	susp	suspension
prn	when required or whenever necessary	T or tbs	tablespoon
Pt	patient	t or tsp	teaspoon
pt	pint	T	temperature
q	every *(quaque)*	t.i.d.	three times a day *(ter in die)*
qh	every hour *(quaque hora)*	tab	tablet
q2h	every two hours	TPN	total parenteral nutrition
q3h	every three hours	USP	United States Pharmacopeia
q4h	every four hours	V/S	vital signs
q6h	every six hours	wt	weight

Appendix D

Units of Measurement in Metric and Household Systems

Abbreviations

Volume

Metric		Household	
milliliter	*mL*	microdrop	*mcgtt*
liter	L	drop	*gtt*
cubic centimeter	cc	teaspoon	*t* or tsp
		tablespoon	*T* or tbs
		fluid ounce	*oz*
		pint	*pt*
		quart	*qt*

Weight

Metric		Household	
microgram	*mcg*	ounce	*oz*
milligram	*mg*	pound	*lb*
gram	*g*		
kilogram	*kg*		

Length

Metric		Household	
millimeter	*mm*	inch	*in*
centimeter	*cm*	foot	*ft*
meter	*m*		

Area

Metric	
square meter	m^2

Appendix E

Celsius and Fahrenheit Temperature Conversions

Reading and recording a temperature is a crucial step in assessing a patient's health. Temperatures can be measured using either the Fahrenheit (F) scale or the Celsius or centrigrade (C) scale. Celsius/Fahrenheit equivalency tables make it easy to convert Celsius to Fahrenheit, or vice versa. Still, it is useful to be able to make this conversion yourself.

You can use the following formulas to convert from one temperature scale to the other:

$$C = \frac{F - 32}{1.8} \text{ and } F = 1.8\,C + 32$$

For those unfamiliar with algebra, the following rules are equivalent to the algebraic formulas.

First rule: To convert to Celsius. Subtract 32 and then divide by 1.8.

Second rule: To convert to Fahrenheit. Multiply by 1.8 and then add 32.

NOTE

Temperatures are rounded to the nearest tenth.

EXAMPLE E.1

Convert 102.5°F to Celsius.

Using the first rule, you subtract 32.

$$
\begin{array}{r}
102.5 \\
-32.0 \\
\hline
70.5
\end{array}
$$

Then you divide by 1.8.

$$
\begin{array}{r}
39.17 \\
1.8\overline{)70.5000}
\end{array}
$$

So, 102.5°F equals 39.2°C.

EXAMPLE E.2

Convert 3°C to Fahrenheit.

Using the second rule, you first multiply by 1.8.

$$
\begin{array}{r}
1.8 \\
\times\, 3 \\
\hline
5.4
\end{array}
$$

Then you add 32.

$$
\begin{array}{r}
5.4 \\
+32.0 \\
\hline
37.4
\end{array}
$$

So, 3°C equals 37.4°F

For those unfamiliar with the Celsius system, the following rhyme might be useful:

> *Thirty is hot*
> *Twenty is nice*
> *Ten is chilly*
> *Zero is ice*

Appendix F

Diluting Stock Solutions

A stock solution is one in which a pure drug is already dissolved in a liquid. The strength of each stock solution is written on the label. If the order is for a stronger solution, you will need to prepare a new solution. However, if the order is for a weaker solution, you can dilute the stock solution to the prescribed strength. To find out how much stock solution to take, use the following formula.

$$\frac{\text{Amount prescribed} \times \text{Strength prescribed}}{\text{Strength of stock}} = \text{Amount of stock}$$

EXAMPLE F.1

How would you prepare 1 L of a 25% solution from a 50% stock solution? Because this example does not indicate whether the drug in the solution is a solid or a liquid in its pure form, you may choose either *grams* or *milliliters* for the amount of the pure drug, and the choice will have no effect on the answer. *Grams* are chosen in the following solution.

Given: Amount prescribed: 1,000 *mL*

Strength prescribed: 25% or $\dfrac{25\ g}{100\ mL}$

Strength of stock: 50% or $\dfrac{50\ g}{100\ mL}$

Find: Amount of stock: ? *mL*

$$\frac{\text{Amount prescribed} \times \text{Strength prescribed}}{\text{Strength of stock}} = \text{Amount of stock}$$

Substituting the given information into the formula, you get

$$\frac{1{,}000\ mL \times \dfrac{25\ g}{100\ mL}}{\dfrac{50\ g}{100\ mL}} = ?\ mL$$

This complex fraction may be written as a division problem as follows:

$$1{,}000\ mL \times \frac{25\ g}{100\ mL} \div \frac{50\ g}{100\ mL} = ?\ mL$$

This division problem may be changed to a multiplication problem by inverting the last fraction. Now, cancel and multiply.

$$1,000 \ mL \times \frac{25 \ g}{100 \ mL} \times \frac{100 \ mL}{50 \ g} = 500 \ mL$$

So, you would take 500 mL of the 50% stock solution and add water to the level of 1,000 mL.

EXAMPLE F.2

How would you prepare 2,500 mL of a 1:10 boric acid solution from a 40% stock solution of this antiseptic?

Given: Amount prescribed: 2,500 mL

     Strength prescribed: 1:10 or $\dfrac{1 \ mL}{10 \ mL}$

     Strength of stock: 40% or $\dfrac{40 \ mL}{100 \ mL}$

Find: Amount of stock: ? mL

$$\frac{2,500 \ mL \times \dfrac{1 \ mL}{10 \ mL}}{\dfrac{40 \ mL}{100 \ mL}} = \text{Amount of stock}$$

$$2,500 \ mL \times \frac{1}{10} \div \frac{40}{100} = \ ? \ mL$$

$$\overset{250}{2,500} \times \frac{1}{\underset{1}{10}} \times \frac{100}{40} = 625 \ mL$$

So, you would take 625 mL of the 40% stock solution of boric acid and add water to the level of 2,500 mL.

EXAMPLE F.3

How would you prepare 500 mL of a 1:25 solution from a 1:4 stock solution of the antiseptic Argyrol?

Given: Amount prescribed: 500 mL

     Strength prescribed: 1:25 or $\dfrac{1 \ mL}{25 \ mL}$

     Strength of stock: 1:4 or $\dfrac{1 \ mL}{4 \ mL}$

Find: Amount of stock: ? mL

$$\frac{500 \; mL \times \dfrac{1 \; \cancel{mL}}{25 \; \cancel{mL}}}{\dfrac{1 \; \cancel{mL}}{4 \; \cancel{mL}}} = \text{Amount of stock}$$

$$500 \; mL \times \frac{1}{25} \div \frac{1}{4} = ? \; mL$$

$$\overset{20}{\cancel{500}} \; mL \times \frac{1}{\underset{1}{\cancel{25}}} \times \frac{4}{1} = 80 \; mL$$

So, you would take 80 mL of a 1:4 stock solution of Argyrol and add water to the level of 500 mL.

Exercises

1. How would you prepare 200 mL of a 5% solution from a 20% stock solution?

2. How would you prepare 500 mL of a 1:4 solution from a 1:3 stock solution?

3. How would you prepare 1 L of a 0.45% solution from a 0.9% stock solution?

4. How would you prepare 200 mL of a 25% solution from a 35% stock solution?

5. How would you prepare 2 L of a 1:5 solution from a $\frac{1}{2}$ strength stock solution?

Answers

1. Take 50 mL of the stock solution and add water to the level of 200 mL.

2. Take 375 mL of the stock solution and add water to the level of 500 mL.

3. Take 500 mL of the stock solution and add water to the level of 1 L.

4. Take 143 mL of the stock solution and add water to the level of 200 mL.

5. Take 800 mL of the stock solution and add water to the level of 2 L.

Appendix G

Apothecary System

The apothecary system is one of the oldest systems of drug measurement. Although the apothecary system was used in the past to write prescriptions, it has largely been replaced by the metric system. Apothecary units are rarely used on drug labels, but when they are, the metric equivalents are also provided.

Liquid Volume in the Apothecary System

The equivalents for the units of measurement for liquid volume in the apothecary system are shown in Table G.1 along with their abbreviations.

Table G.1 Common Equivalents for Apothecary Liquid Volume Units

$$ounce\ (oz)\ 1 = drams\ (dr)\ 8$$
$$dram\ (dr)\ 1 = minims\ 60$$

> **NOTE**
>
> In the apothecary system, the abbreviation or symbol for the unit is placed before the quantity (as in drams 8). Ounces are used for liquid volume in both the household and apothecary systems. To avoid errors, the abbreviations dr and oz are preferred over the formerly used abbreviations ℥ and ʒ.

EXAMPLE G.1

How many minims would be equivalent to dr $\frac{1}{6}$?

$$dr\ \frac{1}{6} = minims\ ?$$

Because $dr\ 1 = minims\ 60$, the unit fraction is $\frac{minims\ 60}{dr\ 1}$

$$\frac{dr\ 1}{6} \times \frac{minims\ 60}{dr\ 1} = minims\ 10$$

So, minims 10 are equivalent to $dr\ \frac{1}{6}$.

> **NOTE**
>
> Decimal numbers are never used in the apothecary system.

EXAMPLE G.2

How many ounces would be equivalent to dr 4?

$$dr\ 4 = ounces\ ?$$

Because $dr\ 8 = ounce\ 1$, the unit fraction is $\frac{oz\ 1}{dr\ 8}$

$$\frac{dr\ 4}{1} \times \frac{oz\ 1}{dr\ 8} = ounce\ \frac{1}{2}$$

So, dr 4 is equivalent to oz $\frac{1}{2}$.

Weight in the Apothecary System

The grain (gr) is the only unit of weight in the apothecary system that is used in administering medications.

Roman Numerals

Dosages in the apothecary system are sometimes written using Roman numerals. Table G.2 shows Roman numerals.

Table G.2 Roman Numerals

	Roman Numerals		Roman Numerals		Roman Numerals
1	I	7	VII	$\frac{1}{2}$	ss
2	II	8	VIII	$1\frac{1}{2}$	iss
3	III	9	IX	$7\frac{1}{2}$	viiss
4	IV	10	X		
5	V	15	XV		
6	VI	20	XX		

NOTE

Here are some useful equivalents:
$1\,t = 5\,mL = dr\,1$
$2\,T = 30\,mL = oz\,1 = dr\,8$

Equivalents of Common Units of Measurement

Tables G.3 and G.4 list some common equivalent values for weight, volume, and length in the metric, household, and apothecary systems of measurement. Although these equivalents are considered standards, many of them are approximations.

Table G.3 Equivalent Values for Units of Weight

Metric		Apothecary		Household
60 *milligrams (mg)*	=	grain *(gr)* 1		
1 *gram (g)*	=	grains *(gr)* 15		
1 *kilogram (kg)*			=	2.2 *pounds (lb)*

Table G.4 Equivalent Values for Units of Volume

Metric		Apothecary		Household
1 *milliliter (mL)*	=	*minims* 15		
5 *milliliters (mL)*	=	*dram (dr)* 1	=	1 *teaspoon (t)*
15 *milliliters (mL)*	=	*ounce (oz)* $\frac{1}{2}$	=	1 *tablespoon (T)*
30 *milliliters (mL)*	=	*ounce (oz)* 1	=	2 *tablespoons (T)*
500 *milliliters*	=	*ounces (oz)* 16	=	1 *pint (pt)*
1,000 *milliliters*	=	*ounces (oz)* 32	=	1 *quart (qt)*

Metric–Apothecary Conversions

EXAMPLE G.3

Convert 40 *milligrams* to grains.

$$40 \; mg = gr \; ?$$

Because $60 \; mg = gr \; 1$, the unit fraction is $\dfrac{gr \; 1}{60 \; mg}$

$$\frac{40 \; \cancel{mg}}{1} \times \frac{gr \; 1}{60 \; \cancel{mg}} = gr \; \frac{2}{3}$$

So, 40 *milligrams* are equivalent to grain $\frac{2}{3}$.

EXAMPLE G.4

Convert 0.12 *milligrams* to grains.

$$0.12 \; mg = gr \; ?$$

Because $60 \; m = gr \; 1$, the unit fraction is $\dfrac{gr \; 1}{60 \; mg}$

$$\frac{0.12 \; \cancel{mg}}{1} \times \frac{gr \; 1}{60 \; \cancel{mg}} = \frac{gr \; 0.12}{60} \times \frac{100}{100} = \frac{gr \; 12}{6000} = gr \frac{1}{500}$$

So, 0.12 milligrams are equivalent to grain $\frac{1}{500}$.

EXAMPLE G.5

Convert 1.5 *grams* to an equivalent weight in grains.

$$1.5 \; g = gr \; ?$$

Because $1 \; g = gr \; 15$, the unit fraction is $\dfrac{gr \; 15}{1 \; g}$

$$\frac{1.5 \; \cancel{g}}{1} \times \frac{gr \; 15}{1 \; \cancel{g}} = gr \; 22.5$$

A decimal number cannot be used in the apothecary system. Therefore, 22.5 must be written in fractional form as $22\frac{1}{2}$. So, 1.5 grams are equivalent to grains $22\frac{1}{2}$.

NOTE

Grains are apothecary units and are expressed as fractions or whole numbers. Therefore, grains 22.5 should be expressed as grains $22\frac{1}{2}$.

EXAMPLE G.6

Convert grain $\frac{1}{300}$ to milligrams.

$$gr \frac{1}{300} = ? \, mg$$

Because $1 \, gr = 60 \, mg$, the unit fraction is $\dfrac{60 \, mg}{gr \, 1}$

$$\frac{\cancel{gr} \, 1}{300} \times \frac{60 \, mg}{\cancel{gr} \, 1} = 0.2 \, mg$$

So, grain $\frac{1}{300}$ is equivalent to 0.2 milligrams.

EXAMPLE G.7

Convert grains $7\frac{1}{2}$ to grams.

$$gr \, 7\frac{1}{2} = ? \, g$$

Because $gr \, 15 = 1 \, g$, the unit fraction is $\dfrac{1 \, g}{gr \, 15}$

$$\frac{\cancel{gr} \, 15}{2} \times \frac{1g}{\cancel{gr} \, 15} = \frac{1}{2} g = 0.5g$$

So, grains $7\frac{1}{2}$ are equivalent to 0.5 gram.

> **NOTE**
>
> Grams are metric units, so they are expressed as decimals or whole numbers. Therefore, $\frac{1}{2}$ gram is expressed as 0.5 gram.

Household–Apothecary Conversions

EXAMPLE G.8

Convert ounces 2 to tablespoons.

$$oz \, 2 = ? \, T$$

Because $oz \, 1 = 2T$, the unit fraction is $\dfrac{2T}{oz \, 1}$

$$\frac{\cancel{oz} \, 2}{1} \times \frac{2 \, T}{\cancel{oz} \, 1} = 4T$$

So, ounces 2 is equivalent to 4 tablespoons.

Exercises

1. $oz\ 1 = dr\ ?$
2. $dr\ 1 = minims\ ?$
3. $dr\ 12 = oz\ ?$
4. $dr\ 1\frac{1}{2} = minims\ ?$
5. $oz\ 64 = dr\ ?$
6. $dr\ 1 = ?\ t = minims\ ? = ?\ mL$
7. $oz\ 1 = ?\ T = dr\ ? = ?\ mL$
8. $1\ cup = ?\ glass = oz\ ? = ?\ pt$
9. $gr\ 1 = ?\ mg$
10. $1\ g = gr\ ?$
11. $0.006\ mg = gr\ ?$
12. $gr\ 3\frac{3}{4} = ?\ mg$

Answers

1. $dr\ 8$
2. $minims\ 60$
3. $oz\ 1\frac{1}{2}$
4. $minims\ 90$
5. $dr\ 512$
6. $dr\ 1 = 1\ t = minims\ 60 = 5\ mL$
7. $oz\ 1 = 2\ T = dr\ 8 = 30\ mL$
8. $1\ cup = 1\ glass = oz\ 8 = \frac{1}{2}\ pt$
9. $60\ mg$
10. $gr\ 15$
11. $gr\ \frac{1}{10,000}$
12. $225\ mg$

Index